PRINCIPLES *of*
ICD-10-CM
CODING WORKBOOK

FOURTH EDITION

Deborah J. Grider, CPC, COC, CPC-I, CPC-P, CPMA, CEMC, CCS-P, CDIP

AHIMA Approved ICD-10-CM Trainer

AHIMA Certified Clinical Documentation Improvement Practitioner

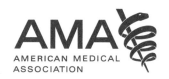

The American Medical Association ("AMA") and its authors and editors have consulted sources believed to be knowledgeable in their fields. However, neither the AMA nor its authors or editors warrant that the information is in every respect accurate and/or complete. The AMA, its authors, and editors assume no responsibility for use of the information contained in this publication. Neither the AMA, its authors or editors shall be responsible for, and expressly disclaims liability for, damages of any kind arising out of the use of, reference to, or reliance on, the content of this publication. This publication is for informational purposes only. The AMA does not provide medical, legal, financial, or other professional advice, and readers are encouraged to consult a professional advisor for such advice.

The contents of this publication represent the views of the author(s) and should not be construed to be the views or policy of the AMA, or of the institution with which the author(s) may be affiliated, unless this is clearly specified.

This publication introduces the reader to the principles of ICD-10-CM coding for outpatient and physician services incorporating information provided by the National Center for Health Statistics (NCHS). The NCHS maintains the ICD-10-CM code set and continues to update the draft version of ICD-10-CM. This publication is designed to provide accurate and authoritative information. The content highlights important changes excerpted from the latest published version of ICD-10-CM available at the time of publication and in no way suggests or infers that the published content represents all instructions and guidelines associated with the use of ICD-10-CM. Every reasonable effort has been made to ensure the accuracy of the information provided. However, the ultimate responsibility for correct coding lies with the provider pertaining to the use of ICD-10-CM. The most recent version of the ICD-10-CM code set has been updated every year since 2007. ICD-10-CM is located on the website of the Centers for Medicare and Medicaid Services (CMS) and can be downloaded at www.cms.gov/ICD10.

Additional copies of this book may be ordered by calling 800 621-8335 or from the secure AMA Web site at www.amastore.com. Refer to product number OP103716.

AMA publication and product updates, errata, and addendum can be found at **amaproductupdates.org.**

ISBN 978-1-62202-557-2
BQ41:12/16

Internet address: www.ama-assn.org

Contents

Preface

Coders, students, and instructors request practical real-life coding case studies with rationales to help ensure accurate interpretation of ICD-10-CM diagnosis coding. The American Medical Association (AMA) has produced several coding products, including *Principles of ICD-10-CM Coding*, Fourth Edition, to assist medical practices in transitioning to ICD-10-CM.

This workbook, the companion to *Principles of ICD-10-CM Coding*, Fourth Edition, is an introduction to intermediate and advanced coding skills incorporating basic to difficult coding case studies to build skills with ICD-10-CM. It has been developed using actual documentation derived from evaluation and management services, surgical procedures, and diagnostic services. Once the reader has a good understanding of the ICD-10-CM Official Guidelines for Coding and Reporting and the chapter-specific guidelines, the workbook cases will be a valuable resource for building ICD-10 coding skills.

The workbook is designed to be used by community colleges, career colleges, and vocational school programs for training coders, medical assistants, medical insurance specialists, medical coders, and other health care providers. It can also be used as an independent study training tool for new medical office personnel, physicians, independent billing service personnel, medical coders, and others in the health care field who want to build additional skill with ICD-10-CM diagnosis coding.

In *Principles of ICD-10-CM Coding Workbook* you will find:

- Information about ICD-10-CM format and conventions

- General coding guidelines in a summarized format

- Chapter-specific diagnosis coding guidelines in each chapter

- Real-life case studies to build ICD-10-CM coding skill

- An answer key (Chapter 12) with rationales to check your answers

How to Use This Workbook

In order to use this workbook, it is important to have the following resources available:

- ICD-10-CM Codebook

- A medical terminology reference

- An anatomy and physiology reference

It is also recommended that you use *Principles of ICD-10-CM Coding*, Fourth Edition, as a reference.

The workbook provides a brief overview of the general guidelines and chapter-specific guidelines for each chapter in ICD-10-CM, followed by several case studies in each chapter to help you practice your knowledge. After reading each chapter, code the case studies. Make certain you reference the ICD-10-CM Official Coding Guidelines when coding the case studies. Read the official guidelines in the ICD-10-CM codebook for further guidance. Also, when working on the coding cases, it might be necessary to reference your medical terminology and anatomy and physiology resources in order to code the cases. Once you have finished coding the case studies, check your progress with the answers and rationales in Chapter 12.

Reviewers

Suzan Hauptman, MPM, CPC, CEMC, CEDC
President
ACE Med Group
Pittsburgh, Pennsylvania

Christina Wear, CPC, CPC-H
Tucson, Arizona

About the Author

Deborah J. Grider is a nationally sought after leader in the industry and is passionate about assisting physicians and hospitals in improving their coding, documentation, and business operations to maintain compliance and improve revenue. She will go above and beyond to help industry leaders, physicians, and others achieve excellence. Her motto is "documentation excellence is the key to improving revenue."

Ms Grider brings more than 35 years of experience as a practice administrator, medical record auditor, and clinical documentation improvement practitioner to the healthcare industry. She has worked with a variety of medical specialties and with hospitals and outpatient facilities both small and large to provide practice assessments, revenue cycle guidance, coding, auditing, CDI development, continuing education, and project management. She also provides litigation support to attorneys nationwide on behalf of their physician and health system clients. She is considered a top ICD-10 implementation expert and routinely appears on ICD-10 Monitor's "Talk Ten Tuesday." She has also written many articles for various healthcare publications including *Medical Economics, Journal of Medical Practice Management, Physician Practice Magazine*, and *Businessweek*, to name a few.

Ms Grider combines teaching with practical advice on coding and revenue cycle issues to many national organizations. She has numerous books and publishing credits and has developed coding program curricula for the American Academy of Professional Coders (AAPC), Indiana University Health, and Martin University in Indianapolis. In addition to her work at Karen Zupko & Associates (KZA) as a Senior Consultant, Deborah was a Senior Manager of Revenue Cycle at Blue and Co., where she oversaw the consulting division for physician services and worked closely with hospitals and hospital-owned physician groups assisting with coding reviews, practice operations, ICD-10 implementation, and consulting. She has held the role of Vice President of Strategic Development and President of the American Academy of Professional Coders where she oversaw the Association's operations. She owned her own full-service consulting firm for 12 years, leading her team to provide coding, auditing, and revenue cycle guidance to hospitals and physician groups. Prior to entering consulting, she was a practice administrator at Indiana University Health.

Ms Grider has a BA in Business Administration from Indiana University. She holds multiple coding, auditing, and clinical documentation credentials. She currently serves on the ICD-10 Monitor Editorial Board and Indiana Health Information Management Association Executive Board of Directors as a delegate. She is the past president of the Indiana Health Information Management Association and the past president of the AAPC National Advisory board and served on the board for seven years. Deborah has served on the CPT Editorial panel representing AAPC, served on the editorial board of Contexo Media, and currently serves on the editorial board of the ICD-10 Monitor.

Ms Grider has authored, among other titles, *Principles of ICD-10-CM Coding,* Fourth Edition (AMA, 2017), *Coding with Modifiers,* Fifth Edition (AMA, 2013), *Medical Record Auditor,* Fourth Edition (AMA, 2014), and *Preparing for ICD-10-CM* (AMA, 2010).

viii

Introduction to ICD-10-CM Coding

Basics of the ICD-10-CM Codebook

The ICD-10-CM codebook is divided into the following seven sections:

1. ICD-10-CM Conventions

2. ICD-10-CM Official Guidelines for Coding and Reporting

3. Index to Diseases and Injuries (Alphabetic Index)

4. Neoplasm Table

5. Table of Drugs and Chemicals

6. ICD-10-CM External Cause of Injuries Index

7. Tabular List by Chapter and Disease Classification

It is important to understand the ICD-10-CM Official Guidelines for Coding and Reporting and coding conventions when coding with ICD-10-CM. Following is a review of those conventions.

CODING CONVENTIONS

Format of ICD-10-CM

ICD-10-CM is divided into two main parts: the Index to Diseases and Injuries and the Tabular List. The Index, typically referred to as the Alphabetic Index, contains diseases, conditions, and injuries. It is important to be able to identify the main term in a diagnostic statement in order to find the correct code classification in the Alphabetic Index. For example, in the diagnostic statement, "the patient has allergic rhinitis," the main term is "rhinitis."

The Tabular List is organized by chapter and contains categories, subcategories, and valid codes. For example, Chapter 10 of ICD-10-CM contains Diseases of the Respiratory System. Within this chapter is the diagnosis, Acute sinusitis (J01). This condition is further subdivided into a fifth-character classification that identifies whether the acute sinusitis is:

- Acute maxillary sinusitis (J01.0-)

- Acute frontal sinusitis (J01.1-)

- Acute ethmoidal sinusitis (J01.2-)

- Acute spenoidal sinusitis (J01.3-)

- Acute pansinusitis (J01.4-)

- Other acute sinusitis (J01.8-)

- Acute sinusitis, unspecified (J01.9-)

The Tabular List includes a three-character category. Some categories in ICD-10-CM are only three characters; however, ICD-10-CM always begins with an alpha character. If the code cannot be further subdivided into the fourth, fifth, sixth, or seventh characters, the three-character code is a valid code. Codes that can be further subdivided must be selected. Codes must always be selected to the highest level of specificity.

When coding in ICD-10-CM, begin with the main term and locate the term in the Alphabetic Index and follow by selecting the correct code in the Tabular List. Never code directly from the Alphabetic Index—especially in ICD-10-CM—because the complete code is not always indicated when additional digits such as a sixth or seventh character are required. This information, including additional instructional notes, is only found in the Tabular List.

Neoplasm Table

The Neoplasm Table is organized by anatomical site and is divided into six columns:

1. Malignant Primary

2. Malignant Secondary

3. Cancer In Situ

4. Benign

5. Uncertain Behavior

6. Unspecified Behavior

The Neoplasm Table should be used only as a reference; the final code should be selected from the Tabular List. The diagnostic statement should indicate which column in the table should be referenced.

For example, if the patient has cancer in situ of the vermilion border of the lip, the coder would reference lip–vermillion border, reference code D00.01 in the Neoplasm Table, and verify the code in the Tabular List. In the Tabular List, code D00.01 is specified as "Carcinoma in situ of labial mucosa and vermilion border."

Table of Drugs and Chemicals

The Table of Drugs and Chemicals lists drugs and chemicals with the codes that identify the intent. ICD-10-CM is different from ICD-9-CM in that the external cause of the injury and poisoning is not coded in ICD-10-CM. The Table of Drugs and Chemicals is divided into the following six columns:

1. Poisoning, Accidental (unintentional)

2. Poisoning, Intentional (self-harm)

3. Poisoning Assault

4. Poisoning Undetermined

5. Adverse Effect

6. Underdosing

As with the Neoplasm Table, never code from the Table of Drugs and Chemicals. Always reference the drug or chemical in the table and then select the appropriate code from the Tabular List, which provides more specificity, instructional notes, and guidance. It is recommended that the coder also have a drug reference book to assist in identifying generic or chemical names, because some brand-name drugs are listed not by the brand name but by the generic name of the drug or chemical.

External Cause of Injuries Index

The External Cause of Injuries Index lists injuries alphabetically. An External Cause code should be reported when an accident or injury occurs, including the place or activity related to the injury. As with the Alphabetic Index, the External Cause of Injuries Index should be used only as a reference. The appropriate diagnosis code should be selected from the Tabular List.

Punctuation

- **Brackets** ([ ])—Used in the Tabular List to enclose synonyms, explanatory phrases, and alternative words. Brackets are used in the Alphabetic Index to identify manifestation codes.

- **Parentheses** (( ))—Enclose supplementary words that may be present or absent in the statement of a disease without affecting the code assigned and are found both in the Alphabetic Index and Tabular List. The terms within the parentheses are nonessential modifiers.

- **Colon** (:)—Used after a complete term when one or more of the modifiers following the colon provide more guidance to assigning the code in the category. The colon is used only in the Tabular List.

Placeholder Character

In ICD-10-CM, "x" is used as a placeholder character for future expansion. In some cases the "x" is included in the code. However, if a code must be coded to the seventh character, and the code is subdivided into a fourth or fifth character, the placeholder "x" must be added to the code in order to code to the highest level of specificity and to validate the code.

Abbreviations Used in Both the Alphabetic Index and the Tabular List

- **NEC**—Not Elsewhere Classifiable. Represents "other specified." Used in the code when a more specific code is not available for the condition.

- **NOS**—Not Otherwise Specified. Equivalent to "unspecified."

Instructional Notes

- **Includes**—Provides guidance to conditions or diseases included in the category. This note appears immediately under a three-character code to further define or provide examples in the category.

- **Excludes**—There are two types of "excludes" notes in ICD-10-CM: Excludes1 and Excludes2.

  - **Excludes1**—The codes or conditions are excluded in the category when two conditions cannot occur together, such as congenital and acquired. For example, a patient coded as having type 1 diabetes mellitus would never be reported with type 2 diabetes mellitus. (Rule of thumb: Never code two conditions that have an Excludes1 note.)

  - **Excludes2**—Represents "Not included here." This note indicates that the condition excluded is not part of the condition represented by the code. A patient may have both conditions, and if the diagnostic statement indicates that both conditions exist, both may be coded. For example, if a patient has a condition of acute bronchitis (J20.-) and the condition is also chronic (J42), both conditions may be coded because there is an Excludes2 note under category J20.

- **Inclusion terms**—This is a list of terms included under the code. Terms may be synonyms of the code for which the code is to be used. The terms are not exhaustive. Additional terms located in the Alphabetic Index may also be assigned to a code.

Etiology/Manifestation Conventions

Two instructional notes are important in ICD-10-CM code reporting. Many conditions have an underlying etiology or might have manifestations due to the underlying etiology. These instructional notes indicate the proper sequencing: etiology followed by the manifestation. In the Alphabetic Index, the manifestation code is listed in brackets. In the Tabular List, follow the instructional notes:

- **Code First**—The codes should be reported as the first-listed diagnosis code.

- **Use Additional Code**—An additional code is required to explain the diagnostic statement.

Other Instructional Notes

- **And**—Means either "and" or "or" when it appears in the title.

- **With**—Means "associated with" or "due to."

- **See**—Indicates that another term should be referenced before going to the Tabular List. (Located in the Alphabetic Index.)

- **See also**—Indicates that another main term should be referenced that may provide additional information. This instruction is optional when the main term provides the necessary guidance. (Located in the Alphabetic Index.)

- **Code also**—Indicates that two codes may be required to fully describe the condition.

- **Code first if applicable, any causal condition first**—Indicates that a code may be assigned as the first-listed or principal diagnosis when the causal condition is unknown or not applicable. If the causal condition is known, the code for the causal condition should be sequenced as the first-listed diagnosis.

- **Default code**—Indicates that the code listed next to the main term in the Alphabetic Index is the default code, which is the condition most associated with the main term or the unspecified code for the condition. If no further information is available, the default code is assigned.

Other and Unspecified Codes

- **Other Specified**—Codes are for use when the information in the medical record provides detail in which a specific code does not exist. Alphabetic Index entries that designate NEC designate "other" codes in the Tabular List.

- **Unspecified Codes**—These codes are used when the information in the medical record is insufficient to assign a more specific code.

CODING TIP It is important that the medical record documentation contain specificity to assign a more specific ICD-10-CM code. Before selecting a code that is "unspecified," query the practitioner for more information.

Be sure to reference the General Coding Guidelines before selecting an ICD-10-CM code. These guidelines are located in the ICD-10-CM Official Guidelines for Coding and Reporting 2017.

1. Always code to the highest level of specificity. If a three-character code cannot be further subdivided into a fourth, fifth, sixth, or seventh character, it is acceptable to report the code. If the code can be further subdivided, the coder must report the full number of characters required for the code.

2. Signs and/or symptoms are reported when a diagnosis is not confirmed. Signs or symptoms that are associated with the confirmed diagnosis should not be assigned. If a definitive diagnosis has not been established by the end of the encounter, it is appropriate to assign a code for the signs and/or symptoms. It is not appropriate to assign a specified diagnosis when it is not supported in the medical record documentation.

3. Signs and/or symptoms that are not associated with the disease or condition may be reported if documented in the diagnostic statement.

4. Multiple coding for a single condition is used when two codes are required to fully describe a single condition that affects multiple body systems or an underlying cause. The instructional notes "Code First" and "Use Additional Code" are used to identify this guideline. Multiple diagnosis codes may be needed to report late effects, complications, or obstetrics to fully describe the condition.

5. When the same condition is both acute (subacute) and chronic, the acute condition is sequenced first followed by the chronic condition.

6. Combination codes are codes that report a single condition that indicates two diagnoses: a diagnosis that includes the manifestation and a

diagnosis that includes an associated complication. If the combination code lacks the specificity in describing the manifestation or complication, an additional code may be reported.

7. The term "sequelae" is a residual effect of the acute phase of an illness or injury. For example, a malunion of a fracture is considered a late effect. There is no time limit on when a late effect code can be reported. Coding of sequelae generally requires two codes: the condition or nature of the sequelae (sequenced first) and the late effect code (sequenced second). (The exception to the rule: When the code for sequelae is followed by a manifestation code, or when the late effect located in the Tabular List includes the manifestation at the fourth, fifth, sixth, or seventh character to include the manifestation. Keep in mind that the code for the acute phase of the illness or injury leading to the late effect is never used with a code for the late effect. In certain conditions the seventh character "S" is reported as the seventh character for the late effect.)

8. If the condition is described in the documentation as "impending" or "threatened" and the condition occurred, code as a confirmed diagnosis. However, if the condition did not occur, reference the Alphabetic Index and look for the subentry terms "impending" and "threatened." If the subterms are listed, follow the guidance in the Index and assign the code; if the subterms are not listed, code only the underlying condition.

9. In general, each diagnosis should be reported only once for each patient encounter. This rule applies to bilateral conditions when a code identifying laterality is not available. In ICD-10-CM many categories and subcategories indicate laterality. The final character of the code indicates laterality. In many categories, there is a separate code for left side, right side, and bilateral. Only if a bilateral code is not available in the category, report separate codes for the left side and right side. If the side is not specified in the documentation, and the provider cannot be queried, use the unspecified side code.

10. Medical record documentation dictates assignment of Body Mass Index (BMI) for pressure ulcer stage codes, which is required when coding pressure ulcers. The patient's primary physician typically will document the BMI when the patient is admitted to the hospital. The BMI codes should only be reported as secondary diagnoses. Additional diagnoses should be reported if the condition affects the patient's care. In addition, the associated diagnosis such as overweight, obesity, and so

on, must be documented in the medical record and should be coded.

11. History codes may be used as secondary diagnoses if the historical condition, personal history, or family history has an impact on care or influences treatment. For example, a patient's personal history of tobacco use would impact or influence the patient's treatment.

12. Patient encounters for circumstances other than diseases or injuries are reported with Chapter 21, "Factors Influencing Health Status and Contact with Health Services (Z00-Z99)."

13. Never code "rule out," "suspected," or "probable." If a confirmed diagnosis cannot be established or is not documented in the medical record, the signs and/or symptoms are reported. This rule differs from the coding guidelines for the inpatient setting.

14. Chronic diseases may be coded as many times as a patient is treated for the condition. For example, if a patient has acute bronchitis that is chronic, the chronic bronchitis should be reported in addition to the acute condition. If the condition is not treated or does not affect patient care during the encounter, do not report the condition.

15. Do not code conditions previously treated that no longer exist. If the condition coexists, report the condition at the time of the encounter that affects treatment or management of the patient. History codes may be reported as secondary diagnoses if the historical condition or family history has an impact or influences treatment.

16. If the patient received only diagnostic services, sequence the reason for the encounter chiefly responsible for the outpatient service being provided. Other conditions such as chronic conditions treated may be reported as additional diagnoses.

17. For routine laboratory/radiology testing when signs and symptoms are not present, assign code Z01.89, Encounter for other specified special examinations. If other non-routine signs, symptoms, diseases, or conditions are treated during the patient encounter, it is appropriate to assign both the Z code and the other diagnoses.

18. For diagnostic tests that have been interpreted and a confirmed diagnosis documented, and a final report is available at the time of coding, code the definitive diagnosis, not the signs or symptoms related to the confirmation. Note: This instruction differs from the coding practice in the inpatient hospital setting.

19. For therapeutic services, code the reason chiefly responsible for the therapeutic service(s) provided during the patient encounter. The exception is when the primary reason for the visit is chemotherapy and/or radiation therapy. The Z code for the chemotherapy or the radiation therapy is listed first, followed by the condition that supports the therapy. For example, if a patient receives chemotherapy for breast cancer, the Z code for the chemotherapy is listed first followed by the appropriate code for the breast cancer.

20. If the purpose of a patient's visit is to receive preoperative evaluations or preoperative clearance, report a code from subcategory Z01.81-, Encounter for preprocedural examinations. The code for the condition/diagnosis that is the reason for surgery should be sequenced as the second-listed diagnosis. If additional findings are documented, such as other diseases or conditions, they may also be reported.

21. For surgical procedures, if the preoperative diagnosis is different from the postoperative diagnosis, code the postoperative diagnosis.

22. For a general medical examination with abnormal findings, a code from category Z00.0- should be assigned as the first-listed diagnosis. A secondary diagnosis for the abnormal finding should also be coded.

23. A screening code may be reported as the first-listed code if the reason for the patient encounter is specifically the screening examination. It may be used as an additional diagnosis code when the screening is performed during the patient encounter for other health problems. A screening code is not required if the screening is inherent to a routine examination. Screening codes are reported with category Z11, Z12, Z13, and Z36.

24. For routine outpatient prenatal visits when no complication is present, report a code from category Z34, Encounter for supervision of normal pregnancy, as the first-listed diagnosis code.

References

1. Centers for Medicare & Medicaid Services ICD-10 website. Available at: www.cms.gov/ICD10.

2. ICD-10-CM Official Guidelines for Coding and Reporting 2017.

CHAPTER 1

Certain Infectious and Parasitic Diseases (A00-B99)

ICD-10-CM Chapter 1 Guideline Review

In this chapter you will find a summary of the chapter-specific coding guidelines for Chapter 1 of the ICD-10-CM codebook followed by case studies to build ICD-10-CM diagnosis coding skills in this area.

Many medical specialties reference Chapter 1 of the ICD-10-CM codebook for human immunodeficiency virus (HIV) infection, other infections, and parasitic diseases. Keep in mind that you should always reference the ICD-10-CM Official Guidelines for Coding and Reporting in its entirety when making a code selection.

Human Immunodeficiency Virus (HIV) Infection Guidelines

Code only confirmed cases of the HIV infection or illness. The first-listed or principal diagnosis should be coded as B20 if the condition is confirmed and the reason for the patient encounter is the HIV infection or illness. The condition should be clearly documented in the patient's medical record. Any related conditions are reported in addition to code B20.

The following guidelines apply to HIV infections:

- Confirmation does not require documentation of positive serology or culture for HIV. The provider's diagnostic statement in the medical record that the patient is HIV positive is sufficient.

- If the patient is treated for an unrelated condition and the patient has HIV disease, the unrelated condition is reported as the first-listed diagnosis followed by code B20 for a patient who has acquired immune deficiency syndrome (AIDS) or the active HIV virus. Any additional diagnoses relative to the patient encounter may be reported.

- If the patient is admitted or treated for an HIV-related condition, the first-listed diagnosis is B20 followed by the diagnosis codes for the related HIV conditions. Any additional conditions treated should also be reported.

- If the patient is asymptomatic, meaning no symptoms or related HIV conditions, code Z21 is reported for the HIV-positive status. This code is not used if the documentation states "AIDS," or if the patient is treated for an HIV-related illness.

- When there is inconclusive evidence or inconclusive HIV serology, report code R75, Inconclusive laboratory evidence of human immunodeficiency virus (HIV).

Once a patient has been diagnosed with any HIV-related illness, code B20 should always be assigned; codes R75 or Z21 (Asymptomatic HIV) should never be assigned.

- If a patient is treated for an HIV-related illness during pregnancy, childbirth, or the puerperium, the first-listed diagnosis should be reported with code O98.7-, Human immunodeficiency (HIV) disease complicating pregnancy, childbirth and the puerperium, followed by code B20 for the HIV-related illness.

For a patient who is treated for asymptomatic HIV during pregnancy, childbirth, or the puerperium, code O98.7- should be the first-listed diagnosis followed by code Z21 for the asymptomatic HIV status.

- For a patient who is being screened for HIV status, report code Z11.4, Encounter for screening for human immunodeficiency virus (HIV), followed by any associated diagnosis for high-risk behavior.

When the patient encounter is for HIV testing and the patient has signs and/or symptoms, report code Z11.4 for the testing and the signs and symptoms. If HIV counseling is provided, report code Z71.7, HIV counseling, as an additional diagnosis.

When the patient who has been tested returns for his or her HIV test results and the test is negative, report code Z71.7 for the HIV counseling. If the results are positive, codes should be selected based on the circumstance.

Infectious Agents as the Cause of Diseases Classified in Other Chapters

Some infectious agents are classified in other chapters of the ICD-10-CM codebook and cannot be identified as part of the infection code. Instructional notes guide the coder to use a required additional code to identify the agent in Chapter 1. Other infectious agents include:

- Organisms, including Streptococcus, Staphylococcus, and Enterococcus (B95)

- Other bacterial agents (B96)

- Viral agents (B97)

Infections that are resistant to antibiotics should be reported with code Z16, Resistance to antimicrobial drugs, followed by the infection code for the patient encounter if the infection does not identify drug resistance.

Sepsis, Severe Sepsis, and Septic Shock

The following guidelines apply when reporting sepsis:

- The underlying systemic infection should be reported. If the type of infection is unknown or causal and is not further specified, report code A41.9, Sepsis, unspecified organism.

Code R65.2, Severe sepsis, should only be reported if severe sepsis or an associated acute organ dysfunction is present. Severe sepsis should not be reported under the following circumstances:

- Negative or inconclusive blood cultures and sepsis

  - Urosepsis

  - Sepsis with organ dysfunction

- Acute organ dysfunction that is not clearly associated

The provider should be queried if it is not evident that the condition is associated with sepsis. Severe sepsis requires two codes: (1) a code for the underlying systemic infection followed by (2) a code from subcategory R65.2, Severe sepsis.

If the causal organism is not documented in the medical record, unspecified code A41.9 is reported. Additional diagnosis codes must be reported for any associated acute organ dysfunction. It is important that the provider is queried if the coder is uncertain as to the complex nature of the severe sepsis.

Septic shock is generally referred to as circulatory failure associated with severe sepsis and is considered a type of organ dysfunction. Following are the guidelines for reporting septic shock:

- When the documentation indicates septic shock, the code for the underlying systemic infection is reported as the first-listed diagnosis followed by code R65.21, Severe sepsis with septic shock, or code T81.12, Postprocedural septic shock. Any acute organ dysfunctions should be assigned an additional code. Septic shock indicates the presence of severe sepsis. When septic shock is documented in the patient's medical record, code R65.21 is assigned even if severe sepsis is not documented. **Note:** The code for septic shock cannot be the principal or first-listed diagnosis.

- When severe sepsis is the principal diagnosis present on admission or develops during the hospitalization, a code for the underlying systemic infection is reported with the appropriate infection code followed by a code from category R65.2. Code R65.2 should not be assigned as the first-listed or principal diagnosis but may be reported as a secondary diagnosis.

- If a localized infection is present on admission and the patient has sepsis or severe sepsis, the code for the underlying systemic infection should be reported first, followed by the localized infection (eg, pneumonia, cellulitis). When the patient has severe sepsis (in the absence of septic shock), a code from category R65.2 should also be reported.

- When sepsis or severe sepsis does not develop until after admission and if the reason for admission is the localized infection, the localized infection should be reported first, followed by a code for the sepsis or severe sepsis.

Sepsis that results in a post-procedural infection is a complication of medical care. To report the infection:

- Report the post-procedural infection codes (T80.2, T81.4, T88.0, or O86.0) followed by the code for the specific infection.

- If the patient has severe sepsis, report a code from category R65.2 along with an additional diagnosis for any acute organ dysfunction. In cases where a post-procedural infection has occurred and has resulted in severe sepsis and post-procedural septic shock, the code for the precipitating complication, such as code T81.4, Infection following a procedure, or O86.0, Infection of obstetrical surgical wound, should be coded first followed by code R65.21, Severe sepsis with septic shock and a code for the systemic infection.

As with all post-procedural complications, code assignment is based on the provider's documentation of the relationship between the infection and the procedure. In some cases, a non-infectious condition may lead to an infection that may result in sepsis or severe sepsis. For example, if a patient suffers a third-degree burn of the trunk and is hospitalized, he or she may develop an infection, which could result in sepsis or severe sepsis. The following coding rules apply:

- When a non-infectious condition such as burn, trauma, or injury is the reason for treatment and meets the criteria for principal or first-listed diagnosis, the non-infectious condition is reported first. When severe sepsis is present, a code from category R65.2 should be reported as a secondary diagnosis along with any associated organ dysfunction codes.

- When the infection is the principal diagnosis and meets the criteria for principal or first-listed diagnosis, it should be reported first followed by the non-infectious condition (eg, burn, trauma).

- When both infectious and non-infectious conditions meet the definition of principal diagnosis, either can be sequenced first.

- Only one code from category R65.- should be assigned for the patient encounter. When a non-infectious condition leads to infection and severe sepsis, a code from category R65.2 is assigned. Do not report a code from category R65.1, Systemic Inflammatory Response Syndrome (SIRS) of non-infectious origin, under this circumstance.

Methicillin-Resistant *Staphylococcus aureus* (MRSA) Conditions

Methicillin-resistant *Staphylococcus aureus* (MRSA) infection is caused by a strain of staph bacteria that's become resistant to the antibiotics commonly used to treat ordinary staph infections.

Most MRSA infections occur in people who have been in hospitals or other health care settings, such as nursing homes and dialysis centers. MRSA infections typically are associated with invasive procedures or devices such as surgeries, intravenous tubing, or artificial joints. MRSA can also occur in healthy people. This form often begins as a painful skin boil. It is spread by skin-to-skin contact.

When a patient is diagnosed with the MRSA infection due to *Staphylococcus aureus*, and that infection includes the causal organism (pneumonia, sepsis, etc), assign a combination code for the condition along with the associated organism. For example, A41.02, Sepsis due to MRSA, along with J15.212, Pneumonia due to Methicillin-resistant *Staphylococcus aureus*, would both be reported. Do not assign B95.62, Methicillin-resistant *Staphylococcus aureus* infection as the cause of diseases classified elsewhere, as a combination code because B95.62 does not identify the type of infection. Furthermore, do not assign Z16.11, Resistance to penicillin, as an additional diagnosis.

When documentation indicates the patient is carrying the condition or the condition has colonized the carrier, code Z22.322 is reported for MRSA colonization. When the patient is suspected to be a carrier of the condition, assign Z22.321, Carrier or suspected carrier of Methicillin-susceptible *Staphylococcus aureus*. When the documentation indicates the patient as having both MRSA colonization or a suspected carrier and the infection during a hospital admission, Z22.322 is reported along with the appropriate code for the MRSA infection.

Zika Virus Infection

Code only a confirmed diagnosis of Zika virus (A92.5), as documented by the provider. This is an exception to the hospital inpatient guideline Section II, H. Confirmation does not require documentation of the type of test performed; the physician's diagnostic statement that the condition is confirmed is sufficient. This code should be assigned regardless of the stated mode of transmission.

If the provider documents "suspected," "possible," or "probable" Zika, do not assign code A92.5. Assign a code(s) explaining the reason for encounter (such as fever, rash, or joint pain) or Z20.828, Contact with and (suspected) exposure to other viral communicable diseases.

Now that you have a good understanding of the general ICD-10-CM coding guidelines and the chapter-specific guidelines for Certain Infectious and Parasitic Diseases, build skill and knowledge by coding the following exercises. Be sure to reference the ICD-10-CM codebook and the ICD-10-CM Official Guidelines for Coding and Reporting, along with the instructional notes, when coding these conditions.

Case Studies

CASE STUDY 1

A 5-year-old boy was brought to the physician's office by his parents. This is the patient's first visit. He has been running an elevated temperature for the past 12 hours; the high was 102°F. He also complains of stomach pains and vomiting. The parents are very concerned. No allergies or medications. Patient lives with his parents.

PHYSICAL EXAMINATION: Well-developed, well-nourished child who is lethargic and pale. His temperature is 101°F; pulse 110; and respiration 28.

Eyes are normal. There is a minimal amount of inflammation of the tonsils. Ears, nose, and mouth are normal. Neck is supple. Skin examined—negative.

CHEST: Lungs sounds are normal.

HEART: Normal rhythm with no murmurs appreciated.

ABDOMEN: Diffuse tenderness. No masses or organomegaly noted.

LABORATORY: Labs normal except for urinalysis (UA) dip performed in the office, which was positive. Urine culture is pending at this time. Blood drawn in office and sent to ABC Lab.

ASSESSMENT AND PLAN: Ordered renal X ray, UA, and labs. Urine culture is pending at this time. Acute pyelonephritis. Nausea with vomiting. Patient to return in two days.

ADDENDUM: Urine culture shows *E. coli* >100,000. Renal X ray indicates acute pyelonephritis.

Patient's mother notified; begin antibiotic regimen and patient will return in one week unless condition worsens. Prescription called into Super K Pharmacy.

ICD-10-CM Code(s) _____

CASE STUDY 2

HISTORY OF PRESENT ILLNESS: This is a 56-year-old white male who underwent coronary artery bypass grafting on 04/20/20xx. His postoperative course was uneventful and he was discharged to home on 04/25/20xx. He felt like he was progressing fairly well; however, on 05/10/20xx, he noted the onset of fever, as well as significant pain in the region of the sternal incision as well as on the right side of the chest. He was noted to have some purulent-appearing drainage from the sternal incision and was ultimately transferred to the Mount Murphy Cardiovascular Care Center for further evaluation and treatment. He was taken to the operating room by the cardiovascular surgeons on 5/11/20xx and underwent incision and drainage of his sternal wound. A significant amount of purulent-appearing fluid was evacuated from the superior aspect of the sternal incision. It was the surgeon's opinion at the time that this fluid was confined to the superficial soft tissues and that the underlying fascia appeared to be intact. There were no exposed wires. The wound was then packed with gauze. Cultures from that external wound have since grown *S. aureus*. Blood cultures also are growing *S. aureus* in four out of four bottles. He was placed empirically on Vancomycin IV. He does state today that his fever and chest pain are improved. His white blood cell count has also decreased.

PAST MEDICAL HISTORY:

- Coronary artery disease
- Hypertension
- Hyperlipidemia
- Depression
- Gastroesophageal reflux disease
- Obstructive sleep apnea
- Chronic low back pain
- History of back surgery

PAST SURGICAL HISTORY:

- Umbilical hernia repair
- Disc surgery in the back
- Coronary artery bypass grafting as mentioned above

MEDICATIONS:

- Lopressor
- Pepcid
- Prozac
- Celebrex
- Zocor
- Humulin 70/30
- Oxycontin
- Vancomycin

SOCIAL HISTORY: He is married, denies any alcohol use, and has never smoked.

FAMILY HISTORY: Significant for coronary artery disease and diabetes.

PHYSICAL EXAMINATION:

VITAL SIGNS: He is currently afebrile, with a blood pressure of 114/64, heart rate 80, and respiration 18.

GENERAL: He is alert, oriented ×3, and has a PICC line.

CHEST: Clear to auscultation. Examination of the sternal wound finds that it is now open and packed. There is still some purulent drainage in the wound bed, although certainly decreased in amount.

CARDIOVASCULAR: Regular.

ABDOMEN: Obese, but soft and nontender.

EXTREMITIES: No edema.

LABORATORY: Cultures are as described above. His white blood cell count has decreased from 7.9 to 15.8; hemoglobin is 11.2; and platelet count is 186,000. His creatinine is 1.5 on admission. A chest X ray shows no acute changes.

IMPRESSION:

1. Surgical wound infection, sternal, secondary to *S. aureus*

2. Septicemia, secondary to *S. aureus*

3. Leukocytosis

4. Anemia

5. Diabetes mellitus; Type 1; good insulin control

PLAN:

1. Continue Vancomycin, 1 g IV every 12 h, at the present time. We will obtain a pharmacokinetics consultation for assistance with dosing.

2. Add Rifampin 300 mg po, bid.

3. Follow up on *S. aureus* susceptibilities. If this is found to be Methicillin-resistant *S. aureus*, then we will leave him on the Vancomycin and Rifampin; however, if this is a Methicillin-susceptible *S. aureus*, we would likely switch him to a continuous infusion of Nafcillin instead of using Vancomycin IV.

4. Continue wound care. We will consider the use of a VAC dressing after discussion with the cardiovascular surgeons.

ICD-10-CM Code(s) _____

CASE STUDY 3

PREOPERATIVE DIAGNOSIS: Dyspepsia and dysphasia.

POSTOPERATIVE DIAGNOSIS: Candida esophagitis confirmed by pathology.

ANESTHESIA: Demerol 50 mg intravenous; Versed 6 mg intravenous.

PROCEDURE: The risks and benefits of the procedure were explained to the patient and informed consent was obtained. The patient was placed in the left lateral decubitus position. Flexible video endoscope was gently advanced through the cricopharyngeus into the esophagus. There are typical changes of Candida esophagitis in the mid and distal esophagus. Photographs and biopsies were taken. The gastro-esophageal (GE) junction is located at 38 cm from the incisors. Retroflexed views in the cardia showed no fundic mass. The endoscope was placed in the forward viewing position and advanced from the greater curvature to the antrum and there is no evidence of ulceration or mass. The pylorus is patent. The duodenal bulb is nondeformed and free of ulceration. Post-bulbar duodenum is unremarkable. The endoscope was then withdrawn back into the stomach. Gastric biopsies were taken to exclude *Helicobacter pylori* and the procedure was terminated. The patient tolerated the procedure well without evident complications.

ICD-10-CM Code(s) _____

CASE STUDY 4

The patient is a 25-year-old male who has had AIDS for the past year complicated with Kaposi's sarcoma (KS). He also complains of pain at the KS lesions on the right leg and left thigh, especially when touched. He indicates his pain is a 5 on the pain scale of 0–10.

MEDICATIONS: See medication sheet in chart.

EXAMINATION: Blood pressure 140/80; pulse 120; and respiration 28. Temperature 103.9°F. General appearance: Ill-looking young man, diaphoretic. Oral mucosa moist without lesions. Lungs: Diminished breath sounds in the right middle lower lobe. Heart: RRR without murmurs. Abdomen: Soft and nontender. Extremities: Without cyanosis or edema. There is a large Kaposi's sarcoma on the right medial leg and left medial proximal thigh, which is somewhat tender. Neurological exam: Cranial nerves II through XII are grossly intact. Mental status: The patient is depressed and withdrawn over his illness.

ASSESSMENT AND PLAN: AIDS complicated with multiple opportunistic infections with poor performance status, which suggested a limited prognosis of less than six months. The patient is experiencing pain from the Kaposi's sarcoma lesions. We will start patient on oxycodone 5 mg q2h as needed for cough and pain. Counseled patient on coping with illness. Patient will return in two weeks for follow-up or sooner if needed.

ICD-10-CM Code(s) _____

CASE STUDY 5

This 34-year-old female patient presents to the office today, complaining of small, open lesion-like sores on her ears. They burn and have been present for two days. The patient has AIDS and has been treated in this office for the past six months.

REVIEW OF SYSTEMS: She notes shortness of breath with walking. She has a frequent cough. She notes a history of bruising easily. Review of systems is otherwise negative.

PAST MEDICAL HISTORY: Developed AIDS via a needle stick. The patient was a nurse at ABC Hospital for eight years prior to her illness.

PHYSICAL EXAMINATION: This is an adult female who is alert and oriented ×3. Temperature is 97.6°F; pulse 118/80; weight 203 pounds; height 6 feet. HEENT: Viral vesicular dermatitis noted in ears. Extraocular movements are intact. PERRLA: Neck is supple. Lungs are clear to auscultation bilaterally. Heart is regular without murmur. Abdomen: Soft, nontender, nondistended. I detect no mass, organomegaly, or hernia. Extremities: No cyanosis, rashes, or edema. Evidence of previous left lower extremity bypass surgery.

ASSESSMENT: Herpesviral vesicular dermatitis

PLAN: Prescribed antibiotic to treat otitis externa. Patient will come back to the office in 10 days for follow-up. Continue same medication regimen.

ICD-10-CM Code(s) _____

CASE STUDY 6

Mary is a 12-year-old girl who comes here for follow-up appointment after her recent emergency room (ER) visit. The patient was seen initially in our office one week ago with fever of 102.8°F and vomiting. She was sent to our ER, was told she was having a simple viral illness, and was sent home with symptomatic treatment. Today she presented to our office indicating she is significantly better. Her fever resolved. She does not have any symptoms such as cough, vomiting, or decreased appetite.

PHYSICAL EXAMINATION: Temperature 98.7°F; weight 78 pounds; height 42 inches. General: In no acute distress. Neck: Supple; no mass, no lymphadenopathy. Oral cavity: Reveals normal oral mucosa, no erythema, no exudate. Lungs: Clear to auscultation bilateral; no rales, no wheezing, no rhonchi. Heart: Regular S1-S2; no murmurs, no gallops, no rubs. Abdomen: Soft, nontender, no distention. Positive bowel sounds in all four quadrants. Ears: Examination reveals normal tympanic membrane, bilateral.

ASSESSMENT AND TREATMENT PLAN: Acute viral infection. Resolved. We will see Mary for a follow-up appointment in one month for her well visit.

ICD-10-CM Code(s) _____

CASE STUDY 7

A 45-year-old female presents to her family practice physician with headache, chills, and myalgia for the last 14 days. She recently returned from her daughter's house in Texas. Her daughter had two dogs and a cat.

While interceding in what sounded like a struggle with the cat, it turns out the cat had trapped a mouse. When she went to move the cat, the patient said she was bitten by the mouse on the index finger. On examination she has a rash with truncal macules and papulae that have spread to the extremities. There is a centrifugal nature to the rash; however, Rocky Mountain spotted fever is ruled out. Lab tests reveal mild thrombocytopenia.

ASSESSMENT: Murine typhus.

PLAN: Ciproxin 500 mg po q 12 hours for 14 days. Return in five days for recheck, or sooner if needed.

ICD-10-CM Code(s) _____

CASE STUDY 8

A 25-year-old male, while hunting last week, stepped on a jagged piece of metal that lodged in his right foot. He was seen in the ER later that day and now six days later has a swollen, red, painful foot that is not relieved with over-the-counter medications. He has no other medical problems and has no allergies.

On examination he is pleasant, alert, and oriented; vital signs are normal with exception of a temperature of 101°F; lungs clear; cardio is negative to mrg's; and abd is benign. He does have some lymphadenopathy and groin tenderness. His extremities are benign except for his right foot that is edematous and has a red appearance. The foot is warm to touch.

ASSESSMENT: Deep infection of the foot from penetrating wound

PLAN: Cultures obtained. Pending these results, I have placed the patient on Vibramycin 100 mg tid for the next ten days. Culture was positive for Madura foot.

ICD-10-CM Code(s) _____

CASE STUDY 9

This is a 52-year-old rancher who raises sheep. He presents today with a history of three weeks of fatigue, weakness, and aching all over his body. He has tried some over-the-counter drugs with no relief and seeks a medical opinion at this time. He denies any n/v/d, cough, abdominal discomfort, or urinary problems. History is significant for his occupation as a sheep farmer and recently lost 25 ewes to some "weird virus" the vet told him about. He is an otherwise healthy male with no other illnesses and no medications. He is single and likes to "dabble in the drink" once

in a while, but otherwise denies any other risks. An old mountain rancher and his wife who are both deceased due to old age adopted him as a child. On exam he is quite pleasant with a slightly disheveled appearance. His vital signs are 136/85; 98.6°F; 88/20; and oriented ×3. HEENT: PERRLA, o/p and mm are clear. Respiration: Clear to auscultation. Heart: RRR S1, S2 normal. Abdomen: Slightly tender with good bowel sounds. Urinary: Negative, no hematuria. Musculoskeletal: DTRs slightly sluggish, no edema in all four extremities. Skin: Very dry and weathered, reflective of his lifestyle.

ASSESSMENT AND PLAN: Virus infection from sheep. Labs reviewed and cultures sent. Start antibiotic therapy and await blood tests and lab. Labs confirm patient suffers from *Brucella melitensis*.

ICD-10-CM Code(s) _____

CASE STUDY 10

A return visit by a 60-year-old male who presents today with a history of joint pain, muscle pain, and malaise for two weeks. He has tried exercise as well as some "pain medication" he had left over from his back surgery two years ago. He has some "funny sensations" in his arms at times that feel like pinpricks. He denies any shortness of breath, but does have some "fluttering sensations in his heart." He has no allergies, takes no other medications, and does not drink or smoke. He is divorced with a son. His mother died at 84 with congestive heart failure, and his dad died of an acute MI last spring. He has one sister who lives in a small town in Oklahoma and is well. Significant history: He went on a fishing trip with his son a month ago and found a very large tick on his arm when he returned to camp the last night of the trip. He lit a match and the tick released and dropped to the floor.

EXAM: Const: He is a pleasant well-nourished male in NAD. HEENT: Negative. Cardio: Slightly irregular; no rubs, gallops, murmurs. Respiration: Breath sounds slightly diminished on the left. Abdomen: No tenderness, bowel sounds present. Skin: He has some erythema-type lesions on both arms and on the bottom portions of his leg.

ASSESSMENT AND PLAN: Possible tick fever. Labs: CBC, Chem 7, H/H. Labs returned with positive diagnosis of Boutonneuse fever. Patient was given appropriate antibiotics and will be checked back in seven days.

ICD-10-CM Code(s) _____

CASE STUDY 11

A 33-month-old girl with history of asthma presents to the ER with vomiting and diarrheal illness. Diarrhea started three days ago with more than 40 episodes during that time, all non-bloody stools. Patient's mother describes these as water green with some mucus. The illness is also associated with vomiting over 20 times in the last three days (non-bilious and non-bloody), low-grade fevers as high as 100°F, decreased po intake, decreased urine output the last 24 hours, abdominal pain, and more sleepy per parents. All other review of systems was negative. Denies, rash, fevers, cough, wheezing, and breathing problems. History of being treated for bronchitis/sinusitis last week by pulmonologist and was started on Azithromycin. Completed a five-day course of Azithromycin three days prior to admission. The patient was taken to the ER for evaluation and found to have a bicarbonate of 11 and to be severely dehydrated. The patient was admitted to the pediatric ward for further management of dehydration with IV fluids and supportive care.

Past medical history includes history of asthma diagnosed July 2014 and is followed by pulmonology.

PAST SURGICAL HISTORY: None.

SOCIAL HISTORY: Lives with parents.

A comprehensive examination was performed.

ASSESSMENT:

1. Dehydration, resolved

2. Viral gastroenteritis, resolving

3. Asthma

4. Diaper rash

A 33-month-old girl with history of asthma with vomiting and diarrhea consistent with viral gastroenteritis complicated by dehydration. Satting well on room air in ER. Chest X ray was negative. Rotavirus screen and strep screen, negative. Symptomatomethlogy consistent with viral gastroenteritis. No emesis or diarrhea prior to discharge.

The patient received a normal saline bolus at 20 ml per kilo in the ER. The patient also received D5/normal saline at one and a half times maintenance, which is 72 ml per hour. Initial bicarbonate was 11. Repeat Chem 7 in am. Strict ins and outs. Age-appropriate diet. Zofran 2 mg IV q eight hours prn, nausea, vomiting.

PLAN: Patient with history of asthma. Will continue on albuterol 2.5 mg nebulizers every four hours. The patient will be continued on home Qvar BID, Veramyst, and ipratropium bromide nasal spray. Spot check pulse and oxygen monitoring. Chest X ray negative. Diaper rash: Riley Butt Cream prn, along with battier wipes.

ICD-10-CM Code(s) _____

References

1. Centers for Medicare & Medicaid Services ICD-10 website. Available at: www.cms.gov/ICD10.

2. ICD-10-CM Official Guidelines for Coding and Reporting, 2017.

Neoplasms (C00-D49) and Diseases of the Blood and Blood-Forming Organs and Certain Disorders Involving the Immune Mechanism (D50-D89)

ICD-10-CM Chapters 2 and 3 Guidelines Review

In this chapter you will find a summary of the chapter-specific coding guidelines for Chapter 2 of the ICD-10-CM codebook followed by case studies to build ICD-10-CM diagnosis coding skills in this area.

There are currently no chapter-specific guidelines for Chapter 3 of the ICD-10-CM codebook (Diseases of the Blood and Blood-Forming Organs and Certain Disorders Involving the Immune Mechanism). In addition to the general coding guidelines, the Index to Diseases and category/subcategory–specific instructions should be followed when coding from Chapter 3 of the ICD-10-CM codebook.

Many medical specialties reference Chapters 2 and 3 of the ICD-10-CM codebook for coding neoplasms and blood disorders. Keep in mind that you should always reference the ICD-10-CM Official Guidelines for Coding and Reporting in its entirety when making a code selection.

Neoplasm Guidelines (C00-D49)

Codes in Chapter 2 include codes for most benign and malignant neoplasms. Some benign neoplasms such as adenomas can be located in the specific-chapter body areas. Neoplasms should first be referenced in the neoplasm table in the Index to Diseases and referenced in the Tabular List. Codes are selected based on the following:

- **Malignant primary**—Where the cancer or neoplasm originated.

- **Malignant secondary**—Where the cancer metastasized or spread to.

- **Cancer in situ**—Neoplasms contained in one area that rarely spread.

- **Uncertain behavior**— Histology cannot confirm benign or malignant.

- **Unspecified behavior**— Information not available to code either benign or malignant.

If the documentation indicates "adenoma," reference the Index to Diseases and review the entries under the term "adenoma" for the specific body area. Neoplasms are referenced in the Neoplasm Table by site (anatomical) and by the type of neoplasm.

CODING TIP Always reference the Tabular List for the correct code verification and to ensure that a more specific code is not available.

Following is a summary of how to code neoplasms based on the ICD-10-CM Official Guidelines for Coding and Reporting:

- When treatment is directed at the malignancy, the malignancy is the first-listed diagnosis. The code selected as the first-listed diagnosis is the condition treated. It could be a primary malignancy or a secondary malignancy.

- If treatment is directed at the secondary site, code the secondary malignancy as the first-listed diagnosis even though the primary malignancy is still present. Code the primary site if the secondary diagnosis is known. For example, if the physician is treating breast cancer that has metastasized from the colon, the malignancy of the breast is coded as the first-listed diagnosis from the malignant secondary column and the secondary diagnosis is coded as a neoplasm of the colon as the secondary diagnosis (malignancy, primary site).

Complication Coding

When coding for anemia that is associated with a malignancy and the treatment is for anemia, follow these guidelines:

- The malignancy is reported as the first-listed diagnosis followed by a code for anemia in neoplastic disease (D63.0).

- When managing anemia associated with the adverse effect of chemotherapy administration, the adverse effect code is reported first followed by the code for anemia (secondary). The malignancy should also be reported along with the adverse effect (T45.1x5, Adverse effect of antineoplastic and immunosuppressive drugs).

- When managing anemia associated with the adverse effect of radiotherapy, the anemia code is sequenced first followed by the appropriate malignancy code (eg, code Y84.2, Radiological procedure and radiotherapy as the cause of abnormal reaction of the patient, or of later complication, without mention of misadventure at the time of the procedure).

- When managing dehydration due to malignancy, if only dehydration is being treated via an IV rehydration, the dehydration code is sequenced first, followed by the malignancy code.

- If a complication results from a surgical procedure, the complication is the first-listed diagnosis if treatment is for the complication.

- When the primary malignancy has been previously excised or eradicated and no further treatment is directed at the site, and there is no other evidence of any existing primary malignancy, a personal history code is reported from category Z85. If documentation indicates that a secondary site is being treated, report the malignancy secondary site as the first-listed diagnosis, with code Z85 for the history of the primary site as the secondary diagnosis.

Encounters for Chemotherapy, Radiation Therapy, and Immunotherapy

Following is a summary of the guidelines used to report patient encounters when a malignancy results in treatment of chemotherapy, immunotherapy, or radiation therapy:

- The code for the neoplasm should be sequenced first when the surgical removal is followed by chemotherapy, immunotherapy, or radiation therapy during the same episode of care regardless of whether the neoplasm was removed from the primary or secondary site.

- When the patient is admitted only for the administration of chemotherapy (Z51.11), immunotherapy (Z51.12), or radiation therapy (Z51.0), the appropriate therapy code is reported. If a combination of more than one of these therapies is performed during the same encounter or admission, the therapies can be sequenced in any order. The malignancy should be assigned as a secondary diagnosis.

- When complications arise following the admission or patient encounter for chemotherapy, immunotherapy, or radiation therapy, the first-listed diagnosis is the therapy followed by the code for the complications. Common complications include dehydration, nausea, and vomiting.

- When the patient encounter or admission is to make a determination of the extent of the malignancy, the first-listed diagnosis is the malignancy or metastatic site even if chemotherapy or radiation therapy is administered.

- Symptoms and/or signs or ill-defined conditions associated with the existing primary or secondary malignancy cannot be used to replace the malignancy code(s). They are reported as additional diagnoses if applicable.

- When the patient encounter is to treat neoplasm-related pain, code G89.3 is reported when the patient is associated with the cancer, primary or secondary malignancy, or tumor. This code is assigned regardless of whether the pain is acute or chronic. When the reason for the encounter is the pain or pain management, G89.3 is assigned as the first-listed diagnosis, with the neoplasm assigned as the secondary diagnosis.

- When the reason for the encounter is the neoplasm and pain associated with the neoplasm, the neoplasm is reported as the first-listed diagnosis, and the pain, G89.3, is reported as an additional diagnosis. It is not necessary to code the site of the pain.

- When there is more than one malignancy in the same organ, the documentation should be specific as to which is the primary malignancy and which is the secondary malignancy. Often the documentation is unclear and the provider must be queried.

- When the patient has advanced metastatic disease and the primary or secondary sites are not known, report code C80.0, Disseminated malignant neoplasm, unspecified.

- Cancer unspecified is reported as code C80.1, Malignant (primary) neoplasm, unspecified. This code is reported rarely in the inpatient setting and is only used when the determination cannot be made as to the primary site of the malignancy.

Sequencing of neoplasms is important for diagnosis reporting purposes. The following rules apply:

- Treatment of the primary malignancy is reported as the first-listed diagnosis followed by any metastatic sites if they exist.

- Treatment of the secondary malignancy is reported as the first-listed diagnosis code followed by the malignancy of primary site (if known).

- When a patient is pregnant and has a malignant neoplasm, code first a pregnancy complication code from category O9A.1- followed by the appropriate neoplasm code.

- When a neoplasm is associated with a complication, and treatment is directed toward the complication, the complication is reported as the first-listed diagnosis followed by the appropriate neoplasm code. One exception is anemia. When the patient has been treated for a malignancy and the patient encounter is directed at the complication, the malignancy is reported as the first-listed diagnosis and the secondary code is the complication for the anemia (D63.0-, Anemia in neoplastic disease).

- When the patient has a surgical procedure due to or as a result of the malignancy and is being treated for a complication, the complication code is the first-listed diagnosis code followed by the malignancy or personal history of the malignancy, whichever is applicable.

- When the patient is treated for a pathological fracture due to a neoplasm and treatment is directed toward the fracture, a code from category M84.5- is reported as the first-listed diagnosis followed by the neoplasm.

- If the focus of treatment is the neoplasm and the patient has an associated pathological fracture, the neoplasm is reported first, with a code from category M84.5- sequenced as the secondary diagnosis.

Current Malignancy versus Personal History of Malignancy

When the provider is treating a patient for a primary malignancy, whether or not surgery, chemotherapy, immunotherapy, or radiation therapy is being provided, report the primary malignancy code until treatment is finished. The following guidelines apply:

- If the primary malignancy has been completely excised or eradicated from the site of the malignancy and no further treatment is necessary, the personal history of the malignancy is reported with category Z85.

- When the patient has been treated for multiple myelomas, leukemia, or malignant plasma cell neoplasms and is in remission, codes from category Z85.6, Personal history of leukemia, or Z85.79, Personal history of other malignant neoplasms of lymphoid, hematopoietic and related tissues, are reported. The physician should be queried if the documentation as to the remission status of the patient is unclear.

- Follow-up care codes are used to explain continued surveillance following the completed treatment of a disease, condition, or injury. The condition in these instances has been completed and no longer exists. Follow-up codes can be used in conjunction with history codes to provide a clear picture of the healed condition and its treatment. The follow-up code should be sequenced first, followed by the history code. Codes to report in this category include Z08, Encounter for follow-up examination after completed treatment for malignant neoplasm. An additional code for any absence of organ removal (Z90.-) and/or history of the malignant neoplasm (Z85.-) can also be reported.

- When a neoplasm is associated with a transplanted organ, the patient encounter should be reported as a transplant complication with a code from category T86.-, Complications of transplanted organs and tissue, as the first-listed diagnosis followed by the code C80.2, Malignant neoplasm associated with transplanted organ, and the code for the malignancy. An additional code should be reported for the specific malignancy.

- When reporting follow-up care after treatment of malignancy, removal of a prophylactic organ for prevention, or provision of aftercare following surgery of a neoplasm, use a code in Chapter 21 in ICD-10-CM (Factors Influencing Health Status and Contact with Health Services).

Now that you have a good understanding of the chapter-specific guidelines for Neoplasms, it is time to build skill and knowledge by coding the following exercises. Be sure to reference the ICD-10-CM codebook and the guidelines when coding these exercises. There are no chapter-specific coding guidelines for Diseases of the Blood and Blood-Forming Organs and Certain Disorders Involving the Immune Mechanism. Reference the ICD-10-CM Official Guidelines for Coding and Reporting along with the instructional notes in the categories and subcategories when reporting these conditions.

Case Studies

CASE STUDY 1

A 52-year-old male with a nine-month history of progressive otalgia and constant otorrhea was noted to have a 1.8-cm ulceration along the floor of his left external auditory canal. The tympanic membrane was intact. A 1.5-cm, mobile, nontender, jugulodigastric lymph node was palpated. Biopsy confirmed the presence of a well-differentiated squamous cell carcinoma. High-resolution CT demonstrated: (1) limited erosion of the tympanic bone, but no extension to the mastoid or middle ear; and (2) several high cervical lymph nodes that were suspicious for metastatic disease.

ICD-10-CM Code(s) _____

CASE STUDY 2

CHIEF COMPLAINT: Spots right chest.

HISTORY OF PRESENT ILLNESS: This patient has had a spot on the right chest for months that itches constantly.

PAST SURGICAL HISTORY: Hand repair, neck surgery, 20xx.

ALLERGIES: NKDA.

CURRENT MEDICATIONS: Evista, Voltaren, MVI, Calcium, Vitamin C, Lysine.

FAMILY HISTORY: Father and sister with melanoma. Mom and sister with unusual moles.

SOCIAL HISTORY: Alcohol; Occupation: Administrative assistant.

REVIEW OF SYSTEMS:

GENERAL: No fatigue.

HEENT: No sinus symptoms.

CARDIOVASCULAR: Denies chest pain, SOB with exertion, palpitations, murmur, leg swelling.

RESPIRATORY: Denies cough, SOB, hemoptysis.

GI: Denies nausea, vomiting, diarrhea, change in bowel habits, melena.

GU: Denies kidney problems, problems urinating, UTI.

MUSCULOSKELETAL: Denies joint pain, muscle weakness.

NEUROPSYCHIATRIC: Denies seizures, memory problems, depression.

ENDOCRINE: Denies cold or heat intolerance, polyuria, polydipsia.

ALLERGY/IMMUNOLOGY: Denies unusual allergic reactions, asthma, hay fever.

HEMATOLOGIC: Denies unusual bleeding, bruising, anemia, lymph node enlargement.

PHYSICAL EXAMINATION:

GENERAL APPEARANCE: Well developed, well nourished, no acute distress.

EYES: Normal conjunctiva and eyelids.

EXTREMITIES: Digits normal.

JOINTS: DJD hands.

NEUROLOGICAL: Balance and gait normal.

PSYCHIATRIC: Oriented ×3; mood and affect normal.

SKIN: Scalp and body hair normal.

ECCRINE AND APOCRINE GLANDS: Normal.

HEAD AND FACE: Normal.

NECK: Normal.

CHEST AND AXILLAE: BCC 8 mm right chest.

BACK: Normal.

ABDOMEN: Normal.

RIGHT UPPER EXTREMITY: Normal nevus each arm; left upper extremity normal.

ASSESSMENT: Basal cell carcinoma right chest wall, 8 mm.

PLAN: The lesion was anesthetized with 1% Xylocaine with 1/100,000 epi, biopsied, and then the base was treated with electrodessication and curettage ×3. Bacitracin and a bandage were applied. The specimen was sent for histology. The patient was counseled concerning skin cancer, monthly self-exams, and the significant risk of developing new skin cancers because the patient has already had skin cancer. The patient should call if he/she identifies any new or unusual spots or moles and return sooner than the scheduled appointment. Patient will return in three months.

ICD-10-CM Code(s) _____

CASE STUDY 3

PROCEDURE: Removal of right internal jugular Port-A-Cath.

ADMITTING DIAGNOSIS: Port-A-Cath removal.

CLINICAL HISTORY: Primary ovarian carcinoma, no longer requiring chemotherapy.

RESULT: Following the usual sterile preparation and local anesthetic, an incision was made over the Port-A-Cath chamber site. Using blunt dissection, the chamber was dissected free of the subcutaneous pocket. The catheter was then pulled out. Manual pressure was held at the base of the neck. The incision site was closed with two layer 4-0 Vicryl sutures. The patient tolerated the procedure without immediate complication.

IMPRESSION: Successful removal of Port-A-Cath.

ICD-10-CM Code(s) _____

CASE STUDY 4

The patient has metastatic colon cancer and is in need of a port.

HISTORY OF PRESENT ILLNESS: I was asked by Dr Meadows to see this patient in the office today. The patient was diagnosed recently with colon carcinoma invasive/metastatic. She had a colectomy and had chemotherapy for about six months. She had a good course after that. Just recently she started to have back pain and epigastric pain. CT scan was performed, which showed metastatic disease to the liver and also to the abdominal cavity. For this reason, I was asked to place a Port-A-Cath for palliative chemotherapy treatment.

PAST MEDICAL HISTORY: Colon cancer stage III.

PAST SURGICAL HISTORY:

- Colon resection
- Hernia repair
- Cholecystectomy
- Appendectomy
- Hysterectomy

SOCIAL HISTORY: The patient is married and has three children. The patient denies alcohol abuse. The patient has not smoked for approximately 15 years; she used to smoke a half a pack a day.

ALLERGIES: Vicodin and Zofran.

MEDICATIONS:

- Morphine
- Phenergan
- Ativan

PHYSICAL EXAMINATION:

GENERAL: She is awake, alert, and oriented ×3.

VITAL SIGNS: Stable; she is afebrile.

LUNGS: Clear.

HEART: Regular.

CHEST: She has a scar on her left chest from a previous port; there is another scar on her right side.

ABDOMEN: Soft and nontender; no hepatosplenomegaly.

ASSESSMENT: This is a patient with metastatic colon cancer.

PLAN: We will place a Port-A-Cath tomorrow. We discussed the risks and complications with the patient including bleeding, infection, and pneumothorax related to the port. She understands and wants to proceed.

ICD-10-CM Code(s) _____

CASE STUDY 5

HISTORY OF PRESENT ILLNESS: John is seen for further follow-up of severe factor VIII deficient hemophilia with a history of a high responding inhibitor. He infuses 1000 units of Recombinate daily. His last infusion was this morning at 6 am. He is also followed by Dr Combs for septic arthritis requiring removal of a left total knee arthroplasty (TKA) in 2005 and removal of a right total hip arthroplasty (THA) in 2004. Currently he is doing well. His protein levels are low and he is working on dietary modification to bring those to an acceptable level for replacement of joints soon and is followed closely by Dr Combs in this regard. He receives physical therapy two times a week. He has not been taking Fosamax due to waking up in the morning with pain, requiring pain medication with a little bit to eat, so he is taking a multivitamin with calcium. Monday he woke up with a left elbow bleed. He infused with Recombinate 2000 units bid. It lasted through Friday. He is feeling significantly better. He does know whenever he wakes up feeling sore, he needs to infuse more than his usual prophylactic dose. Approximately one month ago he had a small, red area close to the catheter, a little inferior to the insertion site. It only lasted a couple of days and he did not have any fever or chills; no night sweats, nausea, or vomiting.

REVIEW OF SYSTEMS: No recent illnesses; no fever or chills, nausea, or vomiting; no diarrhea, constipation, shortness of breath, or chest pain.

MEDICATIONS: Mephyton 5 mg qd; Pepcid 20 mg qd; multivitamin 1 qd; docusate sodium 2 capsules bid; EQ Allergy Relief D Tab 1 qd; Lorazepam 1 mg 1-2 qhs; Methadone 10 mg 5 tablets qid; Flonase 1 spray each nostril qd; calcium with vitamin D 600 mg 1 qd.

PHYSICAL EXAMINATION: HEENT: Mucous membranes moist. Respiratory: CTAB. Cardiovascular: Regular rate, rhythm; no MGR. Abdomen: Positive bowel sounds, no bruits audible. Extremities: Left, lower extremity immobilizer intact. Removed for exam. No open areas, no erythema near incisions on lateral

aspect of knee. A slight amount of skin discoloration due to hemosiderin deposition on lateral aspect of knee; nontender. Integumentary: Right subclavian Hickman. Dressing removed for assessment. No areas of erythema noted. Insertion site clean, dry and intact. Suture intact. No tenderness.

ASSESSMENT AND PLAN:

1. Severe factor VIII deficient hemophilia with resolved left elbow bleed. Instructed him with elbow bleed to infuse 3000 units bid and if it does not resolve within three days to call the office and we will obtain a factor VIII level six hours post infusion.

2. Hickman catheter. The erythematous area near the Hickman catheter is somewhat concerning for possible resurgence of an infection. At this time there was nothing visible and it is nontender. We will continue to monitor catheter.

3. Had scheduled patient for next comp clinic. Has not been to comp clinic in a long time and he declined a comp clinic appointment. Will return in three months for follow-up.

ICD-10-CM Code(s) _____

CASE STUDY 6

HISTORY OF PRESENT ILLNESS: Alan is a 60-year-old African-American male seen in follow-up with hemoglobin sickle cell (SC) disease and history of type 2 diabetes. Chief concern today, "nothing out of the ordinary."

Sickle cell: The patient reports some minor VOC pain approximately two days ago in the morning upon rising. He states the pain is usually an achiness in his left shoulder that tends to resolve as he progresses through the day. He states these symptoms tend to be exacerbated by changes in the weather. He is presently taking Percocet and Oxycontin for pain management. Overall, he continues to do well with home pain management.

Diabetes: The patient continues to see his primary care physician on a monthly basis. He states his random blood sugars have been running between 95 and 102. His primary physician would like to keep this lower and will consider a medication change at the next visit if the blood sugars remain higher than the preferred range. Alan has had intermittent bouts of paresthesia of the left foot. There is no pattern to the onset of episodes and he notes an increase in episodes approximately two to three weeks ago. He thinks that it is probably related to his diabetes and he will be talking with Dr Ogula about the episodes. He is scheduled to see Dr Ogula again in early March.

The patient consistently has increased shortness of breath with any activity, especially walking any distance. Regarding his diet, on the last visit I had encouraged him to try to make his last meal earlier in the day and to eat small meals more frequently. He states that he is beginning to eat his last meal earlier in the evening and has begun to pay closer attention to the amount of food as well as the time of the day and frequency of his meals.

REVIEW OF SYSTEMS: Weight, energy, and appetite remain stable. He is positive for chronic shortness of breath, especially with increased activity. He is negative for chest pain or headaches. He is also negative for any changes in bowel or bladder habits. He denies any changes in his vision and he also denies any sore throat, cough, cold, flu-like symptoms, chills, or fever.

PHYSICAL EXAMINATION: Vital Signs: Weight 135.3 kg; temperature 36.6°C; heart rate 98; respiratory rate 18; blood pressure 146/77 mmHg. General: Alert and oriented ×3, obese African-American male in fair condition, without respiratory distress at this time. He is ambulatory with the aid of a cane. He presents with difficulty upon rising from his chair to move to the examination table. HEENT: Normocephalic and atraumatic. PERRLA: EOMs intact. Moist mucous membrane. There was no conjunctival or mucosal pallor and the oropharynx was clear. Neck: There was no lymphadenopathy and the neck was supple. Chest: There were expiratory wheezes heard throughout. Cardiovascular: Regular rate and rhythm with a systolic ejection murmur. No gallops or rubs were noted. Abdomen: Soft, obese, and bowel sounds in four quadrants. I was not able to appreciate or palpate the liver. Skin: Warm and dry. Extremities: The upper extremities were without edema, pain, or changes in coloration. The lower extremities were with minimum trace edema. Neurological: The lower legs were negative for any changes in sensory. Soft and sharp touch was equal bilaterally.

ASSESSMENT AND PLAN:

1. Hemoglobin SC disease with infrequent vaso-occlusive crisis: Generally, he has some early morning achiness without control with po pain management.

2. Vaso-occlusive crisis: No pain today. We will refill his pain meds of Percocet and Oxycontin.

3. Diabetes: Blood sugar doing well. A limited examination of the bilateral lower extremities and feet revealed no sensory deficits to sharp or soft tough.

4. Physical activity and diet: He has been encouraged to walk as much as possible and try to resume his treadmill use. Regarding his diet, he is encouraged to take small meals more often during the day and to eat his last meal earlier as well.

5. Labs today: CBC with differential V-MET and reticulocyte count. Discussed with Dr Cooper the patient's consistent elevated BUN. I am referring the patient to Dr Cooper for further evaluation. Nonetheless he presented with only trace edema of the lower legs; no UE edema.

6. The patient is to return to the office in one month.

ICD-10-CM Code(s) _____

CASE STUDY 7

HISTORY OF PRESENT ILLNESS: The patient is a 35-year-old African-American woman with hemoglobin SC disease. She has fairly frequent vaso-occlusive symptoms. Currently, the symptoms are reasonably stable. She is on chronic outpatient opioid therapy.

PHYSICAL EXAMINATION: On examination at the time of this visit, she was afebrile. There were no localized areas of bone tenderness.

IMPRESSION/PLAN: The patient's prescriptions were refilled. She is on Duragesic 25 mcg patches, sustained release morphine 60 mg every 12 hours, and immediate release morphine 15 mg every four to six hours prn. I will see her again in four weeks and we will continue to follow her on a monthly basis or sooner as necessary.

ICD-10-CM Code(s) _____

CASE STUDY 8

HISTORY OF PRESENT ILLNESS: Kathryn is a 45-year-old accountant who comes in today for routine follow-up. She had a right lower extremity deep vein thrombosis in 20xx with subsequent compartment syndrome and fasciotomy. She is on indefinite Coumadin and at this time is taking 4 mg daily. She is doing well with no specific complaints. She has had minimal pain that she rates 3 on the 0–10 pain scale.

REVIEW OF SYSTEMS: Her type 1 diabetes is well controlled with Lantus. Her fasting blood sugars in the morning have been running 95 to 110.

PHYSICAL EXAM: General: Pleasant-appearing female in no distress. HEENT: Conjunctiva is pink; neck is supple. There is no palpable cervical adenopathy, no scleral icterus. Cardiovascular: Heart had a regular rate and rhythm, with no appreciable murmurs, gallops, or rubs. There were no carotid bruits. Pulmonary: Breath sounds were equal bilaterally without crackles or wheezes. Extremities: Significant fasciotomy scar on her right lateral lower leg. Smaller scar medially. No ankle edema. Her peripheral pulses were strong and intact bilaterally. She has had some numbness of her right toes since the fasciotomy.

LABORATORY: INR by CoaguChek in office today was 3.8.

ASSESSMENT AND PLAN: Deep vein thrombosis right lower extremity worsening. She will decrease her dose to 3.5 mg daily, as her last three INRs have been elevated. She has a home monitor and emails the results to the office. She will return in six months for follow-up.

ICD-10-CM Code(s) _____

CASE STUDY 9

HISTORY OF PRESENT ILLNESS: Ginger comes in today for follow-up of her acute onset chronic superficial thrombophlebitis. She was started on Lovenox last week with a transition to Coumadin. She feels that her leg pain is better since she started on the Lovenox last week. A thrombosed varicose vein behind her right knee is less tender.

REVIEW OF SYSTEMS: Endocrine: Diabetes mellitus, very well controlled with Lantus and metformin. Vascular: History of multiple vein stripping procedures. GI: Ulcerative colitis under great control with diet and exercise.

PHYSICAL EXAMINATION: Vital Signs: Temperature 36.2°C; heart rate 102; respiration 18; and blood pressure 126/88. Abdomen: Ecchymotic areas in various stages of healing from Lovenox injections. Right lower quadrant subcutaneous hard area approximately 2 to 3 cm secondary from injection. Extremities: Trace edema, with hemosiderin deposits and evidence of chronic venous insufficiency over bilateral lower extremities.

LABORATORY: INR by CoaguChek was 5.6 today.

ASSESSMENT AND PLAN:

1. Superficial thrombophlebitis bilateral: She will stop Lovenox and continue on Coumadin with recommendations given for elevated INR.

2. Follow up in four weeks or sooner if problems.

ICD-10-CM Code(s) _____

CASE STUDY 10

PREOPERATIVE DIAGNOSIS: Nodular basal cell carcinoma, right lower lip and chin.

POSTOPERATIVE DIAGNOSIS: Same.

OPERATION PERFORMED: Excision of basal cell carcinoma and adjacent scar with complex linear repair.

SURGEON: Carl Morrison, MD.

ANESTHESIA: Local.

DESCRIPTION OF PROCEDURE: With the patient in the supine position, the face was prepared with chlorhexidine and draped in the usual manner. The tumor measured 1.5 × 1.0 cm arising in the right lateral lower lip skin and adjacent chin. Just medial and slightly superior to the tumor was an atrophic scar from a previous basal cell cancer removed nine years earlier. Proposed lines of excision were drawn around the tumor to include the adjacent scar and the area was anesthetized with 1% Xylocaine with 1:100,000 epinephrine, buffered with sodium bicarbonate. The tumor was excised down to orbicularis oris muscle, resulting in a defect measuring 2.1 cm wide × 3.0 cm in height in the shape of an inverted teardrop. Bleeding vessels were controlled with bipolar electrocoagulation. Adjacent skin was undermined at the deep subcutaneous level medially and laterally. Consideration was given to a rotation flap repair versus a complex linear repair. It was elected to do the defect extending to the vermilion border to convert the original defect to a lazy-S ellipse. Additional undermining was accomplished and the defect was approximated with layers of 5-0 Polyglactin suture deep. Final skin repair was accomplished and the defect was approximated 6-0 nylon sutures, supported by sterile strips over surgical adhesive followed by sterile occlusive dressing.

The specimen was submitted to pathology, after staining its superior margin red, its medial and deep margin black, and its lateral margin blue for pathologic orientation. The patient tolerated the procedure well and received one gram of acetaminophen (po) postoperatively.

PATHOLOGY REPORT: Confirms nodular basal cell carcinoma right lower lip and chin.

ICD-10-CM Code(s) _____

CASE STUDY 11

PREOPERATIVE DIAGNOSIS: Cavernoma, right cerebellar hemisphere.

POSTOPERATIVE DIAGNOSIS: Same.

PROCEDURE(S) PERFORMED: Right suboccipital craniectomy for resection of cavernoma.

FINDINGS: Old clot. Brain clot cavity was stuck tightly to the dural surface. The cavernoma was easily identified and was purple in color. There was a glottic plane around it.

INDICATIONS: Severe head pain.

DESCRIPTION OF PROCEDURE(S): The patient was brought to the operating room and general endotracheal anesthesia was induced. She was rolled into the prone position after placement of the head holder. Care was taken to pad all pressure points, including elbows and hands. Following this, standard prep and drape were performed. A right-sided incision was planned halfway between the mastoid and the inion running in a cranial-caudal direction. Following sterile prep and drape, local anesthesia was infiltrated into the wound and the skin was opened. The dissection was carried down onto the bone of the occiput, and the foramen magnum and the arch of C1 were exposed. Following this, the perforator and the Black-Max drill were used to drill down the bone and the bone was resected with a Kerrison punch. There was one small incidental durotomy. Following this, the dura was opened in a cruciate fashion and the cisterna magna was opened releasing a large amount of cerebrospinal fluid. The old blood clot, discolored brain, and a tip of the lesion were clearly visible on the surface of the brain. Once adequate hemostasis was obtained, dissection was carried on around the cavernoma within the gelotic space. This was a relatively straightforward maneuver and the lesion was resected in total. Inspection of the bed revealed no residual clot or lesion. Following this procedure, careful hemostasis was obtained. Avitene was placed in the wound and allowed to sit for several minutes. The Avitene was washed out and the lesion bed remained clear. A piece of Surgicel was placed in the craniotomy defect. The overlying muscle and fascia layers were closed with 0-Vicryl sutures, the subcutaneous tissues with 3-0 Vicryl sutures and the skin with a running 3-0 nylon. The patient tolerated the procedure well and was taken to the recovery room, then to the neurological ICU in critical condition.

ICD-10-CM Code(s) _____

CASE STUDY 12

HISTORY OF PRESENT ILLNESS: The patient is a 59-year-old white male who was brought into the hospital by his wife for problems associated with weakness, illness, general inability to ambulate, swollen calf, confusion, and a 25-pound weight loss. This has been ongoing for two months. Initial intake X ray showed evidence of mass lesions in the right lung. The patient was admitted. A Doppler ultrasound of the legs failed to reveal phlebitis. We are asked to see this patient in consultation by Dr Williams at this time, to try to assess how we can achieve diagnostic certainty for what looks like a large cavitary squamous-cell carcinoma with metastases to the brain.

MEDICAL HISTORY: The patient denies any history of coronary disease, diabetes, or hypertension but has had a past history of gastrointestinal abnormalities.

SURGICAL HISTORY: Fractured right hip about 10 years ago, with internal fixation.

SOCIAL HISTORY: The patient's industrial history is somewhat in construction and has some asbestos dust and biological exposures. There is an 80-pack-a-year exposure for smoking.

REVIEW OF SYSTEMS: Review includes some headache, loss of memory, loss of appetite, nausea, and dyspepsia. He reports that he has coughed up a modest amount of sputum and occasionally sees some blood. He has noted that his lower extremities have been progressively more edematous.

LABORATORY: Data includes a CT scan which shows a cavitary lesion of the right upper lobe about 6 cm in diameter, moderately thick-walled in character, with cavitary center. There is extension to the hilum in a 1.5 × 2 cm course. There is also a soft irregular density in the lateral aspect of the middle lobe 1 × 3 cm. The remainder of the CT scan is unremarkable except for a kidney cyst.

The patient's laboratory data show evidence of leucocytosis, significantly elevated D-dimer, mild decrease in albumin, mild elevation in alkaline phosphatase. Hemoglobin is unremarkable. The patient's C-reactive protein is 23.8, suggesting a dramatic inflammatory process.

PHYSICAL EXAMINATION:

GENERAL: The patient is a somewhat distant gentleman, lightly confused, with some problems of short-term memory. His wife reports that his memory is much worse than he will admit. He seems somewhat terrified of his inability to recall things.

VITAL SIGNS: Pulse is 100; blood pressure 150/70; respiratory rate 16; oxygen saturation 95% on room air.

HEENT: No acute pathology; pupils are equal and reactive to light.

NECK: Supple, without thyromegaly or jugular venous distention.

CHEST: Resonant, quiet, and clear.

CARDIAC: Tones are distant, without murmur or gallop.

ABDOMEN: Round and soft, bowel sounds are active.

EXTREMITIES: There is trace swelling over the right lower extremity, and 2+ swelling of the left lower extremity.

NEUROLOGIC: The patient is somewhat confused but has no focal neurologic defects.

IMPRESSION:

1. Cavitary lesion of the patient's right upper lobe, with hilar nodes and a cavitary lesion in the middle lobe, cavitary carcinoma.

2. Weight loss, probably related to malignancy.

3. Confusion, related to brain metastasis.

4. Swollen left leg, which is certainly suspicious for phlebitis, although that has not been documented.

5. Bilateral knee pain, which is suggestive of pulmonary hypertrophic osteoarthropathy. This patient has chronic obstructive lung disease that has not been quantified and is an 80-pack-year smoker.

PLAN: First, this patient needs to be placed in respiratory isolation with acid fasts obtained and category obtained. If the patient does not have evidence of tuberculous organisms in his sputum, a bronchospastic evaluation might be reasonable. The patient is scheduled for a CAT scan of the brain to evaluate the level of brain metastasis.

ICD-10-CM Code(s) _____

CASE STUDY 13

A 49-year-old patient with stage IIB endocervical cancer has completed her external beam radiation and is now scheduled for placement of tandems and ovoids for brachytherapy for completion of her radiation therapy. The patient is placed in the lithotomy position, prepped, and draped. The cervix is dilated using Hegar dilators and the uterus is sounded. A tandem (hollow cylinder) is inserted into the uterus, the other end of which protrudes through the vaginal opening. Two ovoids are placed in the upper part of the vagina, the other end of which protrudes through the vaginal opening. The ovoids and tandem are packed carefully in place to protect the bladder and rectum from radiation damage and to prevent any movement of the devices. Subsequent loading of the radioelement(s) into the cylinders at a later time will deliver a high dose of potentially curative radiation to the cervix from an intracavitary location.

ICD-10-CM Code(s) _____

CASE STUDY 14

PREOPERATIVE DIAGNOSIS: Lentigo maligna of the right neck.

POSTOPERATIVE DIAGNOSIS: Same.

PROCEDURE: Excision of 8-cm lesion, right neck, layered primary closure.

DESCRIPTION OF PROCEDURE: The patient was placed in the supine position. She was prepped and draped in the usual sterile fashion. Her previous biopsy indicated positive margins anteriorly and, therefore, the anterior extent of the lesion was drawn out. Beyond this marking, a 0.5-cm margin was drawn out. This was infiltrated with 1% Lidocaine with epinephrine. A #15 blade scalpel was used for full excision of the lesion. The specimen was sent for permanent histopathologic examination. Light undermining of all margins was performed. Primary closure was obtained with layered closure using 3-0 and 4-0 Monocryl followed by 5-0 nylon. The patient tolerated the procedure well, no complications were encountered.

ICD-10-CM Code(s) _____

CASE STUDY 15

Patient presents today for follow-up after mammogram. A 38-year-old female patient had mammogram after two nodules were found during a breast self-exam two weeks ago. There is no family history of breast cancer or cancer of any type.

EXAMINATION: Breast normal alignment, no drainage from nipple area. Palpation of upper-inner quadrant of the right breast identified two small nodules found in the 3 o'clock position of her breast.

We reviewed the mammogram results that confirmed malignant neoplasm of the right breast.

PLAN: Discussed surgical procedure and radiation therapy to follow. Patient is prepared and understands next steps.

IMPRESSION: Malignant neoplasm of upper-inner quadrant of right female breast.

ICD-10-CM Code(s) _____

Endocrine, Nutritional, and Metabolic Diseases (E00-E89) and Mental Behavioral and Neurodevelopmental Disorders (F01-F99)

ICD-10-CM Chapters 4 and 5 Guidelines Review

In this chapter you will find a summary of the chapter-specific coding guidelines for Chapters 4 and 5 of the ICD-10-CM codebook followed by case studies to build ICD-10-CM diagnosis coding skills in these areas.

Many medical specialties reference Chapters 4 and 5 of the ICD-10-CM codebook for coding endocrine, nutritional, and metabolic diseases and mental, behavioral, and neurodevelopmental disorders. Keep in mind that you should always reference the ICD-10-CM Official Guidelines for Coding and Reporting in its entirety when making a code selection.

ICD-10-CM Coding Guidelines for Endocrine, Nutritional, and Metabolic Diseases

DIABETES MELLITUS

The diabetes mellitus codes in ICD-10-CM are combination codes that include the type of diabetes with any associated complications or manifestations. Sequencing of complications is based on the reason for the patient encounter. The ICD-10-CM Official Guidelines for Coding and Reporting indicate to use as many codes as necessary from categories E08-E13 to identify all of the associated conditions or complications.

TYPE OF DIABETES

Even though most type 1 diabetic patients (ie, insulin dependent) develop diabetes prior to reaching puberty, which is why type 1 diabetes is also referred to juvenile diabetes, the age of the patient is not the sole determining factor in defining the type of diabetes. When the type of diabetes is not documented, the default code is code E11.-, Type 2 diabetes mellitus; however, for accurate coding, query the provider if possible. The most common type is type 2 diabetes mellitus.

DIABETES AND THE USE OF INSULIN

When the documentation does not specify the type of diabetes but does indicate that the patient uses insulin, the diagnosis code to report is E11.-, Type 2 diabetes mellitus.

Code Z79.4, Long-term (current) use of insulin, or Z79.84, Long-term (current) use of oral hypoglycemic drugs, should also be assigned to indicate that the patient uses insulin or hypoglycemic drugs. Code Z79.4 should not be assigned if insulin is given temporarily to bring a type 2 patient's blood sugar under control during an encounter. When the patient is pregnant and has type 1, type 2, or gestational diabetes, the first-listed diagnosis should be selected from Chapter 15 of the ICD-10-CM codebook.

Complications due to insulin pump malfunction include both underdosing and overdosing of insulin. The following guidelines apply:

- Underdosing of insulin due to insulin pump failure should be reported with a code from subcategory T85.6, Mechanical complication of other specified internal and external prosthetic devices, implants, and grafts, as the first-listed diagnosis followed by a poisoning code from category T38.3x6-, Underdosing of insulin and oral hypoglycemic (antidiabetic) drugs. The seventh-character extension will identify whether the encounter is Initial (A), Subsequent (D), or Sequela (S). Any additional codes for the type of diabetes mellitus and any complications should be reported as additional diagnoses.

- When an insulin pump malfunction results in an overdose of insulin, the first-listed diagnosis is reported with code T85.6- followed by code T38.3x1-, Poisoning by insulin and oral hypoglycemic (antidiabetic) drugs, accidental, unintentional, as the secondary diagnosis. The type of diabetes mellitus and any associated complications may be reported as additional diagnoses. Again, as with underdosing, the seventh character for the poisoning depends on the type of encounter.

SECONDARY DIABETES MELLITUS

Secondary diabetes mellitus is reported with codes from categories E08, E09, and E13. Category E08 is used to report diabetes mellitus due to underlying conditions; category E09 is used to report drug- or chemical-induced diabetes mellitus, and category E13 is used to report other specified diabetes mellitus. Category E13 is used to identify complications/manifestations associated with secondary diabetes mellitus. Secondary diabetes is always caused by another condition or event. The Official Guidelines cite examples of possible conditions or events such as cystic fibrosis, malignant neoplasm of the pancreas, pancreatectomy, adverse effect of a drug, or a poisoning. As with type 2 patients, code Z79.4, Long-term (current) use of insulin, or Z79.84, Long-term (current) use of oral hypoglycemic drugs, should also be assigned to indicate that the patient uses insulin or hypoglycemic drugs. Code Z79.4 should not be assigned if insulin is given temporarily to bring a type 2 patient's blood sugar under control during an encounter.

SEQUENCING RULES FOR SECONDARY DIABETES MELLITUS

Sequencing of the secondary diabetes codes is based on the Tabular List instructions for categories E08, E09, and E13.

SECONDARY DIABETES MELLITUS DUE TO PANCREATECTOMY

For post-pancreatectomy diabetes mellitus (ie, lack of insulin due to the surgical removal of all or part of the pancreas), code E89.1, Post-procedural hypoinsulinemia, is reported. A code from categories E13 and

Z90.41-, Acquired absence of pancreas, may be reported as additional diagnoses.

SECONDARY DIABETES DUE TO DRUGS

Secondary diabetes may be caused by an adverse effect of correctly administered medications, poisoning, or sequelae of poisoning, and are reported using the Table of Drugs and Chemicals. Use the Guidelines for Coding External Causes of Injuries, Poisonings, and Adverse Effects of Drugs for external cause code reporting.

Now that you have a good understanding of the chapter-specific guidelines for the Endocrine, Nutritional, and Metabolic Diseases, it is time to build skill and knowledge by coding the following exercises. Be sure to reference the ICD-10-CM codebook and the ICD-10-CM Official Guidelines for Coding and Reporting, along with the instructional notes, when coding these conditions.

Case Studies

CASE STUDY 1

CHIEF COMPLAINT: Unresponsiveness.

The patient is a 77-year-old female diabetic who had an insulin reaction and hypoglycemia. Her husband could not awaken her enough to give her orange juice, so he called the ambulance. She said her blood sugar has been fluctuating a lot more recently since she got a steroid shot because of back pain. When the EMTs arrived, they started an IV and gave D50. The patient awakened. When they re-checked the blood sugar, it was 149. She was brought to the emergency department by ambulance.

VITAL SIGNS: Afebrile, normal. Temperature was 96.9°F.

GENERAL: The patient is moving all extremities. Finger stick blood sugar was 140.

ASSESSMENT: Episode of hypoglycemia.

PLAN: The patient was discharged to home with her husband.

ICD-10-CM Code(s) _____

CASE STUDY 2

This is a follow-up visit for this 65-year-old female IDDM (type 1) patient. She was admitted to the hospital four days ago with cellulitis of the left foot. She was started on IV therapy for her cellulitis. She is recovering well, and the infection is almost gone. She has a history of IDDM. She denies chest pain or shortness of breath. Patient is positive for pain in the left foot that is sometimes severe in nature.

CURRENT MEDICATIONS: 70/30 insulin in the morning and 20 units in the evening; Cardizem CD 180 once daily; Imdur 60 mg once a day; Lasix 80 mg one a day; Pepcid 20 mg twice a day; Paxil 10 mg three times a day; Nitrostat as needed.

Well-developed, well-nourished female in no acute distress. Blood pressure 128/75; pulse: 80, regular and strong; respiration: 12, unlabored and regular. Temperature: Normal. Height: 5 feet. Left foot shows slight reddening on the upper surface. Infection had decreased significantly. All other areas are normal.

Patient is doing well and will be taken off IV Vancomycin. She will be discharged home tomorrow and will be given a prescription for penicillin. She is to follow up in my office in one week.

ICD-10-CM Code(s) _____

CASE STUDY 3

This patient is a pleasant, 67-year-old white female with a history of lower GI bleeding. She was scoped by Dr Barnes and found to have a rectal mass. She came into my office and we decided to perform surgery.

Her preoperative laboratory work found that she had hyponatremia, hypochloremia, and hypokalemia. She has an electrolyte abnormality.

CURRENT MEDICATIONS:

- Synthroid
- Toprol
- Effexor

SOCIAL HISTORY: She is a nonsmoker. She also has a history of drinking beer. She drinks about four beers every other day. She was in alcohol rehab before. No history of drug abuse.

FAMILY HISTORY: Positive for cancer.

REVIEW OF SYSTEMS:

CONSTITUTIONAL: No fevers; she has some weight loss but does not know how much.

CARDIOVASCULAR: No heart attack or high blood pressure.

RESPIRATORY: No asthma or cancer.

GASTROINTESTINAL: No gastric ulcers or gastro-esophageal reflux disease.

GENITOURINARY: No hematuria or dysuria.

MUSCULOSKELETAL: No fractures or dislocations.

INTEGUMENTARY: No new skin lesions or rashes.

NEUROLOGIC: No seizure or stroke.

PSYCHOLOGIC: No history of anxiety or depression.

ENDOCRINE: No diabetes but she does have a history of hypothyroidism and she has taken Synthroid for approximately 10 years.

PHYSICAL EXAMINATION:

GENERAL: She is awake and alert ×3.

LUNGS: Clear.

HEART: Regular.

ABDOMEN: Soft, nondistended and nontender.

RECTUM: There are no palpable masses.

LYMPHATIC: Neck and groin lymph nodes normal.

PSYCHIATRIC: Mood and affect appear to be normal.

ASSESSMENT: This is a patient with rectal cancer, hypochloremia, hyponatremia, and hypokalemia. Will admit her for IV fluid hydration for correction of her hyponatremia. Also, will start a bowel prep today for surgery tomorrow.

ICD-10-CM Code(s) _____

CASE STUDY 4

PREOPERATIVE DIAGNOSES: Acute respiratory failure and protein-caloric malnutrition.

POSTOPERATIVE DIAGNOSES: Same.

PROCEDURE(S) PERFORMED: Tracheostomy and percutaneous gastrostomy tube placement.

INDICATIONS: Respiratory failure and malnutrition.

DESCRIPTION OF PROCEDURE(S): The patient, who is 52 years of age, underwent induction with general anesthesia. After having placed a shoulder roll, the neck was prepared and draped in the usual sterile fashion. An open cutdown to the trachea was performed using a #10 blade scalpel. Dissection was undertaken utilizing Bovie cautery. The strap muscles were divided in the middle and the thyroid was pulled superiorly. A tracheal hook was placed in the trachea and the endotracheal tube was backed up to approximately 15 to 11 cm in distance. The percutaneous rhino technique was then utilized and the needle was introduced into the trachea. The wire was fed and the appropriate steps utilizing the dilators were undertaken. A tracheostomy was placed. Placement was confirmed and the trachea was secured into place utilizing interrupted nylon sutures. The incision was closed with an additional interrupted nylon suture.

Attention was then turned toward the placement of a feeding tube. An esophagogastroduodenoscope was placed via the mouth and the esophagus was viewed. It was felt to be normal; therefore, the stomach was entered. There was no evidence of abnormality and the pylorus was well visualized. The abdominal wall was also prepped and draped at this time. The patient was morbidly obese, and I was not able to gain adequate transillumination after entering the stomach and duodenum. By pushing on the abdominal wall, after determining location, a cutdown was made through the skin overlying the stomach utilizing a scalpel and Bovie cautery.

A retractor was placed. I was then able to transilluminate through the abdominal wall. A standard percutaneous endoscopic gastrostomy tube placement was performed. The needle was introduced and visualized as it passed. The wire was fed in and the grasper was utilized to grasp the wire. It was pulled out of the patient's mouth along with the scope. The tube was secured to the wire and the wire was pulled back out through the abdominal wall, placing the percutaneous endoscopic gastrostomy tube. At this time, the scope was reintroduced and the percutaneous endoscopic gastrostomy tube placement was confirmed.

The abdominal wall was closed utilizing 3-0 Vicryl sutures in an interrupted fashion followed by interrupted 3-0 Ethilon sutures.

All sponge, needle, and instrument counts were correct. The patient left the operating room in good condition and there were no complications. Blood loss was minimal.

ICD-10-CM Code(s) _____

CASE STUDY 5

Patient here for follow-up in the office for hyperlipidemia and some musculoskeletal pain she is concerned about. She has some left shoulder pain that started about two weeks ago. It is not related to any increased activity, however. She points between her scapula and her spine when she brings her elbows back. No weakness in the upper extremities or numbness. No cough, no chest pain, no shortness of breath.

PHYSICAL EXAMINATION: Weight 241 pounds; BP 134/82; pulse 68; respiratory rate 16; temperature 97°F. Eyes: anicteric; ears: clear; throat: normal. Neck: no JVD, no bruits. Abdomen reveals a flesh-colored lesion along the bra line, which is slightly irritated and erythematous. Extremities: no cyanosis, clubbing, or edema. Shoulder reveals good range of motion, some tenderness and spasm along the medial scapula on the left compared to the right. Distal neuro and vascular supply is grossly intact.

ASSESSMENT AND PLAN: Hypercholesterolemia and shoulder pain. Today her lipids revealed LDL of 131, total cholesterol 220. We will continue with the Zocor, given her two risk factors and her age. Recommended ibuprofen for muscle pain. Patient will return in three weeks for follow-up.

ICD-10-CM Code(s) _____

CASE STUDY 6

This established patient of the practice was referred back for consultation by his nurse practitioner regarding a problem with his left third toe. This has been a problem for several weeks. He is not certain what initially happened to the toe. He does have type 1 neuropathic arthropathy. His past medical history is significant for hypertension and diabetes. He denies any heart, liver, lung, or kidney problems; asthma; cancer; seizures; or blood disorders. Past surgical history: None. Medications: Insulin, 30 units in the morning and 20 units in the evening; Allopurinol, 300 mg daily; Lasix, 40 mg daily; Diovan, 80 mg daily; Norvasc, 10 mg daily. Allergies: None. Social history: He is single and disabled, denies tobacco, alcohol, or illicit drug use. Review of systems outlined as above. He denies any other specific complaints.

EXAMINATION: Temperature 97.9°F; heart rate 64; BP 142/79. Focused exam of the area in question reveals an ulcer and extensive callus formation on the distal end of the left third toe. There is no evidence of cellulitis. He has a good dorsalis pedis pulse in this foot.

PROCEDURE: After obtaining consent, extensively debrided the callus and sleuthing nail on the distal phalanx of the left third toe. I cauterized a few minor points of oozing with silver nitrate and applied mercurochrome to this. I instructed him to keep a light dressing on the toe, and we will see him again in two weeks.

ICD-10-CM Code(s) _____

CASE STUDY 7

Lisa comes in for her monthly OB check-up. She is at 30 weeks (third trimester). She has been having headaches, nausea, and vomiting. She thought she was getting the stomach flu. She has no fever, but her blood pressure is 150/90.

Blood sugar indicates gestational diabetes, which is under control with insulin. Gestational diabetes affected her first pregnancy.

Lisa is 5 feet, 4 inches and 175 lb (BMI 30.0) at onset of pregnancy. She now weighs 235 lb.

IMPRESSION: Moderate pre-eclampsia with gestational diabetes; morbid obesity due to excess calories.

ICD-10-CM Code(s) _____

CASE STUDY 8

A 45-year-old female patient is seen today who has type 2 diabetes with chronic kidney disease, stage 3. Her blood sugar is slightly elevated. She has been on insulin for the past seven months. According to the patient, her blood sugars are always elevated during lunchtime. In the am, sugars run between 100 and 120. Patient is undergoing regular dialysis on Monday, Wednesday, and Friday.

No headaches, blood sugar 180. Patient has been compliant with medication and exercising two days a week.

Labs: Microalbuminine.

Follow-up in one month.

IMPRESSION: Type 2 diabetes with chronic kidney disease, stage 3

ICD-10-CM Code(s) _____

Mental, Behavioral, and Neurodevelopmental Disorders (F01-F99)

Mental and behavioral disorders are reported with codes from categories F01-F99. Following are the chapter-specific coding guidelines. Be sure to review the ICD-10-CM Official Guidelines for Coding and Reporting and review all category and subcategory instructional notes when making a code selection.

PAIN DISORDER RELATED TO PSYCHOLOGICAL FACTORS

Pain that is psychological is reported with codes from category F45.41. Diagnosis code F45.41 is reserved exclusively for pain related to psychological factors; pain not elsewhere classified. As indicated by the Excludes1 note under category G89, a code from category G89 should not be assigned with code F45.41.

Code F45.42, Pain disorder with related psychological factors, should be used with a code from category G89, Pain not elsewhere classified, when documentation of a psychological component for a patient with acute or chronic pain.

MENTAL AND BEHAVIORAL DISORDER DUE TO PSYCHOACTIVE SUBSTANCE ABUSE

Several codes from category F10-F19.21 may be used to report tobacco use, cannabis use, and other substance abuse. The codes for "in remission" are only reported if the documentation states that the patient is not actively using the substance or documentation states specifically that the patient is "in remission." Documentation in the medical record should indicate use, abuse, and dependence of the substance (eg, alcohol, opioid, cannabis, and so on). Only one code should be reported for the abuse.

The following guidelines apply to reporting codes from category F10-F19:

- If both use and abuse are documented, assign only the code for abuse.

- If both abuse and dependence are documented, assign only the code for dependence.

- If use, abuse, and dependence are documented, assign only the code for dependence.

- If both use and dependence are documented, assign only the code for dependence.

For psychoactive substance abuse, codes should only be assigned based on documentation in the medical record. The codes are to be used only when the psychoactive substance use is associated with a mental or behavioral disorder, and the relationship is documented in the medical record. These codes include F10.9-, F11.9-, F12.9-, F13.9-, F14.9-, F15.9-, and F16.9-.

Now that you have a good understanding of the chapter-specific guidelines for Mental and Behavioral Disorders, it is time to build skill and knowledge by coding the following exercises. Again, make certain to reference the ICD-10-CM codebook and the ICD-10-CM Official Guidelines for Coding and Reporting, as well as the instructional notes, when coding these exercises.

CASE STUDY 9

This 35-year-old male patient is new to ABC Hospital. He was admitted to this facility on 01/20/20xx with the diagnoses of bilateral lower amputee, ruptured spleen, lacerated liver, and fractured pelvis sustained from a motor vehicle accident. Dr Marcus, his orthopedist, asked that I see the patient in consultation. The patient is admitted for therapy. Patient was healthy prior to the accident. No history of diabetes, hypertension, cardiac, or respiratory disease. Patient has had both legs amputated below the knee; splenectomy; and liver repair. Patient does not smoke or drink. Patient was an avid runner prior to the accident.

REVIEW OF SYSTEMS:

HEENT: normal; Respiratory: normal; Cardiovascular: normal; Hematologic: normal except for splenectomy and repair of lacerated liver; Musculoskeletal: bilateral lower amputee. Healing pelvic fracture. ROS otherwise normal.

PHYSICAL EXAMINATION:

GENERAL: Well-developed, well-nourished, depressed male in no acute distress. BP 128/75; pulse: 90, regular and strong. Temperature: Normal. Height: 5 feet 10 inches.

HEENT: Pupils are reactive to light and accommodations. No vessel changes, exudates, or hemorrhages noted. Oral mucosa is normal. No lesions noted.

NECK: Supple; no masses.

RESPIRATORY: Normal. No wheezes or rubs appreciated; clear to auscultation.

CARDIOVASCULAR: Normal sinus rhythm; no murmurs.

ABDOMEN: Laparotomy scar is healing well. No signs of infection. No evidence of masses or hernias.

MUSCULOSKELETAL: Patient is a bilateral lower amputee. Currently confined to wheelchair. Pelvic fracture is healing according to X rays. Lower leg muscles have not been used since accident and are flaccid. Upper body is within normal limits. Range of motion is good.

NEUROLOGICAL: Cranial nerves are intact. Moves all upper extremities on command without difficulty. Hand grips strong bilaterally. Lower extremities are flaccid and it is unclear if patient is unable to move stumps or will not move stumps.

PSYCHIATRIC: Patient is depressed and this will be a concern that might hinder him in therapy. Patient is orientated to person, place, and time. Judgment is impaired due to depression. Patient does have phantom leg syndrome.

ASSESSMENT AND PLAN: Patient will begin therapy to strengthen his lower stumps. He will be fitted with prostheses and will begin rehabilitative therapy. Psychologist will be obtained to help patient deal with his recurrent major depressive disorder (moderate) and therapy. Patient to continue same medications.

ICD-10-CM Code(s) _____

CASE STUDY 10

This is a 57-year-old new patient, who states she is feeling better than she probably ever had in her life. She has been on Zoloft now and says it really helps. Her PMH shows that she has been depressed off and on for the past two years. This was probably a major depression for her, although it has improved. Also looking at her labs, her total cholesterol is 247 with an LDL of 142 and HDL of 69. These are equivocal results. Her family history is very strong for cardiovascular disease with a brother dying of a heart attack when he was 24 years old. Her mother and father both have heart disease, and it is in both families. She is S/P hysterectomy, and she is on Premarin 1.25 once per day.

PHYSICAL EXAMINATION: This is a 57-year-old female in no acute distress. Eyes PERRLA. She is wearing knee braces. Lungs clear. Heart regular. Abdomen soft. No CVA tenderness. Extremities without clubbing, cyanosis, or edema.

ASSESSMENT:

1. Strong family history of heart disease

2. Elevated cholesterol

3. Mild recurrent major depression

PLAN: We will start her on Zocar 20 mg 1 q day #30 with 1 refill. Check her cholesterol in six weeks with liver function tests and see her back in three months.

ICD-10-CM Code(s) _____

CASE STUDY 11

CHIEF COMPLAINT: Returns today for office visit for medication management.

HISTORY OF PRESENT ILLNESS: Patient's PMSH remains unchanged from previous visit. Patient is a 55-year-old female who lost her husband eight months ago in an industrial accident. She was released from ABC Hospital three weeks ago due to a suicide attempt. She is suffering from a moderate major depressive disorder, which is recurrent. At that time the patient stated she no longer wished to live without her spouse. She has been monitored once per week since her release. Last visit her medications were slightly changed and she was started on Luvox. Patient states feeling better and mood improving slightly. She has no current thoughts of suicide.

CURRENT MEDICATIONS:

- Buspar 5 mg tid

- Luvox 50 mg a day

- Beclovent 10 mg tid

- Relafen 500 mg bid

PLAN: Continue current medications without adjustment. She will be followed by me and Ivan Prentiss, MD, her internist. Return in one week.

ICD-10-CM Code(s) _____

CASE STUDY 12

CHIEF COMPLAINT: To cope with lifestyle changes that are causing depression. The patient stated, "I have had a bad week, I am still having crying spells and tension." Patient states crying spells have decreased in frequency. States depression worsening. Patient discussed her anger, need for distraction, angry at loss of travel opportunity. She is currently going through a divorce. She reports a solid block of sleep at night and adds that she has been spending a lot of time in bed.

ASSESSMENT: Patient presents in a depressed state after 4 of 12 planned counseling sessions.

PLAN: Will continue therapy as planned. Her next session is in two weeks. Continue current meds.

ICD-10-CM Code(s) _____

CASE STUDY 13

CHIEF COMPLAINT: This is a 9-year-old male who came in to recheck his ADHD medicines. We placed him on Adderall—the first time he has been on a stimulant medication—last month. Mother said the next day he had a wonderful improvement and has been doing very well with the medicine. She has two concerns. It seems like first thing in the morning after he takes the medicine, it takes a while for the medicine to kick in. It wears off about 2 pm, and they have problems in the evening with him. He was initially having difficulty with his appetite but that seems to be coming back; it is more the problems early in the morning after he takes this medicine than in the afternoon when it wears off. His teachers have seen a dramatic improvement. She did miss a dose this past weekend and said he was just horrible. The patient even commented that he thought he needed his medication.

PAST HISTORY: Reviewed from appointment on 05/16/20xx.

CURRENT MEDICATIONS: Adderall XR 10 mg once daily.

ALLERGIES: None to medicines.

FAMILY AND SOCIAL HISTORY: Reviewed from appointment on 05/16/20xx.

REVIEW OF SYSTEMS: He has been having problems, as mentioned, in the morning and later in the afternoon, but he has been eating well, sleeping okay. Review of systems is otherwise negative.

OBJECTIVE: Weight is 96.5 pounds, which is down just a little bit from his appointment last month. Physical exam itself was deferred today because he has otherwise been very healthy.

ASSESSMENT: At this point, attention deficit hyperactivity disorder (hyperactivity type); doing fairly well with the Adderall.

PLAN: Discussed two options with patient's mother. Switch him to Ritalin LA, which I think has better release of medicine early in the morning, or increase his Adderall dose. As far as the afternoon, if she really wanted him to be on the medication, we could do a small dose of the Adderall, which she would prefer. So, I have decided at this point to increase him to the Adderall XR 15 mg in the morning and Adderall 5 mg in the afternoon. Mother is to watch his diet. We would like to recheck his weight if he is doing very well in two months. But if there are any problems, especially in the morning, we would change his meds to the Ritalin LA. Mother understands and will call if there are problems. Approximately 25 minutes spent with patient, all in discussion.

ICD-10-CM Code(s) _____

CASE STUDY 14

CHIEF COMPLAINT: Martha is a 68-year-old patient who returns today for medication management. Patient has been depressed and I have been managing her care for the past nine months. Current medications include:

- Xanax 0.25 mg tid
- Premarin 1.25 mg 1× day
- Relafen 500 mg bid

Patient not doing well on current medication. She is still not sleeping well and experiencing panic attacks periodically during the day and is still depressed.

PLAN: Increase Xanax dosage from 0.25 to .05 mg tid and I will see her in follow up in two weeks.

ICD-10-CM Code(s) _____

CASE STUDY 15

The patient is an 83-year-old female referred to the hospital by a neurologist in Miami, Florida, for disorientation and illusions. Symptoms started six months ago when the patient complained of vision problems and disorientation. The patient was seen wearing clothes inside out along with other unusual behaviors. In October or November of 20xx, the patient reported having a sudden onset of headaches, loss of vision, and talking sporadically without making any sense. The patient sought treatment from an ophthalmologist. The

Behavior Center referred the patient to a neurologist, who then referred the patient to our office.

According to the daughter, the patient has had no past major medical or psychiatric illnesses. The patient was functioning normally before June 20xx. The daughter reports worsening symptoms, mainly inability to communicate about auditory or visual hallucinations or any symptoms of anxiety. Currently, the patient lives with her youngest daughter and requires her assistance to perform ADLs. The patient has become ataxic since last month. Sleeping patterns and the amount is unknown. Appetite is okay.

PAST PSYCHIATRIC HISTORY: The patient was diagnosed with severe depression at the Behavior Center a few weeks ago, where she was given Effexor. She stopped taking it soon after, as it worsened her vision and balance.

PAST MEDICAL HISTORY: In 20xx diagnosed with Ménière's disease, was treated such that she could function normally in everyday activities including work. No current medications. Denies history of seizures, strokes, diabetes, hypertension, heart disease, or head injury.

FAMILY MEDICAL HISTORY: Father's grandmother was diagnosed with Alzheimer's disease in her 70s with symptoms similar to the patient described by the patient's mother. Both the mother's father and father's mother had "nervous breakdowns" but at unknown dates.

SOCIAL HISTORY: The patient lives with the youngest daughter, who takes care of the patient's ADLs. Denies use of alcohol, tobacco, or illicit drugs.

MENTAL STATUS EXAMINATION: The patient is an 83-year-old female wearing clean clothes. Decreased motor activity, but did blink her eyes often, but arrhythmically. Poor eye contact. Speech illogic. Concentration was not able to be assessed. Mood is unknown. Flat and constricted affect. Thought content, thought process, and perception could not be assessed. Sensorial memory, information, intelligence, judgment, and insight could not be evaluated due to lack of communication by the patient.

MINI-MENTAL STATUS EXAM: Unable to perform.

AXIS I: Rapidly progressing early onset of dementia; rule out dementia secondary to general medical condition; rule out dementia secondary to substance abuse.

AXIS II: Deferred

AXIS III: Deferred

AXIS IV: Deferred

AXIS V: Deferred

ASSESSMENT: The patient is an 83-year-old black female with rapid and early onset of dementia with no significant past medical history. There is no indication as to what precipitated these symptoms, as the daughter is not aware of any factors and the patient is unable to communicate. The patient presented with headaches, vision forms, and disorientation in June of this year. She currently presents with ataxia, vision loss, and delusions.

ASSESSMENT: Senile dementia.

PLAN: Wait for result of neurological tests from neurologist.

ICD-10-CM Code(s) _____

CASE STUDY 16

CHIEF COMPLAINT: This 45-year-old patient has improved in terms of her mood and still has a flat affect. She is tolerating Zoloft, which was increased to 100 mg yesterday, quite well. She had a bad night yesterday. She is not sleeping well and complains of hearing some voices, although it was unclear if she was really hearing them. The patient appeared disorganized and confused. The charge nurse documented that she was wandering in the unit last evening and had to be redirected several times. The patient slept only 1 hour last night. She denies any suicidal/homicidal ideation.

I will continue to monitor her. If she continues to be stable, she may be discharged after she is less confused and does not complain of auditory hallucinations. It should be noted that the pattern seems to be of her hallucinations waxing and waning, and this would be the most logical explanation. More supportive therapy was provided to her about the nature and etiology of these types of symptoms. She will be followed up daily by me, and twice a day by John Taylor (CP). Spent 30 minutes with patient.

ICD-10-CM Code(s) _____

CASE STUDY 17

GROUP THERAPY: Develop awareness of social interaction behaviors. This 17-year-old female patient has developed severe antisocial behaviors since the age of 12, which is worsening.

TREATMENT PLAN GOAL: Patient to demonstrate an increased level of independent functioning as evidenced by improvement in interpersonal skills. Provided opportunity for learning and practicing interpersonal skills.

PATIENT OUTCOME/RESPONSE: Patient again quiet and withdrawn at times; distracted by other peers in group and engaged in side talking with a peer. Patient agreed that social interaction is an important part of one's life. Patient having good eye contact; some confusion with questions being asked.

PLAN FOR FUTURE INTERVENTION WITH GROUP: Role play appropriate behaviors in group and have patient act out interaction to further this skill.

ICD-10-CM Code(s) _____

CASE STUDY 18

This is a 56-year-old female who is having ongoing problems with anxiety attacks, shaking, and palpitations. Apparently she has seen her family doctor and has been placed on some thyroid, estrogen, and progesterone, and for a while felt better. However, a couple weeks later, again she began having shaking attacks during the night and not sleeping well, feeling very jumpy on the inside. She also has some problems with depression. The only thing that seems to help here at this time is Ativan 1 mg, either a quarter-tablet or half-tablet at bedtime. She also feels a constriction in her throat; occasionally she gets hot flashes. She has tried Paxil 20 mg a day and Celexa up to 10 mg a day. She has fear about her health. She has gotten additional counseling from a professional counselor.

PAST MEDICAL HISTORY: She states she does not do well with medications, but has no specific medicines that she cannot take. She has had no major surgeries in the past. She did state she does have allergy to sulfa, which I forgot to mention. She did have tonsils removed as a child.

MEDICATIONS: Ativan 1 mg and Synthroid 88, 0.088 mg a day.

FAMILY HISTORY: Mother is 78 and in good health. Father left when the patient was 8, unknown. There is one grandmother with diabetes and breast cancer, but no strong family history of heart disease.

SOCIAL HISTORY: She does not drink alcohol and is a nonsmoker. She is divorced.

REVIEW OF SYSTEMS:

HEENT: She has neck pain and headaches from time to time, no blurred vision or lack of vision. She does have the constriction in her throat. Pulmonary system: No hemoptysis, fevers, chills, or chronic sputum production. Cardiovascular system: Occasionally she gets a racing heartbeat, but no specific chest discomfort. GI system: She denies heartburn, indigestion, blood in the stools. GU system: No hematuria, pyuria, kidney stones, or kidney infection. Musculoskeletal system: She generally has some upper neck and back discomfort. Endocrine system: She does require thyroid supplementation, but has never been on any kind of medicines for diabetes.

EXAMINATION: Blood pressure 100/60; pulse 72; respiration 16. The patient is afebrile. HEENT: Unremarkable. No carotid bruits or JVD, trachea midline. No thyromegaly. Lungs: Clear to auscultation and percussion, no rales or rhonchi noted. Heart: There is a regular sinus rhythm with a I/VI near holosystolic murmur at the apex. No point tenderness over the costal chondral joints. Abdomen: Soft, no point tenderness. Bowel sounds active. No pulsatile masses. Genitorectal: Deferred. Pulses: Femorals 2+, popliteals 2+, posterior tibial and dorsalis pedis 2+.

IMPRESSION AND PLAN OF CARE: The patient is suffering from generalized anxiety that could be related to her menopausal symptoms. Increased her Ativan from 1 mg to 2 mg per day. Will see the patient in the office in one month. Gave her a referral to a GYN for her hot flashes.

ICD-10-CM Code(s) _____

Diseases of the Nervous System (G00-G99) and Diseases of the Eye and Adnexa (H00-H59)

ICD-10-CM Chapters 6 and 7 Guidelines Review

In this chapter you will find a summary of the chapter-specific coding guidelines for Chapter 6 and Chapter 7 of the ICD-10-CM codebook followed by case studies to build ICD-10-CM diagnosis coding skills in this area.

Many medical specialties reference Chapters 6 and 7 of the ICD-10-CM codebook for coding diseases of the nervous system and diseases of the eye and adnexa. Keep in mind that you should always reference the ICD-10-CM Official Guidelines for Coding and Reporting in its entirety when making a code selection.

ICD-10-CM Coding Guidelines for Diseases of the Nervous System

CODING FOR HEMIPLEGIA AND HEMIPARESIS

Codes from categories G81, G83.1, G83.2, and G83.3 for hemiplegia, hemiparesis, monoplegia of upper and lower limb, and unspecified identify whether a patient's dominant or non-dominant side is affected. When the documentation specifies the site of the condition but does not identify whether the side affected is dominant or non-dominant, the following guidelines apply:

- If the left side is affected, the default is non-dominant.
- If the right side is affected, the default is dominant.
- If the patient is ambidextrous the default is dominant.

To support correct coding, it is recommended that the coder query the provider to code to the proper site as well as to determine whether the patient's dominant or non-dominant side is affected.

PAIN GUIDELINES

Code G89, Pain, not elsewhere classified, may be used with codes from other code categories in the ICD-10-CM codebook to assist in providing more detail about acute, chronic, or neoplasm-related pain. The following pain guidelines apply:

- To report code G89, the pain must be specified as acute, chronic, post-thoracotomy, post-procedural, or neoplasm-related pain, and the pain must be documented. If none of these conditions apply, do **not** report code G89.

- If the definitive diagnosis is known, do not report code G89 unless the reason for the patient encounter is pain control or management of pain and not treatment for the underlying condition.

- Category G89 should not be used when the patient encounter is for a procedure aimed at treating the underlying condition.

A code from category G89 may be reported under the following conditions as the first-listed diagnosis:

- Report a code from category G89 when pain control or pain management is the reason for the patient encounter and it is well documented in the medical record. The underlying condition (ie, the cause of pain) should be reported as an additional diagnosis.

- When a neurostimulator is inserted for pain control, report a code from category G89 as the first-listed diagnosis. Report the underlying condition as an additional diagnosis.

- When the patient encounter is to treat the underlying condition, such as severe back pain, and a neurostimulator is inserted for pain control, the underlying condition is reported as the first-listed diagnosis followed by the appropriate pain code.

- When coding the site of the pain, a code from Chapter 18 of the ICD-10-CM codebook should be assigned for the site. If the pain is documented as acute or chronic, a code from category G89 should also be assigned.

- When sequencing codes from category G89 with site-specific pain codes (eg, from Chapter 18 of the ICD-10-CM codebook), a code from category G89 is reported as the first-listed diagnosis followed by a code for the specific site of the pain if the patient encounter is for pain control or pain management.

- When the patient encounter is for reasons other than pain control or pain management, and a definitive diagnosis has not been confirmed by the provider, assign a code from the site of the pain as the first-listed diagnosis followed by a code from category G89.

- When the patient encounter is for pain for an implant, graft, or medical device left in the surgical site, codes are assigned from Chapter 19, Injury, poisoning, and certain other consequences of external causes. Diagnosis codes for pain due to medical devices are assigned a "T" code. These codes are sequenced first followed by a code from category G89 to identify acute or chronic pain due to presence of the device, implant, or graft using G89.18, Other acute post-procedural pain, or G89.28, Other chronic post-procedural pain.

POSTOPERATIVE PAIN

Documentation is the key factor in selecting codes for postoperative pain. The following guidelines apply:

- Routine or normal expected pain following surgery should not be coded.

- When documentation does not indicate whether post-thoracotomy and other postoperative pain is acute or chronic, the pain should be coded as acute.

- Postoperative pain not associated with a postoperative pain complication is assigned a code from category G89.

- Postoperative pain associated with a specific postoperative complication is assigned a code from Chapter 19 of the ICD-10-CM codebook. If the patient also suffers from acute or chronic pain, select a code from category G89 to identify the acute or chronic pain (eg, G89.18 or G89.28).

NEOPLASM-RELATED PAIN

Code G89.3 is reported for pain related or due to cancer, which includes a primary or secondary malignancy or tumor. The code is assigned even when acute or chronic is not documented. This code is assigned as the first-listed diagnosis when the reason for the patient encounter is pain control or pain management for the cancer or tumor. The underlying neoplasm is reported as an additional diagnosis.

When the reason for the encounter is management of the neoplasm and pain is associated with the neoplasm, the neoplasm code is reported as the first-listed diagnosis followed by code G89.3 for the neoplasm-related pain. The site of pain does not need to be assigned.

CHRONIC PAIN

Chronic pain is reported with codes from subcategory G89.2. Documentation should be specific that the pain is chronic. There is no time frame for the chronic pain in order to report this code. Codes for central pain syndrome (G89.0) and chronic pain syndrome (G89.4) are selected based on the documentation in the medical record.

CHRONIC PAIN SYNDROME

Central pain syndrome (G89.0) and chronic pain syndrome (G89.4) are different than the term "chronic pain," and therefore codes should only be used when the provider has specifically documented this condition.

Now that you have a good understanding of the chapter-specific guidelines for diseases of the nervous system, it is time to build skill and knowledge by coding the following exercises. Be sure to reference the ICD-10-CM codebook and the ICD-10-CM Official Guidelines for Coding and Reporting, along with the instructional notes, when coding these conditions.

Diseases of the Nervous System (G00-G99)

CASE STUDY 1

SUBJECTIVE: This 35-year-old, female patient is 12 days' status post excision of a mass on the left buttock. She has had pain and fever for the past three days.

PHYSICAL EXAMINATION: Her wound looks clean, dry. There is no purulence of her wound. The Penrose drain is intact.

PLAN: We will remove the drain today and perform a CAT scan to see if there is any retained fluid collection in that area. We will arrange wound care to do wet-to-dry dressing changes to the wound daily.

ICD-10-CM Code(s) _____

CASE STUDY 2

PREOPERATIVE DIAGNOSIS: Cerebral spinal fluid (CSF) leak bilaterally.

POSTOPERATIVE DIAGNOSIS: Same.

PROCEDURE: Bilateral frontal sinus endoscopic repair of cerebral spinal fluid leak with layered grafting with SIS tissue replacement as well as temporalis muscle fascial graft harvested from the left post-auricular tissues and local mucosal graft from intranasal left nasal chamber and bilateral endoscopic anterior ethmoidectomies.

OPERATIVE FINDINGS: The patient is a 70-year-old female who in 20xx was involved in a severe motor vehicle accident. At that time, she had sustained a Le Fort II and mandibular fracture that was repaired with interdental wiring. She apparently developed recurrent clear rhinorrhea in 199x and that was initially attempted to be repaired transnasally. This ultimately required an intracranial repair with cranialization of a frontal sinus to repair the leakage. The patient was seen this past fall complaining of recurrent watery rhinorrhea primarily from the left nasal chamber, less so from the right. On radionuclide scanning she was found to have frontal sinus area leakage. At the time of surgery, the patient was found to have fairly normal appearance to the right middle meatus and superior nasal vault area without any obvious acute changes. The anterior ethmoid air cells contained polypoid degeneration changes but the maxillary sinus ostia were widely patent on the right side. On the left side, the patient had partial resection of the middle turbinate with remnants of the anterior portion of the left middle turbinate still in place. There was significant scarring at the frontal recess as well as the ethmoid sinus chambers showing postsurgical changes. The sphenoid sinus was widely patent on the left side and the mucosa in the sphenoid sinus looked normal on endoscopic examination as did the maxillary sinus mucosa. Once the left frontal recess was surgically opened up, it appeared to terminate in a somewhat of blind fact with tissue in its superior aspect, which was

ballotable, and there was CSF fluid coming from this area.

DESCRIPTION OF PROCEDURE: The patient was brought to the operating suite and placed in a supine position under general endotracheal anesthesia. After the patient had already had a lumbar CSF drain placed, the intranasal mucous membranes were treated with 4% cocaine and cotton pledgets. The mucosa of the lateral walls and superior nasal chamber were infiltrated with 1% Xylocaine with 1:100,000 epinephrine. Following this, starting with the right side, the middle turbinate was gently infractured. The uncinate process was taken down and an anterior ethmoidectomy was performed to gain visualization in this area. The superior nasal vault area revealed no evidence of any acute drainage and the frontal recess on this side appeared to be scarred off and completely stenosed off. This area was excoriated as was the superior nasal chamber anteriorly and then an SIS piece of tissue was used to graft this area. This was placed in position and then scaled with Tisseel. Following this, the area was packed with layered Gelfoam packing followed by neurosurgical cottonoids and then a Doyle Merocel sponge pack to complete this side. Following this, attention was turned to the left side, which was the more prominent side of the CSF leakage. With an endoscopic approach, scar tissue from the frontal recess was carefully removed with Blakesley forceps and curettes. The remnant bone of the anterior portion of the remnant middle turbinate was then resected, maintaining the mucosa of the turbinate for use as a flap to cover the surgical site once the remaining grafts were placed. Following this, opening up the frontal recess further with curettes, tissue could be seen in the depths of this area from the previous cranialization of the frontal sinus. This tissue was carefully elevated circumferentially and once this was done there was more CSF leakage noted coming down through this area, verifying this as the location of the leakage. Once this was accomplished, the post-auricular incision was created. A muscle and fascial graft was harvested from the temporalis muscle that measured 2 × 3.5 cm to 4 cm in size. This graft was trimmed and then this was used to pack up into the frontal recess and up into the infundibulum area of the remnant frontal infundibulum to act as the first layer of closure in this region. Following this, a piece of SIS tissue was cut which was 1 × 2 cm in dimension. This was then layered into this area underneath the remnant middle turbinate up into the frontal recess and along the anterior lamina papyracea. This was then sealed into place with Tisseel glue following which the mucosal flap was brought from medial to lateral over this entire area and this likewise was sealed down with Tisseel glue. Following this, the area was packed with layered Gelfoam packing followed by neurosurgical cottonoid packing and then a Doyle Merocel sponge pack was placed in this area. Once this was completed, the left sphenoid was examined and found to be patent with normal-appearing mucosa prior to placement of the Doyle Merocel sponge pack. Following this, the patient was awakened and returned to the recovery area in satisfactory condition.

ICD-10-CM Code(s) _____

CASE STUDY 3

PREOPERATIVE DIAGNOSIS: Carpal tunnel syndrome, left wrist.

POSTOPERATIVE DIAGNOSIS: Same.

DESCRIPTION OF PROCEDURE: Under general anesthesia, the wrist was prepped and draped in the usual fashion. Two arthroscopic portals were introduced into the operating field and the arthroscope was inserted. The median nerve was visualized at the proximal edge of the transverse carpal ligament. The nerve was protected and the transverse carpal ligament was sectioned through the arthroscope to obtain release of the nerve, which was quite compressed. After the ligament had been sectioned, the scope was withdrawn and the wound closed. The patient tolerated the procedure well and circulation to the extremity was intact at the completion of the procedure.

ICD-10-CM Code(s) _____

CASE STUDY 4

PREOPERATIVE DIAGNOSES:

1. Obstructive sleep apnea

2. Tonsillar hypertrophy

3. Pigmented lesion, left temple

POSTOPERATIVE DIAGNOSES: Same

PROCEDURES:

1. Uvulopalatopharyngoplasty

2. Tonsillectomy

3. Excision of pigmented lesion left temple measuring 9 mm in width and 2.4 cm in length

DESCRIPTION OF PROCEDURE: The patient was brought to the operating room and placed supine on the operating room table. The patient was put to sleep by a general technique of anesthesia and incubated

carefully. A Crowe-Davis retractor was inserted in the oral commissure to retract the tongue and mandible. The patient was placed in gentle neck extension and suspended from towels on the chest. A red rubber catheter was inserted through the nostril to retract the soft palate. The tonsils were each grasped and metalized.

Each tonsil was resected from its fossa using a needle-tip Bovie. The tonsils were found to be much smaller than they appeared to be due to the amount of subcutaneous fat in the posterior tonsillar pillar in particular. Homeostasis was obtained with a suction electrocautery. Next, a uvular flap was developed with a longer posterior than anterior edge. A small amount of tissue from the posterior tonsillar pillars was removed on each side and the anterior and posterior pillars were sutured together using 3-0 Vicryl sutures in horizontal mattress fashion after a superiorly based relaxing incision was made. Similar sutures were used to close the uvular flap. A nasal trumpet was placed through the right nostril. The Crowe-Davis retractor was removed. The room was then reset for the clean portion of the case. The wound was cleansed with Betadine. This was infiltrated with 1% Lidocaine with 1:100,000 epinephrine. This was a pigmented lesion on the left temple and approximately 3-mm margins were designed on either side of the approximately 3-mm lesion. The lesion was then sharply excised through the full thickness of the skin. This was marked at 12 o'clock. Hemostasis was obtained with a bipolar electrocautery. The wound edges were reapproximated with 4-0 Vicryl and the skin was closed with a 5-0 fast-absorbing gut. The patient was awakened from anesthesia and extubated without any difficulty. He was brought to the recovery room in stable condition. He did not have any obvious airway problems. The nasal trumpet was maintained.

ASSESSMENT: No significant tonsillar hypertrophy, severe crowding of the pharyngeal airway, and pigmented lesion right temple.

SPECIMENS: Tonsils, uvula, and pigmented lesion right temple marked at 12 o'clock. Estimated blood loss is 3.0 cc.

ICD-10-CM Code(s) _____

CASE STUDY 5

PREOPERATIVE DIAGNOSIS: Left carpal tunnel.

PROCEDURE(S): Left carpal tunnel release; median epineurolysis.

FINDINGS: Median nerve was adherent but no masses.

INDICATIONS: This patient has documented carpal tunnel syndrome based on electromyelogram results and desires elective release.

PROCEDURE: The patient was taken to the operating room, positioned supine on the operating room table, and anesthesia was administered. The limb was prepped and draped in sterile fashion. The limb was elevated using a compressive bandage and the tourniquet was inflated to 225 mmHg. The gauge was tested for oscillation. Local infiltration with 1% Xylocaine into the medial and ulnar positions was performed. An incision was made deep through the subcutaneous tissues. Bleeding points were electrocoagulated using bipolar cautery and the skin edges were handled atraumatically. The palmar fascia was identified and incised and the transverse carpal ligament was exposed. A wide release was achieved by opening its ulnar-most aspect and carrying the dissection distally to crossing the ulnar neurovascular bundle and proximally under vision in the antebrachial fascia of the forearm. The median nerve was adherent and an epineurotomy was carried out. The thenar branch was carefully protected and the wound was irrigated carefully. Hemostasis was achieved and closure was accomplished with 5-0 nylon sutures applied to the skin to ensure good coaptation of the skin edges. A sterile compressive dressing was applied with antibiotic-laden, non-adherent gauze. A volar cock-up wrist splint was applied with the thumb and digits free and the wrist in a moderate dorsification position. All sponge, needle, and instrument counts were correct. There were no operative complications. The tourniquet was deflated and the patient was returned to the recovery room in good condition. Estimated blood loss was less than 50 cc.

ICD-10-CM Code(s) _____

CASE STUDY 6

PREOPERATIVE DIAGNOSIS: Right temporal pain, rule out temporal arteritis.

POSTOPERATIVE DIAGNOSIS: Right temporal pain, vascular headache, rule out temporal arteritis.

OPERATION PERFORMED: Right temporal artery biopsy.

HISTORY: The patient is a 77-year-old, white female who has been bothered with right temporal pain and headaches with some visual changes and has a sedimentation rate of 51. I saw her in the office in consultation and she was scheduled for a temporal artery biopsy to rule out temporal arteritis. The procedure

and operative risks were explained to her and consent was obtained.

OPERATIVE NOTE: The patient was brought to the operating room on 5/27/20xx. She was placed in the supine position and given intravenous sedation. Her right temporal area was prepped with Betadine scrubs and paint. Towels and drapes were placed in the usual sterile fashion. Prior to prepping, a Doppler probe was used to isolate the temporal artery and, using a marking pen, the path of the artery was drawn. 1% Lidocaine was used to infiltrate the skin, and using a #15 blade scalpel, the skin was opened in the preauricular area and dissected down to the subcutaneous tissue where the temporal artery was identified in its bed. It was a medium size artery and we dissected it out for a length of approximately 4 cm with some branches. The ends were ligated with 4-0 Vicryl, and the artery was removed from its bed and sent to Pathology as specimen. The wound was irrigated and we reapproximated the skin with Prolene pullout stitch. Mastisol and half-inch Steri-Strips were placed over the incision. She was awakened and sent to recovery in good condition. She tolerated the procedure well.

ICD-10-CM Code(s) _____

CASE STUDY 7

POSTOPERATIVE DIAGNOSES:

1. Right compressive neuropathy ulnar nerve at the wrist

2. Right lateral epicondylitis

PROCEDURES:

1. Ulnar nerve release at the wrist

2. Celestone injection plus Marcaine, right elbow

INDICATIONS: This is a 46-year-old with a coexistent ulnar neuropathy of the wrist and lateral epicondylitis. She was informed of the risks, benefits, and alternatives to the above procedure including but not limited to those of infection, anesthetic, blood loss, neurologic compromise, wound healing complications, decreased range of motion and strength, possible recurrence or worsening of condition, and consent was obtained.

DESCRIPTION OF PROCEDURE: The patient was brought into the operative suite, placed in supine position, and prepped and draped in the normal routine sterile fashion after successful induction of anesthetic, infusion of IV antibiotic, and exsanguination of the limb to 250 mm Hg. Through an incision in line with the ulnar border of the ring finger from Kaplan's cardinal line heading proximal for 2 to 4 cm, dissection was carried down through the palmar fascia bringing into loupe-magnified view the ulnar nerve and artery as they diverge proximal into the palmar arch. The ulnar nerve was traced proximally back to Guyon's canal with careful fascial dissection completely releasing the ulnar nerve. Revascularization of the epineurium was appreciated. The wound was copiously irrigated and closed. The surgical site was dressed with Xeroform gauze, a 4 × 4, Webril, and a plaster splint.

After the ulnar nerve release was performed at the wrist, the patient underwent a sterile injection of 1 ml of Celestone and 2 ml of Marcaine with a #22-gauge needle at the lateral epicondylar region at the outcropping muscles. She tolerated it well. A Band-Aid dressing was applied. Suture, towel, and instrument counts were correct at the end of the case and the patient was transferred to recovery without incident.

ICD-10-CM Code(s) _____

CASE STUDY 8

DIAGNOSIS: Migraine with aura.

PROCEDURE: Fluoroscopically guided lumbar puncture.

INDICATION: Migraine headache, pseudotumor cerebri.

PROCEDURE: The patient was prepped in the appropriate fashion. 1% Lidocaine was used to anesthetize the skin. Under fluoroscopic guidance, a #20-gauge spinal needle was used to perform the procedure. Opening pressure was measured at 18 cm of H_2O. Approximately 5 cc of clear cerebral spinal fluid were obtained. The patient tolerated the procedure well. There were no immediate complications. Pressure at the end of the procedure was 11 cm of H_2O.

IMPRESSION: Successful fluoroscopically guided lumbar puncture; pseudotumor cerebri.

ICD-10-CM Code(s) _____

CASE STUDY 9

HISTORY OF PRESENT ILLNESS: This is an established patient who has been complaining of left wrist pain for approximately one year. She has been receiving physical therapy for six months and it does not seem to be helping. She is a customer service representative and does repetitive computer work. She

has been wearing bilateral wrist supports, which have helped to some extent.

PAST MEDICAL HISTORY: The patient has a history of T and A; had a hysterectomy two years ago; and has a history of diabetes and hypertension. She does not complain of chest pain, shortness of breath or dizziness.

ALLERGIES: No apparent allergies.

MEDICATIONS: Patient takes Humulin 70/30 and Zestril.

PHYSICAL EXAMINATION: This is a well-developed, well-nourished female in no acute distress. Head is normocephalic. Neck is supple with no masses. Carotid pulse is palpable and trachea is in midline. Chest is clear to auscultation and percussion. Examination of the heart shows no murmurs, gallops, or rubs. Abdomen is negative. Extremities: Patient has left wrist weakness, unable to touch thumb and little finger together. There is a prominent mass on the palmar aspect of the left wrist.

PLAN: Patient has carpel tunnel syndrome in her left wrist and will be seen at the ambulatory surgery center for carpal tunnel surgery in two weeks. In the meantime, I have placed the patient on pain management and she was placed on short-term disability.

ICD-10-CM Code(s) _____

CASE STUDY 10

EXAMINATION: MRI of the brain with and without contrast.

ADMITTING DIAGNOSIS: Left facial weakness/ Bell's palsy.

CLINICAL HISTORY: Comparison. Left facial weakness in a patient with history of Bell's palsy and MS.

RESULT: MRI of the brain was obtained at 1.5 Tesla. Axial T1 weighted pre- and post-Gadolinium, T2 weighted FLAIR, and diffusion images were obtained. Sagittal T1 weighted and high-resolution coronal and axial pre- and post-Gadolinium images of the internal auditory canals were obtained. The old study was available for comparison.

The ventricles and sulci are within normal limits. There is no evidence of mass effect or midline shift. There are no extra-axial fluid collections. There are multiple punctuate areas of abnormal increased T2 weighted signal in the periventricular white matter and in the subcortical white matter of the centrum semiovale. Many of the foci are elongated and oriented toward the ventricles. Since the prior exam, there has been an increase in the number of hyperintense plaques. With contrast enhancement, none of the plaques appears to enhance at this time. The enhancement seen previously has resolved. The pattern and distribution is most characteristic for MS. The pituitary gland and cerebellum are unremarkable. There are multiple punctuate areas of hyperintense signal in the brain stem and brachium pontis. These do not enhance with Gadolinium. There is no edema or mass effect from the lesions. There is a 7-mm focus of increased signal at the left CP angle. No abnormal signal, enhancement of discrete mass lesion is appreciated within the internal auditory canals. This would correlate with the patient's symptoms of a left facial palsy.

IMPRESSION: Multiple hyperintense lesions predominately in the periventricular white matter with positive characteristic pattern for MS. None of the plaques currently enhances. There has been a fairly significant increase in the number of lesions since the last exam. Multiple lesions were also seen in the brain stem and the brachium pontis. Specifically, there is a 7-mm focus in the left CP angle, which is probably the cause of the patient's left facial palsy. No discrete abnormality was seen in the internal auditory canals.

ICD-10-CM Code(s) _____

CASE STUDY 11

This 7-month old baby presents to the emergency room (ER) with his mother. She indicated that the patient fell from her (mother's) bed onto the floor in the bedroom of their apartment while sleeping. Mom states baby has a contusion on the back of his head that is quite large. ER referred patient to neurology.

On exam there was swelling and redness on the baby's scalp with a small contusion. Sent the baby to have an MRI to determine extent of any damage.

IMPRESSION: Encephalopathy and contusion of scalp.

PLAN: MRI results indicate that the patient does have cerebral edema. Will begin anti-inflammatory medications today.

ICD-10-CM Code(s) _____

Guidelines for Diseases of Eye and Adnexa

The guidelines for glaucoma were added to Chapter 7, Diseases of Eye and Adnexa. Glaucoma is coded from category H40. As many codes from H40 should be reported as necessary to identify:

- Type of glaucoma
- Affected eye
- Glaucoma stage

When a patient has glaucoma in both eyes (bilateral), and both eyes are documented in the medical record as the same type and stage, and a code exists for bilateral glaucoma, report only one code for the type—bilateral. The seventh character will identify the stage.

When a patient has glaucoma in both eyes (bilateral), and both eyes are documented in the medical record as the same type and stage, and the classification does not provide a code for bilateral glaucoma (ie, H40.10, H40.11, and H40.20), report only one code for the type and the appropriate seventh character to identify the stage.

When a patient has glaucoma in both eyes (bilateral), and each eye is documented in the medical record as having a different type or stage, and a code exists for laterality, assign a code for each eye with the appropriate seventh character for each eye to identify the stage. Do not report a bilateral code in this instance because the type and/or stage might be different.

When a patient has glaucoma in both eyes (bilateral), each eye is documented in the medical record with a different type or stage, and the classification does not distinguish laterality (ie, H40.10, H40.11, and H40.20), report one code for each type of glaucoma for each eye with the appropriate seventh character to identify the stage.

If a patient is admitted to the hospital with glaucoma, and the stage changes or evolves during the admission or stay, assign a code for the highest stage documented.

When assigning seventh character "4" (Indeterminate stage), assignment should be based on the clinical documentation when the stage cannot be clinically determined.

Note: The seventh character "0" (stage unspecified) should not be confused with the seventh character "4." The seventh character "0" is reported when there is no documentation in the medical record regarding the stage of the glaucoma.

Diseases of the Eye and Adnexa (H00-H59)

ASSIGNING CODES FOR GLAUCOMA

Assign as many codes as necessary to identify the type of glaucoma, the affected area, and stage in category H40.

CASE STUDY 12

INDICATIONS FOR PROCEDURE: The patient presents with a primary malignant lesion involving the right upper eyelid margin verified via biopsy and pathology report.

DESCRIPTION OF PROCEDURE: The patient was taken to the operating room and placed on the table in the supine position where anesthesia was induced. 2% Xylocaine with epinephrine was injected over the surgical site, and the patient was prepped and draped in the usual manner for orbitofacial surgery. A #15 Bard-Parker blade incision was made through the right upper eyelid crease and across the entire horizontal extent of the eyelid. Sharp dissection was carried down to the border of the tarsal plate. A full-thickness en bloc excision of the eyelid margin and tarsus was carried out to the top of the tarsal plate. The lesion was removed in its entirety. The tarsal plate was closed with interrupted 7-0 silk sutures, partially penetrating the tarsus to avoid corneal irritation. The eyelid margin was closed with a 6-0 silk suture through the mucocutaneous junction. The skin muscle flap was closed with 7-0 silk sutures. The eyelid crease was closed with a 7-0 Prolene suture. The patient was then awakened and taken from the operating room in good condition, having tolerated the procedure well. There were no complications, and the estimated blood loss was less than 50 cc.

ICD-10-CM Code(s) _____

CASE STUDY 13

PREOPERATIVE DIAGNOSIS: Cataract of the left eye.

POSTOPERATIVE DIAGNOSIS: Senile cataract, left eye.

OPERATION PERFORMED: Phacoemulsification of left eye cataract with posterior chamber lens implantation, Alcon Model SA6CAT, 18.5 diopters.

INDICATIONS FOR PROCEDURE: The patient is a 65-year-old female with advancing cataract of the left eye. Best corrected vision is 20/400. The cataract of the left eye has developed rapidly. She is experiencing extreme interference with her overall visual performance. Her left eye vision is unable to be improved with spectacles and physical examination suggests that the cataract is the primary cause of the reduced vision. The option of cataract extraction has been presented to her. The risks and benefits have been discussed. She has been provided with up-to-date printed information. The patient wishes to have the left eye cataract removed on the basis of impairment of lifestyle due to reduced vision.

DESCRIPTION OF PROCEDURE: The patient was brought to the operating room on 02/14/20xx. Intravenous anesthesia and retrobulbar and peribulbar block had been administered approximately 30 minutes prior to her arrival in the operating room. The left eye was prepped. A blepharostat was inserted between the lids and the surgical microscope was focused into position. A conjunctival peritomy was performed. The anterior chamber was entered at the 12 o'clock position using a keratome inserted at the end of a self-sealing limbal incision. Viscoelastic material was used as necessary throughout the case. A capsulorhexis was performed. The cataract was removed by phacoemulsification techniques without difficulty. The implant was delivered and inspected. The implant power was confirmed to be 18.5 diopters on the package. The implant was inserted into the capsular bag without difficulty. Viscoelastic material was removed from the eye. The wound was observed to be watertight. A single suture of 10-0 nylon was placed in the wound for additional security. TobraDex ointment was applied to the surface of the eye and a sterile patch taped into place. There were no complications.

ICD-10-CM Code(s) _____

CASE STUDY 14

DIAGNOSIS: Cataract of the right eye.

OPERATION PERFORMED: Phacoemulsification, right eye cataract, with posterior chamber lens implantation, Alcon model SA6CAT, 20.5 diopters.

INDICATIONS FOR PROCEDURE: This patient is a 62-year-old male with advancing cataract of the right eye. Best corrected vision is 20/50. He has a posterior subcapsular polar type of cataract. It is bothering him tremendously when he attempts to do close work, which is required for his occupation. He is also experiencing significant glare. He had undergone cataract surgery to the left eye several years ago with excellent visual recovery. He understands the process. He is being bothered by his symptoms. The risks and benefits of surgery have been reviewed. He has been provided with fresh, up-to-date, pertinent information. The patient decided to have the cataract of the right eye removed on the basis of impairment of lifestyle.

DESCRIPTION OF PROCEDURE: The patient was brought to the operating room on 01/10/20xx as an outpatient. Intravenous anesthesia and retrobulbar block to the right eye were administered. The eye was prepped. The blepharostat was inserted and the surgical microscope was brought into position. Conjunctival peritomy was performed. The anterior chamber was entered at the 12 o'clock position using a keratome inserted at the end of a self-sealing limbal incision. Viscoelastic material was used as necessary throughout the case. A capsulorrhexis was performed. The cataract was removed by phacoemulsification technique. The implant was then delivered and inspected. Implant power was confirmed to be 20.5 diopters on the package. The implant was inserted into the capsular bag without difficulty. Viscoelastic material was removed from the eye. The wound was observed to be fluid tight. A single 10-0 nylon suture was placed for additional security. TobraDex ointment was applied to the surface of the eye. A sterile patch was taped into place. There were no complications.

ICD-10-CM Code(s) _____

CASE STUDY 15

This patient presents with acquired stenosis of the nasal lacrimal duct with obstruction bilaterally. The patient was taken to the operating room and placed on the table in the supine position, where anesthesia was induced. 2% Xylocaine with epinephrine was injected over the surgical site, and the patient was prepped and draped in the usual manner for orbitofacial surgery. A #15 Bard-Parker blade incision was made over the right anterior lacrimal crest. Sharp dissection was carried down to the lacrimal crest periosteum. The periosteum was elevated with a Tenzel periosteal elevator. A rhinostomy was created through the lacrimal sac fossa with a dental burr drill. The rhinostomy was enlarged to a dimension of 10 × 15 mm with Kerrison rongeurs. The nasal mucosa was opened in an "H"-shaped flap with sharp dissection. Purulent material was irrigated from the lacrimal with 5-0 Vicryl suture. Crawford tubing was inserted through the upper and lower canallculi and brought through the rhinostomy with a 5-0 Prolene suture. The skin was closed with 7-0 Prolene suture. An identical procedure was performed on the left side.

A #15 Bard-Parker blade incision was made at the right lateral canthus. Sharp dissection was carried down to the lateral orbital rim periosteum. The inferior ramus of the lateral canthal tendon was identified and severed with sharp dissection. A full-thickness en bloc excision of the lateral aspect of the tarsal plate was carried out with sharp dissection, and bleeding was controlled with electrocauterization. The cut edge of the tarsal plate was advanced to the lateral orbital rim periosteum, where it was sutured with 5-0 Prolene suture to the internal aspect of the lateral orbital rim periosteum. The skin muscle flap was then anchored to the lateral orbital rim periosteum with 5-0 Prolene suture, and the skin was closed with 7-0 Prolene suture. An identical procedure was performed on the left side.

The patient was then awakened and taken from the operating room in good condition, having tolerated the procedure well. There were no complications, and the estimated blood loss was less than 50 cc.

ICD-10-CM Code(s) _____

CASE STUDY 16

PREOPERATIVE DIAGNOSIS: Ptosis.

POSTOPERATIVE DIAGNOSIS: Same.

PROCEDURE: Müllerectomy.

INDICATIONS: The patient had been complaining of a progressive drooping of the left eyelid that was interfering with the patient's ability to watch TV and read. By holding the lid up the patient can see better. Visual field testing, which demonstrated a loss of the superior visual field, was performed. By taping the lid up into its proper anatomic position there was a marked improvement in the field. Neosynephrine 10% instilled into the eye resulted in a good elevation of the lid.

DESCRIPTION OF PROCEDURE: After informed consent was obtained, the patient was brought to the operating room. A supraorbital block of local anesthetic consisting of a 50/50 mixture of 1% Xylocaine with epinephrine mixed with Marcaine .75% with epinephrine. The face was then prepped and draped in the usual sterile fashion. The lid was then everted over a Desmarres retractor. The superior border of the tarsus was then marked with a marking pen. Another line was then marked on the conjunctiva 8 mm superior to this. The conjunctiva and Müller's muscle were then freed up from the underlying levator muscle by pulling on these tissues with an Adson forceps. A Müllerectomy clamp was then placed on the two previously marked lines. The clamp was shut to enclose the 8 mm of Müller's muscle and conjunctiva. A 6-0 plain suture was then run along the underside of the clamp. The clamp and its tissues were then excised by running a #15 Bard-Parker blade along the underside of the clamp. The 6-0 plain suture was then run once again along the length of the wound to close the edge of tarsus to the conjunctiva. The suture was buried temporally. The patient tolerated the procedure well and left the operating room in good condition.

ICD-10-CM Code(s) _____

CASE STUDY 17

PREOPERATIVE DIAGNOSIS: Uncontrolled primary open-angle glaucoma, left eye.

POSTOPERATIVE DIAGNOSIS: Same.

OPERATION: Trabeculectomy of externo with peripheral iridectomy, left eye.

ANESTHESIA: Conscious sedation, peribulbar block.

INDICATIONS: The patient has had progressive visual field deterioration on maximum tolerated medications and pressures in the high teens. To preserve her visual field, it was felt that surgery was necessary given the extensive damage to her optic nerve and visual field already existing.

PROCEDURE: The patient was brought to the operating room where she was given an intravenous sedative and peribulbar block. She was then prepped and draped in customary sterile fashion for intraocular surgery. A wire lid speculum was placed and a 6-0 Vicryl traction suture was put through the superior peripheral cornea. The globe was retracted downward. The conjunctiva was entered 12 mm proximal to the limbus. With a combination of blunt and sharp dissection, it was dissected down to the surgical limbus. The Gill's knife was used to bare the limbus and hemostasis was achieved with bipolar cautery. A 4 × 4 mm rectangular lamellar flap was outlined with the 200- to 300-micron blade, after which Mitomycin C 0.3 mg/cc was applied to the surface of the sclera overlying the outlying trap door for 2 minutes, 30 seconds.

The sponge and all instruments used to manipulate the Mitomycin sponge were removed from the field, and the eye was vigorously irrigated with balanced salt solution (BSS). A paracentesis was then made at the 3 o'clock position and Healon was injected into the anterior chamber. The lamellar flap was then dissected into the peripheral clear cornea, the anterior

chamber was entered with a #75 blade, and a posterior lip sclerectomy was performed with the Kelly-Descemet punch. A superior peripheral iridectomy was already present, but was enlarged to avoid entrapment. The rectangular flap was then closed using five 10-0 monofilament sutures, and the knots were rotated and buried. The conjunctiva was closed using a running, interrupted 8-0 Vicryl suture. Atropine 1% was applied to the eye several times, after which TobraDex ointment and monocular dressing were placed on the eye. The patient tolerated the procedure well and was taken to Phase II in excellent condition with instructions for a follow-up visit at noon on the day after surgery. (An appointment time of 8 am was preferable for the follow-up visit, but the patient indicated that transportation was not available.)

ICD-10-CM Code(s) _____

CASE STUDY 18

This very pleasant 90-year-old gentleman complains of constant tearing from both eyes, with the right eye being worse than the left. This has been going on for approximately one year. It has been painless, he has no foreign body sensation, and he has never had facial bone fractures, but he did have cautery in the right nares approximately 50 years ago.

EXAMINATION: Visual acuity is 20/50 in the right eye and 20/30 in the left eye. The papillary reactions are normal and extraocular motility is full. Confrontational visual fields are full to finger counting. The external examination is significant for moderate bilateral lower eyelid laxity with ectropion and punctual eversion. He has mild punctual stenosis bilaterally and complete nasolacrimal duct stenosis on the right side. The orbital examination is normal. The slit-lamp examination is normal, including conjunctiva, cornea, anterior chamber, iris, and lens.

IMPRESSION: The patient has complete nasolacrimal duct stenosis on the right side and senile ectropion of both lower eyelids.

PLAN: I have recommended dacryocystorhinostomy on the right side and ectropion repair of both lower eyelids. I have fully discussed the risks, benefits, and alternatives of surgery with the patient, his daughter, and his son-in-law. I have answered all of their questions and they all appear to understand. The patient wishes to proceed with surgery.

ICD-10-CM Code(s)_____

CASE STUDY 19

This very pleasant 1-year-old still has a cyst in the right orbit. We had originally scheduled this procedure for last October; however, the child was sick at that time and the parents cancelled the surgery. He is now walking and is very active and running into things, and the patient's parents are very anxious to get this cyst removed.

EXAMINATION: Visual acuity is central, steady, and maintained in each eye. The papillary reactions are normal and extraocular motility is full. Confrontational visual fields and intraocular pressures were not checked. The external examination is significant for a round, freely mobile lesion at the zygomatical frontal suture on the right side. The lacrimal and orbital examinations are otherwise normal. The slit-lamp examination is normal, including conjunctiva, cornea, anterior chamber, iris, and lens. The fundus examination is also normal.

IMPRESSION: The patient has a cyst in the right orbit.

PLAN: I have recommended orbitotomy with removal. I have fully discussed the risks, benefits, and alternatives of surgery with the patient's parents. I have answered all of their questions and they both appear to understand and they wish to proceed with surgery. The surgery has been scheduled for the near future.

ICD-10-CM Code(s) _____

CASE STUDY 20

This very pleasant 64-year-old lady complains of a lesion on the right upper eyelid that has been present for a couple of years. It has exhibited recent growth. The lesion is painless but it does sometime itch. It has never opened or bled or drained any purulent material.

EXAMINATION: Visual acuity is 20/20 in each eye. The papillary reactions are normal and extraocular motility is full. Confrontational visual fields are full to finger counting. The external examination is significant for a large mass approximately 7 × 7 mm in the central portion of the right upper eyelid. The lacrimal and orbital examinations are normal. There are no other eyelid lesions. The slit-lamp examination is normal, including conjunctiva, cornea, anterior chamber, iris, and lens. The lesion on the right upper eyelid does involve the lash follicles. The fundus examination is also normal.

IMPRESSION: The patient has a benign lesion on the right upper eyelid including the canthus. However, this lesion has been growing and it is beginning to cause some difficulties with her vision.

PLAN: I have recommended removal by wedge resection. I have fully discussed the risks, benefits, and alternatives of surgery with the patient and her husband. I have answered all of their questions and they both appear to understand and the patient wishes to proceed with surgery. The surgery has been scheduled for the near future.

ICD-10-CM Code(s) _____

CASE STUDY 21

DATE OF PROCEDURE: June 11, 20xx

PREOPERATIVE DIAGNOSIS: Bilateral upper eyelid dermatochalasis obstructing vision.

POSTOPERATIVE DIAGNOSIS: Same.

OPERATION PERFORMED: Bilateral upper eyelid blepharoplasty.

INDICATIONS: The patient presents with excessive upper eyelid skin obstructing the visual field. Risks, benefits, and alternatives of bilateral upper eyelid blepharoplasty on a medical basis to improve vision were reviewed. He elected to proceed.

DESCRIPTION OF PROCEDURE: After informed operative consent was obtained, the patient was brought to the operating room and laid in the supine position. Intravenous sedation was administered per Dr Crash. Both upper eyelids were infiltrated with 2% Lidocaine with epinephrine mixed with 0.5% Marcaine. The operative area was prepped and draped in the usual manner for eyelid surgery. Tetracaine and corneal protectors were inserted bilaterally. The desired level of postoperative eyelid crease was marked with a marking pen and a pinch test with Adson forceps was used to assess the adequacy and appropriateness of eyelid skin incision. Blepharoplasty markings were completed. Premarked areas were incised with a #15 Bard-Parker blade. The skin was excised with Westcott scissors along with some portions of orbicularis. This was performed on both upper eyelids.

Hemostasis was obtained in both upper eyelids. Inspection revealed good skin excision and symmetry bilaterally. The lid crease was re-formed by placating the cut inferior edge of orbicularis to higher position of orbicularis and levator using 6-0 fast-absorbing gut suture in a buried interrupted fashion ×3 in both eye-lids. The skin was closed with 6-0 Prolene in a simple running fashion in both upper eyelids. The operative areas were clean and dry. The patient was then trans-ferred from the operating room to the recovery room in stable and satisfactory condition. There were no intraoperative complications.

ICD-10-CM Code(s) _____

CASE STUDY 22

The patient presented to the hospital urgent-care cen-ter, complaining of a swollen left upper eyelid for the past two days. She stated that the swelling was increas-ing and putting more and more pressure on her eye. The eyelashes were affecting her vision as the angle of the lashes had changed due to the swelling. She reported a history of surgery to her sinus on the left side about two months ago. On physical examination the physician noted that the left eyelid and surround-ing tissue were severely swollen and had a focal area consistent with an internum hordeolum of the left upper eyelid.

ASSESSMENT AND PLAN: Internum hordeolum of left upper eyelid with secondary orbital cellulitis.

The physician prescribed Keflex 500 mg four times a day for seven days and cortisporin ophthalmic oint-ment twice daily to the eye. The physician advised washing the eyelid with Johnson's No More Tears baby shampoo twice daily, using good handwashing tech-nique and not touching either eye during the healing process, except for treatments as above. The patient was told to follow up in three days for a recheck or sooner if the area increases in size.

ICD-10-CM Code(s) _____

CASE STUDY 23

A 36-year-old patient who has two chalazion lesions in the upper eyelid of the right eye underwent excision in the hospital surgery department. Once the patient was prepped and draped, local anesthesia was administered. The physician uses a chalazion clamp and exposes the posterior surface of the eyelid. Both lesions were excised and the eyelid was explored with curet after both incisions were drained. The wounds were cauter-ized and the clamp released. The patient tolerated the procedure well and was released from the outpatient recovery area two hours later in good condition.

ICD-10-CM Code(s)_____

Diseases of the Ear and Mastoid Process (H60-H95) and Diseases of the Circulatory System (I00-I99)

ICD-10-CM Chapters 8 and 9 Guidelines Review

In this chapter you will find a summary of the chapter-specific coding guidelines for Chapter 9 of the ICD-10-CM codebook (Diseases of the Circulatory System) followed by case studies to build ICD-10-CM diagnosis coding skills in this area. For diseases of the ear and mastoid process (Chapter 8 of the ICD-10-CM codebook), general coding guidelines and instructional notes apply because currently there are no specific guidelines for Chapter 8.

Many medical specialties, including primary care, ear, nose, and throat (ENT), otolaryngology, and cardiology, reference Chapters 8 and 9 of the ICD-10-CM codebook for coding diseases of the ear and mastoid process and diseases of the circulatory system. Keep in mind that you should always reference the ICD-10-CM Official Guidelines for Coding and Reporting in its entirety when making a code selection.

ICD-10-CM Official Coding Guidelines for Diseases of the Circulatory System

The following summarized guidelines apply when coding hypertension and conditions causal to the condition. Hypertension is coded in ICD-10-CM as I10, whether the condition is malignant, benign, essential, or unspecified.

HYPERTENSION WITH HEART DISEASE

The classification presumes a causal relationship between hypertension and heart involvement and between hypertension and kidney involvement, as the two conditions are linked by the term "with" in the Alphabetic Index. These conditions should be coded as related even in the absence of provider documentation explicitly linking them, unless the documentation clearly states the conditions are unrelated. For hypertension and conditions not specifically linked by relational terms such as "with," "associated with" or "due to" in the classification, provider documentation must link the conditions in order to code them as related. The following guidelines apply to coding hypertension with heart disease:

- Hypertension with heart conditions classified to I50.0- or I51.4- are assigned a code from category I11, Hypertensive heart disease. An additional code from category I50, Heart failure, is reported for a patient with heart failure.

- The type of heart failure (if documented) should be reported with codes from category I50.

- The same heart conditions (I50.-, I51.4-I51.9) with hypertension are coded separately if the provider has specifically documented a different cause. Sequencing is guided by circumstances of the admission or patient encounter.

HYPERTENSIVE CHRONIC KIDNEY DISEASE

Hypertensive chronic kidney disease (CKD) is reported with codes from category I12 under the following conditions:

- Unlike hypertension with heart disease, ICD-10-CM coding presumes a cause-and-effect relationship between the two conditions.

- ICD-10-CM classifies CKD with hypertension as "hypertensive chronic kidney disease."

- Hypertensive CKD is assigned in category I12 when both hypertension and a condition classifiable to category N18, Chronic kidney disease, is present.

- CKD should not be coded as hypertensive if the physician had specifically documented a different cause.

- A code from category N18 should be reported as a secondary diagnosis with a code from category I12 to report the stage of the CKD whether it is stage 1–5, or end stage.

- If the documentation indicates the patient has hypertensive CKD with acute renal failure, code the acute renal failure (required) as an additional diagnosis.

HYPERTENSIVE HEART AND CHRONIC KIDNEY DISEASE

Often patients with hypertensive CKD also have hypertensive heart disease. The following guidelines are applicable when reporting a diagnosis from category I13, which is considered a combination code because it combines both hypertensive heart and kidney disease in its descriptor:

- Assign codes from category I13, Hypertensive heart and chronic kidney disease, when there is hypertension with both heart and kidney involvement. Always assume the relationship as stated earlier with hypertension with heart disease and/or CKD whether or not it is clearly stated in the documentation. If heart failure (I50) is specified, it should be reported as an additional diagnosis.

- Assign a code from category N18, Chronic kidney disease, as a secondary diagnosis to identify the stage of the CKD.

- **Do not** report hypertension and heart disease and/or CKD separately as they are considered causal even if a causal relationship is not stated in the documentation.

- For patients with both acute renal failure and CKD, an additional code for acute renal failure is required.

HYPERTENSIVE CEREBROVASCULAR DISEASE

Codes from categories I60-I69 are reported for hypertensive cerebrovascular disease. The appropriate hypertension code is reported as a secondary diagnosis.

HYPERTENSIVE RETINOPATHY

Subcategory H35.0, Background retinopathy and retinal vascular changes, should be reported with a code from category I10-I15 for the hypertensive disease.

- Hypertension is reported as code I10, Essential (primary) hypertension, which includes systemic hypertension.

- Sequencing is based on the reason for the encounter.

HYPERTENSION, SECONDARY

Secondary hypertension is due to an underlying condition. Two codes are required: (1) one code to identify the underlying etiology and (2) one code from category I15 to identify the hypertension. Sequencing of codes is determined by the reason for admission/encounter.

HYPERTENSION, TRANSIENT (ELEVATED BLOOD PRESSURE)

A patient with elevated blood pressure does not necessarily mean the patient is hypertensive. There are many reasons a patient's blood pressure may become elevated. Hypertension should not be reported unless stated clearly in the documentation. Elevated blood pressure is reported with a sign and symptom code R03.0, Elevated blood-pressure reading, without diagnosis of hypertension.

For gestational (pregnancy-induced) hypertension without significant proteinuria, report a code from O13.-, or for pre-eclampsia for transient hypertension use O14.-.

HYPERTENSION CONTROLLED VERSUS UNCONTROLLED

Hypertension controlled indicates good blood pressure control with therapy. Hypertension uncontrolled is when the current therapeutic treatment does not effectively control the patient's blood pressure. Code categories I10-I15 are assigned to both types of hypertension. There is no distinction in ICD-10-CM between controlled and uncontrolled hypertension.

HYPERTENSIVE CRISIS

Assign a code from category I16, Hypertensive crisis, for documented hypertensive urgency, hypertensive emergency, or unspecified hypertensive crisis. Code also any identified hypertensive disease (I10-I15). The sequencing is based on the reason for the encounter.

ATHEROSCLEROTIC CORONARY ARTERY DISEASE AND ANGINA

Code I25.11, Atherosclerotic heart disease of native coronary artery with angina pectoris, and code I25.7, Atherosclerosis of coronary artery bypass graft(s) and coronary artery of transplanted heart with angina pectoris, are combination codes that include angina pectoris. The following guidelines apply:

- A causal relationship is assumed in a patient with both atherosclerosis and angina pectoris unless the documentation indicates the angina is due to something other than atherosclerosis.

- When a patient is admitted for an acute myocardial infarction (AMI) and the patient also has coronary artery disease (CAD), the AMI is sequenced before the CAD.

INTRAOPERATIVE AND POSTPROCEDURAL CEREBROVASCULAR ACCIDENT (CVA)

Medical record documentation should clearly specify the cause-and-effect relationship between the medical intervention and the cerebrovascular accident in order to assign a code for intraoperative or post-procedural CVA. Code assignment depends on the following:

- Whether the accident was an infarction or hemorrhage.

- Whether the accident occurred intraoperatively or postoperatively.

- If it was a cerebral hemorrhage, code assignment depends on the type of procedure performed.

SEQUELAE OF CEREBROVASCULAR DISEASE

Category I69 is used to indicate conditions classifiable to categories I60-I67 as the causes of sequelae (neurologic deficits), which are classified elsewhere. These "late effects" include neurologic deficits that persist after the initial onset of conditions classifiable to categories I60-I67. The neurologic deficits caused by cerebrovascular disease may be present from the onset or may arise at any time after the onset of the condition classifiable to categories I60-I67.

Codes from category I69 may be assigned on a health care record with codes from I60-I67 if the following conditions are met:

- The patient has a current cerebrovascular disease and deficits from an old cerebrovascular disease.

- When no neurologic deficits are present, assign code Z86.73, Personal history of transient ischemic attack (TIA), and cerebral infarction without residual deficits, not a code from category I69, as an additional code for history of cerebrovascular disease.

Category I69 is also used to indicate conditions classifiable to categories I60-I67 as the causes of sequelae

(neurologic deficits) classified elsewhere as described in the following guidelines:

- Sequelae includes neurologic deficits that persist after initial onset of conditions classifiable to categories I60-I67.

- Codes from category I69, Sequelae of cerebrovascular disease, that specify hemiplegia, hemiparesis, and monoplegia identify whether the dominant or non-dominant side is affected. When the affected side is documented but the documentation does not specify dominant or non-dominant, selection of the code is as follows:

  - For ambidextrous patients, the default is dominant

  - If the left side is affected, the default is non-dominant

  - If the right side is affected, the default is dominant

- Neurologic deficits caused by cerebrovascular disease may be present from the onset or may arise at any time after the onset of the condition classifiable to categories I60-I67.

- Codes from category I69 may be reported with codes from I60-I67 if the patient has a current cerebrovascular disease and deficits from an old cerebrovascular disease.

- When no neurologic deficits are present, report code Z86.73, Personal history of transient ischemic attack (TIA), and cerebral infarction without residual deficits, not a code from category I69, as an additional code for history of cerebrovascular disease.

ACUTE MYOCARDIAL INFARCTION

The ICD-10-CM codes for an acute myocardial infarction (AMI) identify the site, such as anterolateral wall or true posterior wall. When coding an acute myocardial infarction, the following guidelines apply:

- Report subcategories I21.0-I21.2 and code I21.3 for ST elevation myocardial infarction (STEMI).

- Code I21.4, Non-ST elevation (NSTEMI) myocardial infarction, is used for non-ST elevation myocardial infarction (NSTEMI) and non-transmural myocardial infarction.

- If NSTEMI evolves to STEMI, assign the STEMI code.

- If STEMI converts to NSTEMI due to thrombolytic therapy, it is still coded as STEMI.

- Code I21 is reported when a patient requires continued care for the myocardial infarction. It may be reported for a duration of four weeks or 28 days or less of onset, regardless of setting even when a patient is transferred from the acute care setting to a post-acute care setting if the patient is within four weeks of onset and requires continued care related to the myocardial infarction.

- After the four-week period, an appropriate aftercare code is reported and not a code from category I21.

- Code I25.2, Old myocardial infarction, may be reported for an old or healed myocardial infarction not requiring further care.

What Do STEMI and NSTEMI Mean?

STEMI (ST elevation myocardial infarction) refers to a transmural infarction of the myocardium—the thickness of the myocardium has undergone necrosis—resulting in ST elevation. This is typically due to a complete block of a coronary artery (ie, occlusive thrombus). NSTEMI (non-ST elevation myocardial infarction) refers to a partial dynamic block to coronary arteries (ie, non-occlusive thrombus). The difference between NSTEMI and unstable angina is that in NSTEMI the severity of ischemia is sufficient to cause cardiac enzyme elevation. The ICD-10-CM codes for acute myocardial infarction identify the site, such as anterolateral wall or true posterior wall.

ACUTE MYOCARDIAL INFARCTION, UNSPECIFIED

Code I21.3, ST elevation (STEMI) myocardial infarction of unspecified site, is the default for the unspecified term acute myocardial infarction. The following guidelines apply:

- If only STEMI or transmural myocardial infarction without the site is documented, query the provider as to the site, or assign code I21.3.

- If an AMI is documented as non-transmural or subendocardial, but the site is provided, it is still coded as a subendocardial AMI.

SUBSEQUENT ACUTE MYOCARDIAL INFARCTION

The following guidelines apply when coding subsequent acute myocardial infarction:

- If a patient suffers a new AMI within four weeks of the initial AMI, two codes are required:

- A code from category I22, Subsequent ST elevation (STEMI) and non-ST elevation (NSTEMI) myocardial infarction.

- A code from category I22 must be used in conjunction with a code from category I21 for the current AMI.

- Sequencing depends on the circumstance of the encounter.

When the patient is admitted due to an AMI and has a subsequent AMI while still hospitalized:

- Report a code from category I21 for the first AMI as the first-listed or principal diagnosis code.

- Report a code from category I22 as the secondary diagnosis.

If the patient suffers a subsequent AMI after the hospital discharge for the initial AMI, is admitted for treatment of the subsequent AMI, and is within the four-week time frame of healing from the initial AMI, the following guidelines apply:

- A code from category I22 is sequenced as the first-listed or principal diagnosis.

- A code from category I21 is reported as the secondary diagnosis.

- The guidelines for assigning the correct I22 code are the same as for the initial AMI.

It is time to build skill and knowledge by coding the following exercises. Be sure to reference the ICD-10-CM codebook and the ICD-10-CM Official Guidelines for Coding and Reporting, along with the instructional notes, when coding these conditions.

Diseases of the Ear and Mastoid Process (H60-H95)

CASE STUDY 1

Thank you for referring this patient who was seen regarding her nasal allergies. She also developed pneumonia and was put on Prednisone, which has in fact improved her nasal function by reducing the polypoid change in the nose. She is breathing quite well through the nose, has a good sense of smell, and ears are feeling well.

EXAMINATION: Revealed a moderate degree of hyperemic change and congestion to the nose, consistent with a viral rhinitis. There are some very high polyps bilaterally, which are certainly not obstructive to her airway. The throat and larynx were clear. Otoscopy shows the left ear to be normal. The previously inserted tube in her right ear has now extruded, the drum has healed, and there is no fluid in this ear either.

DIAGNOSIS: Ongoing allergic rhinitis and polyposis problem with superimposed viral rhinitis.

PLAN: Once her cold settles, I have asked her to start using the Nasacort spray again on a regular basis and to see me again in three months or sooner if she notices a loss of sense of smell again.

ICD-10-CM Code(s) _____

CASE STUDY 2

PREOPERATIVE DIAGNOSIS: Sensorineural hearing loss, left ear.

POSTOPERATIVE DIAGNOSIS: Same.

PROCEDURE: Left middle ear hearing device implantation.

INDICATIONS: Loss of hearing in the left ear. Hearing in right ear is normal.

OPERATION: The patient was taken to the operating room and placed on the operating room table in the supine position. General anesthesia was administered and a laryngeal mask airway was used for ventilation. The left ear was prepped in the usual sterile fashion. Ancef was given preoperatively. Facial nerve monitoring was performed throughout and the patient was infiltrated with Lidocaine and Adrenaline post-auricularly. Standard incisions for implant surgery were performed. The sigmoid sinus, middle fossa, dura, and posterior canal wall were all identified. The antrum was entered and the incus was identified. The horizontal canal was identified; the facial nerve and facial recess were identified and opened. The chordae tympani was sectioned because it was interfering with adequate visualization. Bleeding was controlled as it was encountered, and a bed was created for the implant. Stay sutures of 2-0 Prolene were fixed appropriately. The implant was sent into the bed and the transducer was crimped to the incus without difficulty. The implant was irrigated and a layered closure performed. A Glasscock bubble was placed. The patient was awakened and transported to the recovery room in stable condition with the facial nerve intact. All sponge, needle, and instrument counts were correct. Estimated blood loss was 10 cc.

ICD-10-CM Code(s) _____

CASE STUDY 3

PREOPERATIVE DIAGNOSIS: Recurrent serous otitis media (chronic).

POSTOPERATIVE DIAGNOSIS: Same.

INDICATIONS: This is a 10-year-old who has had multiple episodes of otitis. We did manage to clear chronic serous otitis, but it returned shortly thereafter. It was therefore felt he would benefit from bilateral myringotomy and tubes.

PROCEDURE: The patient was brought to the operating room and placed on the operating room table and a general anesthetic was provided by the anesthesiologist. Following that, the left ear was cleaned of cerumen and debris, an anterior inferior myringotomy incision was made, and a collar button tube was slipped into position after encountering a dry middle ear. The same procedure was completed on the patient's other ear. Cortisporin otic was instilled in both ears, and cotton was placed in the os. The patient was then awakened and taken to the recovery room in good condition. Sponge and needle counts were correct.

ICD-10-CM Code(s) _____

CASE STUDY 4

Thank you for referring this patient who was seen for an evaluation of hearing loss. Hearing allegedly is generally reduced in both ears, but he has always, throughout his entire life, had worse hearing in his left ear, presumably subsequent to childhood otorrhea that he does recall.

EXAMINATION: Revealed an intact right tympanic membrane. He has a relatively small posterosuperior perforation of the left drum, which unfortunately overlies the stapes incus, and to a slight degree, the round window. He also has a bit of otomycosis infection involving the proximal ear canal, although no evident involvement of the middle ear.

DIAGNOSES:

1. Mild to moderately severe bilateral sensorineural hearing loss

2. Perforated left tympanic membrane with moderate conductive deafness

3. Otomycosis, left ear canal

PLAN: The ear was cleaned, and I have applied a Canesten ointment to the entire canal and will follow-up in a month. His option is either to use a hearing aid in the left and/or both ears to improve his hearing or to undergo tympanoplasty surgery to his left ear to close the perforation. He can then see how he feels about his hearing loss, of which the sensorineural component will remain, to see whether subsequent hearing aids are still needed. He will give me his decision on these options when he returns for a recheck of his otomycosis.

ICD-10-CM Code(s) _____

CASE STUDY 5

The patient is a 68-year-old woman who has had approximately a four-month history of blockage, obstruction, fluid, fullness, pressure, and head noise in the right ear. She has had tubes inserted. The last tube was placed by Dr Minor in February, but it did not resolve the problem. On earlier examination today, the tube was noted to have been extruded into the ear canal, and the middle ear was noted to be filled with an amber, straw-colored fluid. The right ear also was noted to be filled with an amber, straw-colored fluid.

With the patient positioned supine with no sedation, a small amount of Lidocaine was injected into the posterior superior vascular strip area. Following this, an anterior inferior quadrant radial myringotomy was performed in the good firm remnant of the tympanic membrane. Fluid was suctioned from the right middle ear space and a fluoroplastic spoon-bobbin was inserted. Following this, the patient was observed for approximately 30 minutes and discharged in good condition.

ICD-10-CM Code(s) _____

CASE STUDY 6

This patient is a 45-year-old gentleman who underwent ligation of the right ethmoid artery and the right internal maxillary artery four years ago for control of a severe posterior epistaxis. Since then, he has been complaining about paresthesia or a numbness sensation on the right mid-face and the right forehead. He also has chronic nasal obstruction since he recovered from the surgery.

EXAM: There is a synechia between the medial surface of the inferior turbinate and the septum.

There is also a small polyp located in the left middle meatus. The postnasal space is clear. X rays of the sinuses revealed cloudiness of the frontal as well as the ethmoid sinuses. The right maxillary antrum is opaque. There is a small air-fluid level in the left maxillary antrum, indicating apparent sinusitis.

DIAGNOSES:

1. Paresthesia of the right face, probably due to injury to the infraorbital nerve and the supraorbital nerve, during the last surgery for control of epistaxis

2. Acute pansinusitis with left-sided nasal polyp

3. Synechia of the right nasal cavity

PLAN: The patient will have a CT scan of the paranasal sinus and will come back to discuss the finding with a view to doing some endoscopic sinus surgery to remove the polyps as well as to release the adhesion in the right nasal cavity.

ICD-10-CM Code(s) _____

CASE STUDY 7

CHIEF COMPLAINT: This 3-year-old female presents today for evaluation of chronic ear infections bilateral.

Associated signs and symptoms include cough, fever, irritability, and speech and language delay. Duration of symptom: 12 rounds of antibiotics for otitis media. Quality of the pain is throbbing.

IMPRESSION: Chronic mucoid OM bilateral; adenoid hyperplasia.

ICD-10-CM Code(s) _____

Diseases of the Circulatory System (I00-I99)

CASE STUDY 8

PREOPERATIVE DIAGNOSES: Superficial venous insufficiency; leg edema.

POSTOPERATIVE DIAGNOSIS: Superficial venous insufficiency; varicose leg ulcer inflammation; varicose veins with inflammation; vascular disorders of skin.

PROCEDURES:

1. Preoperative venous duplex mapping of the right small saphenous vein

2. Ultrasound-guided venipuncture of the right small saphenous vein

3. Introduction of a 5-French catheter into the right small saphenous vein

4. Selective placement of a 600-micron laser fiber at the saphenopopliteal junction

5. Transcatheter occlusion of the right small saphenous vein with endovenous laser set to a power level of 12 with continuous energy, and a total of 842.16 for a length of 11.00 cm averaging 76.56 joules per cm

6. Radiological supervision and interpretation of transcatheter occlusion of the right small saphenous vein

7. Post procedure color duplex imaging of the right small saphenous vein

ICD-10-CM Code(s) _____

CASE STUDY 9

INDICATIONS: This is a 77-year-old male patient with vasculitis and varicose veins of right lower extremity that are associated with aching, itching, edema, and ulcer. Duplex ultrasound revealed an open popliteal vein. The patient reviewed the treatment consent, all questions were answered, and the consent was signed. The patient requested pre-operative medication for anxiety.

RADIOLOGIC INTERPRETATION AND FINDINGS: Preoperative venous duplex mapping revealed an incompetent right small saphenous vein. The course of the vein was marked on the skin with a sterile, indelible marker. Ultrasound was then used to guide the selective placement of a 600-micron laser fiber at the saphenopopliteal junction, and the infiltration of local anesthetic in a subfascial perivenous tumescent technique that compressed the vein around the laser fiber, as well as provided maximum anesthetic efficacy. Finally, color duplex was used at the end of the procedure to confirm occlusion, and it showed the treated vein occluded.

ANESTHESIA:

- 2% Lidocaine, 20 ml given subcutaneously.

- 0.1% Xylocaine with epinephrine in lactated Ringer's solution, 100 ml given in an ultrasound-guided subfascial perivenous tumescent technique.

DESCRIPTION OF PROCEDURE: The patient was taken to the office operating suite where the right leg vein mapping was performed. The right leg was then prepped and draped in the usual fashion. Ultrasound-guided venipuncture was performed on the right small saphenous vein and a guidewire was inserted. A 5-French introducer catheter was inserted over the guidewire using the Seldinger technique. A 600-micron laser fiber was then placed through the introducer catheter and the tip positioned at the saphenopopliteal junction under ultrasound guidance and confirmed with transillumination. The local anesthetic was then infiltrated along the course of the vein in a subfascial perivenous tumescent technique that compressed the vein around the laser fiber as well as provided maximum anesthetic efficacy. The diode laser was set at 12 continuous energy and at a length of 11.00 cm. Laser occluded averaging 76.56 joules per cm. Repeat color duplex imaging confirmed occlusion of the vein by the lack of color flow, and color flow demonstrated an open popliteal vein. A sterile pad was placed over the percutaneous access site. Absorbent dressing and stockings were then placed on the patient. The patient tolerated the procedure well and was ambulating in the office immediately following the procedure.

IMMEDIATE POST-TREATMENT: 30-40 mmHg pressure gradient stockings were prescribed.

DISCHARGE: The patient was given verbal and written instructions, prescriptions for analgesics, and discharged to home. The patient is to continue massage three times daily and ice three to four times daily. He is to continue to wear compression stocking for 48 hours continuously and then thereafter for two weeks. The patient will return for follow-up in one week.

ICD-10-CM Code(s) _____

CASE STUDY 10

PROCEDURE: Ultrasound-guided sclerotherapy to varicose veins.

SUBJECTIVE: Patient presented to our office for limited ultrasound examination of, and possible treatment to, both legs. Patient reported lumpy areas and continued leg pain from previous treatment. The patient reports that she is massaging her legs three times daily. She is no longer taking Asclera. She reported having worn 30-40 mmHg compression stockings daily, as directed.

OBJECTIVE: Ultrasound examination of both lower extremities was performed to identify areas of venous disorder that required treatment and to locate veins that required injection. Ultrasound examination reveals that all varicosities are closed, and no treatment is necessary today. No edema was noted.

ASSESSMENT: Varicose veins with inflammation; peripheral venous insufficiency; restless leg syndrome, bilateral.

PLAN: Patient to call if she experiences additional pain and will return for follow-up in three months.

ICD-10-CM Code(s) _____

CASE STUDY 11

This is a 72-year-old, established patient who has been in the nursing home for the past six months and is being evaluated on a monthly basis. He has a previous history of left-sided cerebrovascular accident with right side paralysis, which is his dominant side. The patient has been demented since his stroke and has been seen by a psychiatrist who diagnosed psychosis and placed him on Risperidone and Lorazepam. Patient will open his eyes to name only. He does not answer any questions. He has been having swallowing problems but has not developed any signs of choking. Unable to obtain a review of systems due to the patient's non-responsiveness.

PHYSICAL EXAMINATION:

GENERAL: BP 125/78; pulse 78; weight 108 lb with a loss of 5 pounds since last month. Laxity of the lower jaw; cataracts bilaterally. The patient responds to name only; right-sided paralysis due to old CVA.

LUNGS: Clear to auscultation and percussion.

HEART: Normal sinus rhythm.

ABDOMEN: No masses or tenderness.

ASSESSMENT AND PLAN: Right-sided paralysis; malnutrition with weight loss; psychosis. Will have speech pathologist evaluate the patient. I will follow up at his next visit in two weeks. The patient will continue same medications.

ICD-10-CM Code(s) _____

CASE STUDY 12

PREOPERATIVE DIAGNOSIS: Atherosclerotic heart disease of native coronary artery with angina pectoris with spasm.

POSTOPERATIVE DIAGNOSIS: Same.

PROCEDURES:

1. Reverse saphenous vein bypass graft from the aorta to the first diagonal and first marginal coronary artery in a sequential fashion; reverse saphenous vein bypass graft from the aorta to the posterior descending coronary artery.

2. Reverse left internal mammary artery to the left anterior descending coronary artery; temporary cardiopulmonary bypass.

3. Cold cardioplegia

DESCRIPTION OF PROCEDURE: A primary median sternotomy incision was used. The saphenous vein was taken from the left leg and the incision closed in the usual manner. The left internal mammary artery was dissected free from its bed. Cardiopulmonary bypass was established at a flow of 2.2 L per minute per meter squared for 120 minutes. A partial occluding clamp was placed on the ascending aorta and two segments of saphenous vein were anastomosed to it using a continuous 5-0 Prolene suture. The aorta was then cross-clamped for 78 minutes and cold cardioplegic solution was infused. The vein was taken to the right and anastomosed end-to-side to the posterior descending coronary artery using 7-0 Prolene sutures. The other one was taken to the left and anastomosed side-to-side to the first diagonal coronary artery using 7-0 Prolene sutures in a sequential fashion. The left internal mammary artery was then brought through a hole in the pericardium and anastomosed end-to-side to the left anterior descending coronary artery using 7-0 Prolene sutures. The aortic cross clamp was then removed and re-warming begun. After an adequate period of re-warming, cardiopulmonary bypass was gradually disconnected with the hemodynamic state becoming good. Wires were left in the right ventricle and right atrium for pacing and a polyvinyl catheter was placed in the left atria. Two pericardial tubes and one pleural tube were placed. Hemostasis was then obtained and the incision closed in the usual manner. The patient was taken to the recovery room in stable condition. There were no complications.

ICD-10-CM Code(s) _____

CASE STUDY 13

PREOPERATIVE DIAGNOSIS: History of anal ulcerations and hemorrhoids.

POSTOPERATIVE DIAGNOSIS: Internal hemorrhoids present posterior aspect, small and stable.

PROCEDURE: Anoscopy performed. No ulcerations, no fissures, hemorrhoids present posterior aspect, and are small. Hemorrhoids are stable.

PLAN:

1. Continue avoiding foods and liquids as recommended in the first visit.

2. Can restart suspended food and liquids, one at a time, for 10 days. If there is no recurrence, add a second food, and so on.

3. Follow-up visit in three months.

ICD-10-CM Code(s) _____

CASE STUDY 14

HISTORY OF PRESENT ILLNESS: The patient is a 42-year-old, Caucasian male with no prior cardiac history. He presented to the emergency room at ABC Hospital complaining of chest pain. This morning he noticed some numbness and pain in his left arm. Later in the day he developed pressure in the chest. This gradually worsened throughout the morning until shortly before lunch when he was rating the pain at 8/10 in severity and decided to go to the emergency room for evaluation. When he arrived at the hospital he was given sublingual nitroglycerin and the pain improved to 4/10 and has stayed at that level since then. He denies any prior cardiac history. Risk factors for coronary disease include hypertension. The patient's lipid status is unknown. He has a history of tobacco abuse. He stopped smoking four years ago. The patient is unaware of any thromboembolic disease in the family. He denies any drug use. The initial EKG at the hospital showed some subtle ST elevation in an inferolateral distribution. His initial cardiac enzymes showed a CK of 253, MB fraction of 36, and troponin 0.24. He was sent here for possible left heart catheterizaton and ongoing care. At the time of his arrival he was rating his pain at 4/10 in severity.

PAST SURGICAL HISTORY: The patient has had an adenoidectomy.

MEDICATIONS: At the outlying hospital the patient was started on heparin and nitroglycerin drips. He was given Lopressor and aspirin.

SOCIAL HISTORY: The patient denies tobacco use now, but smoked previously for 10 years. He drinks alcohol on occasion. He denies drug use.

FAMILY HISTORY: There is no known heart disease in the family.

REVIEW OF SYSTEMS: Significant for the arm and chest pain mentioned above. The patient denies fevers, chills, unusual bleeding, rashes, headache, visual changes, dizziness, syncope, palpitations, dyspnea on exertion, orthopnea, paroxysmal nocturnal dyspnea, cough, shortness of breath, wheezing, abdominal pain, nausea, vomiting, diarrhea, hematochezia, melena, dysuria, or hematuria. No allergies.

PHYSICAL EXAMINATION:

VITAL SIGNS: Pulse is 103 and regular, blood pressure 129/89, respiratory rate 18.

GENERAL APPEARANCE: This is a Caucasian male who is awake, alert, and oriented, and who appears uncomfortable.

HEENT: Pupils are equal, round, and reactive to light. Extraocular movements are intact. Oropharynx is clear.

NECK: There is no jugular venous distention (JVD), thyromegaly, lymphadenopathy, or bruit.

LUNGS: Clear to auscultation bilaterally without wheeze, rhonchi, or crackle.

HEART: Reveals regular rate and rhythm without murmur, rub, or gallop.

ABDOMEN: Soft, nontender, nondistended with good bowel sounds.

EXTREMITIES: Reveals no lower extremity edema. Pulses are 2+ throughout.

NEUROLOGIC: Cranial nerves II–XII are grossly intact. Strength is 5/5 in all four extremities.

LABORATORY: EKG shows normal sinus rhythm with minimal ST elevation in an inferolateral distribution. Chest X ray shows no active disease. Hemoglobin is 12.8; hematocrit 38; white count 16.3; platelets 273; sodium 139; potassium 3.6; chloride 108; bicarbonate 21; BUN 8; creatinine 0.5; glucose 138; calcium 8.8; D-dimer negative; CK 253; CK-MB 36.4; troponin 0.24.

ASSESSMENT AND PLAN: Acute myocardial infarction. The patient is continuing to complain of pain at 4/10. His EKG is certainly abnormal and his enzymes have already bumped. The case was discussed with Dr James who agrees that a left heart catheterization is indicated.

ICD-10-CM Code(s) _____

CASE STUDY 15

HISTORY OF PRESENT ILLNESS: The patient is a 57-year-old, white female with no prior cardiac history who presented to the emergency room complaining of chest pain. The patient reports that she was feeling fine yesterday. When she awoke this morning, however, she noticed some paresthesia and pain in her left shoulder and arm. Later in the day she developed pressure in her chest. This gradually worsened throughout the morning until shortly after lunch when she was rating the pain at a 10/10 in severity and decided to go to the emergency room for evaluation. She did note the pain was worse with inspiration. When she arrived at the outlying hospital she was given sublingual nitroglycerin and the pain improved from 10/10 to 3/10 and has stayed at that level since then. She denies any prior cardiac history. Risk factors for coronary disease include hypertension. The patient's lipid status is unknown. She denies any history of diabetes, family history of heart disease, or history of tobacco abuse. The patient is unaware of any thromboembolic disease in the family. She denies any illicit drug use, specifically cocaine. The initial EKG at the outlying hospital showed some subtle ST elevation in an inferolateral distribution. Her initial cardiac enzymes showed a CK of 253, MB fraction of 36, and troponin 0.24. She was sent here for possible left heart catherization and ongoing care. At the time of her arrival she was rating her pain at 3/10 in severity.

PAST SURGICAL HISTORY: The patient has had a tonsillectomy.

MEDICATIONS: At home Avapro, dose unknown; Seasonale birth control. At the outlying hospital the patient was started on heparin and nitroglycerin drips. She was given Lopressor and aspirin. She is allergic to sulfa.

SOCIAL HISTORY: The patient denies tobacco use. She drinks alcohol occasionally. She denies other drug use.

FAMILY HISTORY: There is no known heart disease in the family.

REVIEW OF SYSTEMS: Significant for the arm and chest pain mentioned above. The patient denies fevers, chills, unusual bleeding, rashes, headache, visual changes, dizziness, syncope, palpitations, dyspnea on exertion, orthopnea, paroxysmal nocturnal dyspnea, cough, shortness of breath, wheezing, abdominal pain, nausea, vomiting, diarrhea, hematochezia, melena, dysuria, or hematuria.

PHYSICAL EXAMINATION:

VITAL SIGNS: Pulse is 100 and regular; blood pressure 120/88; respiratory rate 18.

GENERAL APPEARANCE: This is a white female who is awake, alert, and oriented and who appears uncomfortable.

HEENT: Pupils are equal, round, and reactive to light. Extraocular movements are intact. Oropharynx is clear.

NECK: There is no jugular venous distention (JVD) thyromegaly, lymphadenopathy, or bruit.

LUNGS: Clear to auscultation bilaterally without wheeze, rhonchi, or crackle.

HEART: Reveals regular rate and rhythm without murmur, rub, or gallop.

ABDOMEN: Soft, nontender, nondistended with good bowel sounds.

EXTREMITIES: Reveals no lower extremity edema. Pulses are 2+ throughout.

NEUROLOGIC: Cranial nerves II–XII are grossly intact. Strength is 5/5 in all four extremities.

LABORATORY: EKG shows normal sinus rhythm with ST elevation in an inferolateral distribution. Chest X ray shows no active disease. Hemoglobin is 12.8; hematocrit 38; white count 16.3; platelets 273; sodium 139; potassium 3.6; chloride 108; bicarbonate 21; BUN 8; creatinine 0.5; glucose 138; calcium 8.8; D-dimer negative; CK 253; CK-MB 36.4; troponin 0.24.

ASSESSMENT AND PLAN:

1. Acute myocardial infarction. The patient is continuing to complain of pain at 3/10. Her EKG is certainly abnormal and her enzymes have already bumped. The case was discussed with Dr Wills who agrees that emergent left heart catherization is indicated.

2. Hypertension. The patient is on Avapro at home.

3. Further recommendations to follow pending the patient's course.

ICD-10-CM Code(s) _____

CASE STUDY 16

ADMITTING DIAGNOSIS: Congestive heart failure exacerbation.

CHIEF COMPLAINT: Swelling in both feet.

HISTORY OF PRESENT ILLNESS: This 62-year-old gentleman presented to my office today with complaints of swelling in his feet and increased shortness of breath and workup breathing. He had previously been in my office late in the day on 12/2/20xx with similar complaints. We had increased his Lasix dose and given him a shot of Lasix in the office. This apparently had little effect on his overall condition. He states that he began swelling approximately a week to two prior to presentation when he decreased his dose of Lasix at home. Upon chart review he had called my office on 12/6/20xx with blood pressure around 95/43 and feeling weak with standing. He had just not generally been feeling well so I suspected that he was a bit hypovolemic at the time and advised him to decrease his Lasix to one daily until he felt better. There obviously was some miscommunication and he never resumed his twice-daily Lasix dose. Therefore, he presented to my office with worsening of swelling and difficulty breathing. He states that at home his oxygen saturations had gotten down into the low 70s. He was having a very hard time breathing with any exertion. Just to get ready to come to my office he had to stop getting dressed and rest on the bed several times to catch his breath. He daughter states that his lips had been turning blue. The patient states that he has gained approximately 10 pounds since he decreased his dose of Lasix. He had increased his oxygen to 4 L per nasal cannula just to stay comfortable. His weight differential from the office was approximately a six-pound increase. He states his weight was increased three pounds over the past two days.

PAST MEDICAL HISTORY:

- Coronary artery disease

- COPD, severe end-stage requiring continuous home O_2

- He has a pacemaker inserted

- Colon cancer diagnosed in 20xx

- He had a stroke five years ago that affected his left side and from which he has had full functional recovery

PAST SURGICAL HISTORY:

- Gunshot wound to his right neck and still has a bullet lodged in the base of his right lung

- Right carotid endarterectomy

- Transurethral resection of the prostate (TURP)

- Coronary bypass grafting (×2)

- Pacemaker was inserted

- Colon resection

ALLERGIES: No known drug allergies.

SOCIAL HISTORY: This patient is retired who recently moved from southern Kansas to live with his daughter and son-in-law. He has experienced increasing health problems recently and was unable to independently care for himself at home. He does have a home care nurse who visits a few times a week to help with ADL and just general monitoring of his condition. He has a long history of tobacco use but he quit smoking in 196x. He denies any current alcohol or illicit drug use.

MEDICATIONS:

- Lasix 20 mg one to two po daily

- Lipitor 20 mg one po daily

- Albuterol nebulizer every three to four hours prn

- Aspirin 325 mg daily

- Imdur 60 mg three times a day

- K-Dur 20 mEq with each Lasix dose

- Thero-Dur 200 mg po q 12 hours

- Lanoxin 0.25 mg one po daily (he holds this if his heart rate is less than 60)

REVIEW OF SYSTEMS:

HEENT: Negative without any ear pain or throat pain. No nasal drainage, no facial congestion, no visual or hearing problems.

CARDIOVASCULAR: No chest pain at this time.

LUNGS: As noted above in History of Present Illness.

GU: Denies any heartburn, diarrhea, constipation, or any other problems with bowel movements. He does state that his urine stream has been weak of late and he has had some difficulty starting his urine stream.

SKIN: Without complaints.

MUSCULOSKELETAL: He denies any joint aches or muscle pains.

EXTREMITIES: He is complaining about the swelling as noted above. His feet/toes have also been turning blue occasionally with this increased swelling.

ALL OTHER SYSTEMS: Negative.

PHYSICAL EXAMINATION:

GENERAL: He is seated and appears to be breathing heavier. His lips are pursed with each breath. He is leaning forward as he breathes.

VITAL SIGNS: Weight: 168 pounds; pulse: 101; respiratory rate: 40; Blood pressure: 109/83; His O_2 saturation levels are 84% on 4 L.

HEENT: Pupils are equally round and reactive to light. Sclerae are white. The ear canals are clear. His oropharynx is moist without lesions.

NECK: Supple without thyromegaly or lymphadenopathy. No carotid bruits are audible.

CHEST: Decreased breath sounds throughout as usual for this patient. No crackles are heard at the bases.

COR: Regular rate and rhythm. He has a 3/6 holosystolic murmur.

ABDOMEN: Soft without masses or tenderness. Good bowel sounds.

GU: Evaluation is deferred.

SKIN: Multiple seborrheic keratoses on his neck; otherwise, dry.

EXTREMITIES: With 2 to 3+ pitting edema at the ankles and about midway to the calf. He has no edema of the thighs. His toes are somewhat cyanotic. He has sensation all the way to his toes. His feet are warm to the touch.

ASSESSMENT AND PLAN:

1. Systolic heart failure acute on chronic with exacerbation. The patient has basically failed home therapy for his CHF exacerbation. There was some miscommunication with his home care nurses and he actually did not get his medication at home until the evening of 12/4/20xx. He also was not tripling his Lasix therapy at home as advised. For these reasons, worsening of his breathing, increased swelling, and all the other symptoms above. He will be admitted for aggressive diuresis with IV Lasix. He will also be receiving very small amounts of IV fluids with potassium. We need to carefully watch his BUN and creatinine and his potassium levels with all of the diuretic being administered. I feel very confident that his exacerbation was from a decrease medication. I discussed the possibility of some worsening cardiac function. At this point, given his end-stage COPD, the patient declines any further cardiac workup. This discussion was held with the gentleman and his daughter at the bedside. They both agreed with the plan. The patient will have a chest X ray on admission just to make sure that the rest of the lung fields are clear. Because the majority of his symptoms are swelling and difficulty breathing, I think that CHF can account for all of this. We will carefully monitor labs, I&Os, and daily weights to assess improvement. I would expect that he would need to be hospitalized for two to three days to effect enough diuresis to be comfortable going home.

2. Chronic obstructive pulmonary disease. We will continue his oxygen at 4 L to keep his stats above 88%. He will continue to receive Albuterol nebulizer treatments here every three hours while awake and then through the night prn.

3. Cardiac arrhythmia. The patient has a pacemaker and will continue to receive his Lanoxin.

4. Coronary artery disease. The patient is on Imdur and Lipitor for optimal cholesterol control. He is stable on both of these medications.

ICD-10-CM Code(s) _____

CASE STUDY 17

The patient is a 68-year-old male with a history of coronary disease, atrial fibrillation, and previous bypass surgery in 20xx. Dr Stevens has requested that I evaluate the patient for atrial fibrillation. From the hospital records, he had an echocardiogram done in February 20xx, which was technically difficult but showed overall normal systolic function. He has not been seen by our office in the last three years. He was admitted to the hospital several weeks ago with worsening shortness of breath and a chest X ray concerning for multilobar pneumonia. He worsened, required a period of intubation and mechanical ventilation, and was ultimately extubated and has been improving.

Review of telemetry and electrocardiograms this hospitalization has shown predominant sinus rhythm with frequent premature atrial contractions. They also showed periods of atrial fibrillation and atrial flutter. As far as I can tell, he has not been treated for atrial dysrhythmia this hospitalization or in his past. He was re-hospitalized late yesterday afternoon.

The patient is not able to communicate at this time. He has had a worsening of his mental status recently, treated with Haldol. The etiology for his agitation is not known.

Last night the patient went into atrial fibrillation at a rate of 10 to 160 and it was continuous. He was treated with intravenous Cardizem in increasing doses, and on my arrival he was at 15 mg per hour with a heart rate between 90 and 110, though this increased to greater than 140 beats per minute during periods of agitation. The Cardizem was increased to 20 mg an hour, and when he was quieter, his heart rate was in the 100 to 110 range. Telemetry now shows sinus rhythm frequent premature atrial contractions.

PAST MEDICAL HISTORY:

- Multilobar pneumonia with respiratory failure
- Coronary artery disease with previous bypass surgery; echocardiogram from July 20xx showed an ejection fraction of 55%
- Agitation, questionable toxic metabolic encephalopathy
- Hypertension
- Anemia

CURRENT MEDICATIONS:

- Insulin
- Nebulizers
- Zoloft 100 mg a day
- Protonix 40 mg a day
- Aspirin 81 mg a day
- Lovenox 40 mg a day
- Nitroglycerin patch 0.2 mg per hour
- Lopressor 5 mg intravenous q six hours
- Relafen
- Rhinocort
- Ativan
- Haldol
- Flagyl
- Diltiazem intravenous

FAMILY HISTORY: Father died of CHF at age 56; mother died in car accident at age 30.

REVIEW OF SYSTEMS: Could not be obtained.

PHYSICAL EXAMINATION:

VITAL SIGNS: Blood pressure ranges between 131 and 167 systolic and 57 and 69 diastolic. Heart rate ranges between 90 and 140.

HEENT: The sclerae could not be adequately examined due to his agitation.

NECK: Jugular venous pulse is elevated to the angle of the jaw while he is thrashing in bed. Carotids are +2/4 bilaterally without bruits.

LUNGS: Loud inspiratory and expiratory wheezes.

HEART: Tachycardia and irregular rhythm. Normal S1, S2; no S3 or S4 murmur or rub.

ABDOMEN: Soft with normal active bowel sounds.

EXTREMITIES: No pitting edema.

NEUROLOGICAL/PSYCHIATRIC: He could not cooperate with an examination, but he is clearly agitated. He is not responsive to simple questions, but his last chest X ray obtained on July 24 showed an interval increase in the bilateral alveolar infiltrates.

LABORATORY: No chest X ray has been obtained in the last two days. White count is 21; creatinine 22; potassium 3.7; CPK MB normal at 3 and 4; CPK normal at 76. Troponins are mildly elevated at 0.15 and 0.11. Telemetry and electrocardiogram were dictated in the history of present illness.

IMPRESSIONS: Atrial fibrillation. Since the time of the beginning of this dictation, the patient has changed from intermittent to paroxysmal atrial fibrillation, now into a sinus rhythm with frequent premature atrial contractions. We will try to wean and discontinue use of intravenous Cardizem as long as he remains in sinus rhythm. If atrial fibrillation recurs, the Cardizem should be given when he is able to take orally. Given his loud wheezing, one may want to avoid the use of a beta blocker (on intravenous Lopressor q eight hours). Digoxin 0.25 mg intravenous q day after the appropriate lading dose can be given if his heart rate high on Cardizem, though my impression is that the Cardizem would offer adequate control. It seems that the patient's agitation is the most common precipitant for his poor heart rate control, and unfortunately, his mental status changes at this time are neither well defined nor well treated.

ICD-10-CM Code(s) _____

CASE STUDY 18

This is a 55-year-old, new patient who is having episodes of rapid heartbeats. He is also experiencing shortness of breath, with some severe chest discomfort for three days. He is visiting from out of town and has a history of acute MI in 20xx.

REVIEW OF SYSTEMS:

HEENT: He has had problems with sinus drainage in the past.

PULMONARY: He has a hacking cough, probably from cigarettes. No productive sputum.

CARDIOVASCULAR: He describes a mild chest discomfort, mild chest ache with a rapid heartbeat. He can tell his heart is racing. He has had no peripheral edema.

GI: No nausea, vomiting, constipation, diarrhea, or blood in the stools. No heartburn or indigestion.

GU: No hematuria, pyuria, kidney stones, or kidney infections.

MUSCULOSKELETAL: States he has some weakness in the left arm and left leg from his stroke, which was last year on 12/5/xx. He is seen by Dr John Doe. He also had to have a stomach tube after the stroke because he could not do any swallowing, but the tube has been removed since that time.

ENDOCRINE: No heat or cold intolerance.

NEUROLOGIC: No complaint of headaches.

INTEGUMENTARY: No skin lesions or complaints.

HEMATOLOGIC: No bleeding problems.

PAST MEDICAL HISTORY: He has had no other major hospitalizations or surgeries.

ALLERGIES: He has no known allergies. Tetanus shot gave him local swelling.

MEDICATIONS:

- Plavix 75 mg qd
- Lanoxin 0.25 mg qd

FAMILY HISTORY: Mother has had diabetes and hypertension. Father had three heart attacks and died at 52. Patient has two sisters, one of whom had brain cancer. There is a strong family history of coronary artery disease and heart disease as well as myocardial infarction.

SOCIAL HISTORY: He continues to smoke about a pack a day. He has decreased from three packs a day. He states on some days he will only smoke a pack every four days. Apparently he has also been a fairly heavy drinker in the past. His wife was here with him today and he tends to be somewhat noncompliant.

PHYSICAL EXAMINATION:

VITAL SIGNS: On admission, blood pressure is 120/74; pulse 150 and irregular; temperature 98; and respiration 20.

ENT: Ears and nose unremarkable, oropharynx clear.

NECK: Supple.

LUNGS: Clear to auscultation and percussion. No rales or rhonchi noted. Somewhat decreased breath sounds.

HEART: Irregular rhythm and running fast at a rate of 150.

ABDOMEN: Soft without organomegaly. No point tenderness; bowel sounds active.

PULSES: Femorals are 1+, pedals at the popliteal and distal are faint, but this may be due to the rapid atrial fibrillation. Will have to check this when he is back in sinus rhythm.

ASSESSMENT:

1. Rapid atrial fibrillation with some symptoms of shortness of breath and chest pain.

2. Strong family history of coronary artery disease.

RECOMMENDATIONS: Admit to hospital. We are going to start the patient on IV Cordarone after a bolus. He is going to be started on a heparin drip. If he does not convert by the morning, will probably go ahead and do a TEE cardioversion as he needs to be back in sinus rhythm and then he can continue with his medication.

ICD-10-CM Code(s) _____

CASE STUDY 19

INDICATIONS: A 68-year-old man is hospitalized with unstable angina. He has been treated in the past with coronary bypass surgery. A cardiac catheterization and coronary and graft angiograms are ordered.

PROCEDURE: The surgeon performs retrograde left heart catheterization, left ventriculography, selective coronary angiography, and vein graft angiography. In addition, the cardiologist also injects the internal mammary artery to determine whether it would be a suitable arterial conduit for a second bypass operation.

IMPRESSION:

1. Arteriosclerotic heart disease of native coronary arteries (ASHD)

2. Arteriosclerotic heart disease of autologous venous grafts

3. Left ventricular hypertrophy

ICD-10-CM Code(s) _____

CASE STUDY 20

HISTORY OF PRESENT ILLNESS: This is a 94-year-old, white female who presents with shortness of breath. The patient is unable to tell me what time period she has had her shortness of breath. In the emergency room, the patient had an examination and laboratory data consistent with congestive heart failure. Results from a BNP test were elevated, and a chest X ray demonstrated fluid overload. She is now being admitted as inpatient.

PAST MEDICAL HISTORY: Significant for hypertension, stroke in February 20xx, hypothyroid, diabetes, allergic rhinitis, gastroesophageal reflux disease, depression, and dementia.

MEDICATIONS:

- Synthroid 50 mcg po daily
- Claritin 10 mg po daily
- Pepcid 20 mg po bid
- Amaryl 1 mg po daily
- Diovan 160/12.5 of hydrochlorothiazide po bid
- Zoloft 50 mg po daily
- Aspirin 81 mg po daily
- Aricept 10 mg po daily
- Risperdal 0.5 mg po qpm

PAST SURGICAL HISTORY: The patient has had a TAH/BSO. She has had cataracts. She had her right kneecap removed. Ankle fracture that needed some surgery and rotator cuff repair.

REVIEW OF SYSTEMS: Unable to obtain because patient has dementia.

PHYSICAL EXAMINATION:

GENERAL: This is a well-developed, well-nourished, white female in mild distress.

CHEST: Some coarse crackles throughout the lung fields. She has some inspiratory and expiratory crackles.

HEART: Regular rate and rhythm with a murmur heard.

ABDOMEN: Benign, soft, and with positive bowel sounds. Nontender, nondistended, no hepatosplenomegaly.

EXTREMITIES: Peripheral edema.

NEUROLOGIC: Alert, but somewhat confused. The patient could not answer simple questions and does not know where she is.

ECHOCARDIOGRAM: The patient did have one in July 20xx, which showed LVH with normal left ventricular function.

IMPRESSION AND PLAN: Congestive heart failure. The patient has no underlying heart disease, just her LVH. We will continue aggressive diuresis and Diovan treatment. Repeat her echocardiogram and do blood work-up to try to find the etiology for congestive heart failure. Dementia secondary to vascular dementia with her previous stroke. We will continue the patient with her Aricept, Risperdal, and aspirin therapy.

ICD-10-CM Code(s)_____

CASE STUDY 21

HISTORY OF PRESENT ILLNESS: This is a 60-year-old, white male with history of a large hemispheric stroke two months ago. Since that time, the patient has been aphasic and difficult to ambulate with right-sided weakness. Two days prior to presentation to the hospital, he started to have increased problems with coordination and weakness and therefore presented to the emergency department after the patient also developed a fever at home.

MEDICATIONS:

- Zoloft 100 mg daily

- Senokot as needed for constipation

- Aspirin 325 mg daily

- Colace 100 mg daily as needed for constipation

PAST MEDICAL HISTORY: Significant for left-sided cerebrovascular accident, left hemisphere, in 20xx. At that time, the patient was found to have complete left internal carotid occlusion, felt inoperable at that time. The patient also had a left fem-pop procedure back in 199x. The patient quit smoking and quit his chronic alcohol use when he had the stroke. The patient did not know his parents. The patient is retired. The patient lives with his son. The patient also has two other sons.

REVIEW OF SYSTEMS: Difficult to get because the patient is unable to talk. It is apparent based on my observation he has some left leg pain.

PHYSICAL EXAMINATION:

GENERAL/VITAL SIGNS: The patient was febrile with temperature of 102° F. The rest of the vital signs were stable. This is a well-developed, well-nourished, white male who looks older than his stated age, in no acute distress.

HEENT: No bruits, no thyromegaly, no lymphadenopathy.

CHEST: Crackles at the bases, otherwise sounds clear.

CARDIAC: Regular rate and rhythm without any murmurs heard.

ABDOMEN: Benign, soft, positive bowel sounds, nontender, nondistended, no hepatosplenomegaly.

EXTREMITIES: The patient has palpable pedal pulses but decreased, 1+ edema, greater on the right than the left, with chronic redness. The patient has developed stiffness of his right upper extremity. Keeping a closed fist is difficult. The patient does have some weakness here also.

IMPRESSION AND PLAN:

1. Admit as inpatient.

2. Pneumonia. I am concerned about aspiration with right upper lobe and left lower lobe affected. The patient is on Zosyn, which is the appropriate antibiotic. We will ask Speech also to do a swallowing study on this patient.

3. Hyperglycemia. This was never an issue before but patient was hyperglycemic on admission. We will check his blood sugars throughout the hospital course.

4. With his previous stroke, there is concern that the patient is using his right side even worse than before. We will obtain MRI to see if new thrombotic event has occurred.

5. Deep venous thrombosis right lower extremity. We will use Lovenox to treat.

ICD-10-CM Code(s) _____

CASE STUDY 22

PREOPERATIVE DIAGNOSIS: Sick sinus syndrome with bradycardia/tachycardia.

OPERATION PERFORMED: Pacemaker insertion.

ANESTHESIA: Local with conscious sedation.

DESCRIPTION OF PROCEDURE: Following informed consent, the left subclavian artery was prepped and draped in the usual sterile manner. Following local administration of 1% Xylocaine anesthesia, the left subclavian vein was entered with an 18-gauge thin-wall needle. A J-wire was placed. Transverse incision was created and dissected at the pectoral fascia. A subcutaneous pocket was created and one gauze sponge was placed in the pocket. A 7-French sheath introducer was placed leaving a J-wire in place. A Medtronic 5076 (serial number PJN1629690) bipolar lead was placed in right ventricle apex and measurements taken. This lead screwed into position. A second 7-French introducer was placed. A Medtronic 5076 (serial number PJN1617191) atrial lead positioned in the right atrial appendage using fluoroscopic guidance. Measurements were taken and lead screwed into position. Both leads were then suture-ligated in position. The gauze sponge was extracted from the pocket. The pocket was irrigated with Bacitracin solution. The leads were connected to a Medtronic Adapta (serial number PWB298644H) device. The device was placed in the pocket. The subcutaneous tissue was closed with one row of running 3-0 suture. Subcutaneous tissue was closed with one row of running 4-0 suture.

A sterile dressing was applied. Dermabond dressing was also applied. The patient tolerated the procedure well. At the end of the procedure, the patient was returned in good condition to a room. Initial measures include an R-wave of 10.9 mV with threshold 0.9 volts and resistance of 810 ohms of the V-lead. The atrial lead had a P-wave of 2.0 mV, threshold 0.5 volts, resistance 1184 ohms. Initial settings include the AAIR-DDDR mode with a lower rate of 60, upper rate limit of 130, Paced AV intervals 150 and sensed 120 milliseconds. Pulse amplitude on both leads is 3.5 volts with a pulse width of 0.4 milliseconds. Atrial sensitivity is 0.5 mV. Ventricular is 2.8 mV.

ICD-10-CM Code(s) _____

CASE STUDY 23

This 44-year-old female presented with numbness in her fingers and feet for the last month. She also has complaints of her fingers feeling cold and the color of her feet has changed.

Exam reveals slightly pale female, BP 140/80 mm Hg, HR 80/min, regular. Pulses in the extremities are weakened. Erythema is extended up to the knees, coolness to ankles of both feet. Erythema is noted on the fingers of both hands, warm to touch. After additional testing that included a Doppler ultrasound, the patient was diagnosed with erythromelalgia and Raynaud's syndrome.

ICD-10-CM Code(s) _____

CASE STUDY 24

A 15-year-old male presented with what he describes as a sharp, piercing pain on the left side of his chest in the nipple region. It lasts anywhere from 30 seconds to 2-3 minutes. He says it seems to be worse when he takes deep breaths. After a thorough history, it is noted that he leads a fairly sedentary lifestyle, playing video games, not active in any school sports, etc. Examination reveals a cooperative, anxious teenage male. Blood pressure is 125/79 mmHg; temperature 98.9°F. Lungs clear to auscultation; heart has regular rate and rhythm. Abdomen is nontender, no hepatosplenomegaly. Extremities normal range of motion, no bruising, no edema. After further testing, the patient is diagnosed with precordial chest pain.

ICD-10-CM Code(s) _____

66

CHAPTER 6

Diseases of the Respiratory System (J00-J99)

ICD-10-CM Chapter 10 Guideline Review

In this chapter you will find a summary of the chapter-specific coding guidelines for Chapter 10 of the ICD-10-CM codebook followed by case studies to build ICD-10-CM diagnosis coding skills in this area.

Many medical specialties, including primary care and pulmonology, reference Chapter 10 of the ICD-10-CM codebook for coding diseases of the respiratory system. Keep in mind that you should always reference the ICD-10-CM Official Guidelines for Coding and Reporting in its entirety when making a code selection.

ICD-10-CM Official Coding Guidelines for Diseases of the Respiratory System

CHRONIC OBSTRUCTIVE PULMONARY DISEASE (COPD) AND ASTHMA

Correctly coding asthma and COPD requires an understanding of an acute versus an uncomplicated case:

- An acute exacerbation is a worsening or decompensation of a chronic condition.

- An exacerbation might be triggered by an infection.

- An acute exacerbation is not equivalent to an infection superimposed on a chronic condition.

- Asthma and COPD are reported with codes J44 and J45.

ACUTE RESPIRATORY FAILURE AS THE PRINCIPAL OR FIRST-LISTED DIAGNOSIS

Subcategory J96.0, Acute respiratory failure, and subcategory J96.2, Acute and chronic respiratory failure, may be assigned as the first-listed diagnosis when:

- The respiratory failure after diagnostic study is responsible for admission to the hospital.

- Code selection can be confirmed in the Tabular List.

- Following instructional notes and guidelines when reporting these codes for instructions and sequencing guidance.

ACUTE RESPIRATORY FAILURE AS THE SECONDARY DIAGNOSIS

Respiratory failure may be listed as a secondary diagnosis if:

- Respiratory failure occurs after admission, or if it is present on admission but does not meet the definition of principal diagnosis.

SEQUENCING OF ACUTE RESPIRATORY FAILURE AND ANOTHER ACUTE CONDITION

When a patient is admitted with respiratory failure and another acute condition (eg, myocardial infarction, cerebrovascular accident, aspiration pneumonia), the following guidelines apply:

- The principal diagnosis will not be the same in every situation. (This applies whether the other acute condition is a respiratory or non-respiratory condition.)

- Selection of the first-listed diagnosis will be dependent on the circumstances of admission:

  - If both the respiratory failure and the other acute condition are equally responsible for occasioning the admission to the hospital, and there are no chapter-specific sequencing rules, the guideline regarding two or more diagnoses that equally meet the definition for principal or first-listed diagnosis may be applied in these situations.

- If the documentation is not clear as to whether acute respiratory failure and another condition are equally responsible for occasioning the admission, query the provider for clarification.

INFLUENZA DUE TO CERTAIN IDENTIFIED INFLUENZA VIRUSES

Code only confirmed cases of influenza due to certain identified influenza viruses (category J09) and due to other identified influenza virus (category J10). This is an exception to the hospital inpatient guideline Section II, H. (Uncertain Diagnosis). When coding influenza due to certain identified influenza viruses, the following guidelines apply:

- Confirmation does not require documentation of positive laboratory testing specific for avian or other novel influenza A.

- Coding should be based on the provider's documentation in the medical record confirming that the patient has avian influenza or other novel influenza A, for category J09, or has another particular identified strain of influenza (H1N1 or H3N2), but not identified as novel or variant (category J10).

- If the provider records "suspected or possible or probable avian influenza," the influenza code from category J11, Influenza due to unidentified influenza virus, is reported.

- A code from category J09, Influenza due to certain identified influenza viruses, or category J10, Influenza due to other identified influenza virus, should not be assigned.

VENTILATOR-ASSOCIATED PNEUMONIA

Code assignment for ventilator-associated pneumonia is based on the documentation in the medical record. The following guidelines apply:

- Code J95.851, Ventilator associated pneumonia, is reported when the documentation indicates ventilator-associated pneumonia (VAP).

- A secondary code to identify the organism (eg, code B96.5) should also be reported.

- Do not report an additional code from categories J12-J18 to identify the type of pneumonia.

- Code J95.851 should not be reported when the patient has pneumonia and is on a mechanical ventilator and the provider has not specifically stated that the pneumonia is VAP.

- If the documentation is unclear as to whether the patient has a pneumonia that is a complication

attributable to the mechanical ventilator, query the provider.

VENTILATOR-ASSOCIATED PNEUMONIA DEVELOPED AFTER ADMISSION

When coding ventilator-associated pneumonia developed after the patient was admitted to the hospital, the following guidelines apply:

- A patient may be admitted with one type of pneumonia (eg, code J13, Pneumonia due to Streptococcus pneumoniae) and subsequently develop VAP.

- When VAP develops after hospital admission, the principal or first-listed diagnosis would be the appropriate code from categories J12-J18 for the pneumonia diagnosed at the time of admission. Code J95.851, Ventilator-associated pneumonia, is reported as an additional diagnosis when the provider has documented the presence of VAP in the medical record.

Now that you have a good understanding of the chapter-specific guidelines for diseases of the respiratory system, it is time to build skill and knowledge by coding the following cases. Be sure to reference the ICD-10-CM codebook and the ICD-10-CM Official Guidelines for Coding and Reporting, along with the instructional notes, when coding these conditions.

Diseases of the Respiratory System (J00-J99)

CASE STUDY 1

CHIEF COMPLAINT: Dyspnea.

HISTORY OF PRESENT ILLNESS: This patient has stage IIIB non-small cell lung carcinoma in the right lower lobe and previously completed a round of radiation and chemotherapy. He had been doing well until just today when he became acutely dyspneic and started coughing constantly after eating a large meal. He was taken to the emergency department of the local hospital.

PAST MEDICAL HISTORY:

- Stage IIIB non-small cell lung carcinoma right lower lobe now status post radiation and chemotherapy

- Chronic obstructive pulmonary disease (COPD)

- Esophageal stenosis secondary to lung cancer related mediastinal lymphadenopathy now status post esophageal stent placement
- Bilateral pulmonary emboli now with inferior vena cava filter on Coumadin therapy
- Non-insulin dependent diabetes mellitus, not controlled on last A1c
- Benign hypertension
- Atherosclerotic coronary artery disease
- Anemia
- History of thrombocytopenia

ALLERGIES: NKDA.

MEDICATIONS:

- Lantus U-100 1 x day before breakfast
- Coumadin dosing per Coumadin clinic
- Lortab Liquid 10 mL per G-tube every four hours prn
- Risperdal 0.5 mg per G-tube nightly
- Atrovent nebulizer 0.5 mg four times a day
- Xopenex 0.625 mg three times a day
- Os-Cal with vitamin D 500 mg twice a day
- Combivent inhaler two puffs every four hours prn
- Lipitor 20 mg po every day
- Pulmicort 180 mcg per inhalations two inhalations twice a day
- Remeron SolTab 30 mg per G-tube nightly
- Reglan 10 mg per 10 cc, 10 cc per G-tube before every meal and nightly

SOCIAL HISTORY: Former smoker with multiple pack-year history.

FAMILY HISTORY: Significant for diabetes.

REVIEW OF SYSTEMS: No chest pain at present. Still short of breath on a re-breather mask with high-flow oxygen. He has had some swelling in his lower extremities but no exacerbation recently. This is likely attributable to hypercaloric G-tube feedings he has been receiving. It is improving as the calorie content has been lowered recently. He was intolerant of the 500 calorie G-tube feedings. No fever, chills, or sweats. No abdominal pain. The remainder of the review of systems is negative.

PHYSICAL EXAMINATION:

OBJECTIVE: Temperature 97.4°F; blood pressure 132/82; respirations 12-30; pulse 128; oxygen saturation 94%.

GENERAL APPEARANCE: Pleasant male in no acute distress. Slightly tachypneic on examination.

HEENT: Normocephalic, atraumatic. Mucous membranes are moist. External nose and ears are normal. Oropharynx is widely patent.

EYES: Pupils, iris, conjunctivae, and eyelids all normal. No conjunctival pallor.

NECK: Neck is supple without jugular venous distention, rigidity, bruits, thyromegaly, visible asymmetry, palpable nodularity, or lymphadenopathy.

LUNGS: Lungs reveal coarse crackles in both bases, right worse than left. No wheezing is noted.

HEART: Heart is regular without audible murmur, gallop, rub, carotid bruits, or pedal edema.

ABDOMEN: Abdomen is scaphoid, soft, nontender, and nondistended. Normal bowel sounds. G-tube is secure. No evidence of infection around the G-tube.

MUSCULOSKELETAL: He is able to move all extremities normally. Strength is globally intact. He does have trace ankle edema, nonpitting.

PSYCHOLOGICAL: Mood and affect are normal.

SKIN: Warm, dry, and normal turgor.

LYMPH: No palpable abnormal lymphadenopathy.

LABORATORY: CBC reveals white count elevated at 17,100; hemoglobin 12.7; hematocrit 38.5; platelets 241,000. Differential reveals elevated neutrophil percentage of 90.2%. Elevated bands are also noted. INR is 1.4; D-dimer is 4.7. Blood gas on 100% oxygen reveals a pH of 7.397, pCO_2 of 48.7, and pO_2 of 76.1. Comprehensive metabolic profile reveals albumin slightly low at 2.5. Sodium is low at 131; chloride 90; BUN 4; creatinine 0.54; glucose 208. ALT is slightly low at 14. B-type natruretic peptide is 100. Chest X ray reveals bilateral lower lobe infiltrates.

ASSESSMENT AND PLAN:

1. Aspiration pneumonia. The patient has been started on intravenous antibiotics and appropriate respiratory support.

2. COPD acute exacerbation.

3. Lung cancer stage III right lower lobe—oncologist called in to see patient; watching pulmonary status closely; bilateral lower lobe infiltrates.

4. Non-insulin dependent diabetes mellitus; is currently on insulin and has good control.

5. Bilateral pulmonary emboli; continue anticoagulation.

6. Benign hypertension; well controlled at present.

7. Admit to pulmonary service.

ICD-10-CM Code(s) _____

CASE STUDY 2

A patient with bilateral partial vocal cord paralysis requires removal of the arytenoids cartilage to improve breathing. Following a temporary tracheostomy, a topical anesthetic is applied to the oral cavity, pharynx, and larynx, and the laryngoscope with operating microscope is inserted. After adequate visualization is established, the arytenoid cartilage is exposed by excision of the mucosa overlying it. The procedure is performed in the outpatient surgery center of the hospital.

ICD-10-CM Code(s) _____

CASE STUDY 3

HISTORY OF PRESENT ILLNESS: This is a 60-year-old male who came to the hospital with complaints of dyspnea, shortness of breath, and cough lasting for a week with intermittent productive, pleuritic chest pain. He feels warm periodically and bursts into sweat. No rigors. No nausea, vomiting, abdominal pain, or diarrhea.

ALLERGIES: There are no allergies.

MEDICATIONS:

- Dapsone 100 mg (1 and ½ tablet) daily; Toprol XL 50 mg daily
- Zocor 20 mg daily
- Nasacort AQ, two sprays at bedtime; Naprosyn 500 mg bid
- Trazodone 100 mg po at bedtime

PAST MEDICAL HISTORY: Includes coronary artery disease status post CABG in January 20xx, chronic skin disorder, and dermatitis herpetiformis. He is on Dapsone and follows with dermatologist, Dr

Cardene. Sleep apnea on BiPAP with pressures of 16/6, gastroesophageal reflux disease, post-nasal drip, osteoarthritis, degenerative joint disease, obesity, history of pancreatitis in 199x.

PAST SURGICAL HISTORY: Cholecystectomy and coronary artery bypass grafting. He also had a colonoscopy four years ago that he states was normal.

FAMILY HISTORY: Both parents are dead. Father died of a heart attack.

SOCIAL HISTORY: He is married. Denies alcohol or tobacco use.

REVIEW OF SYSTEMS: No confusion. No visual blurring. No hearing problems. No speech problems. He denies any weight loss or bowel problems. Denies history of blood clots. No stroke. No diabetes or immune system problems. No seizures, no falls, no weakness. Breathing problems are as described above. All other systems are reviewed and negative.

PHYSICAL EXAMINATION:

GENERAL: He is awake, alert, oriented ×3. No distress. Slightly tachypneic.

VITAL SIGNS: Temperature 97.8°F; blood pressure 127/68; pulse 82; regular respirations at 20.

HEENT: Extraocular movements are intact. Throat is clear. Tympanic membranes clear.

NECK: No JVD. No lymphadenopathy. No thyromegaly. No masses.

LUNGS: Shows harsh vesicular breathing. Few sparse rhonchi.

HEART: Regular rate and rhythm. Normal S1 and S2, no S3. No murmur.

ABDOMEN: Soft, obese, nontender. No organomegaly.

EXTREMITIES: Show no cyanosis, clubbing, or edema. Positive varicose veins in both lower extremities.

NEUROLOGIC: He is moving all extremities. Cranial nerves are intact. There is no focal deficit.

LABORATORY: His labs show white count of 13,000. Hemoglobin and hematocrit are normal. Platelets are 142. Electrolytes are normal. BUN 15; creatinine 0.8; glucose 116. Calcium is 8.2. BNP level is 35. Cardiac enzymes: Troponin I level is less than 0.01.

DIAGNOSTIC STUDIES: Chest X ray shows cardiomegaly, but ER physician thought it showed an infiltrate.

IMPRESSION: There is some atelectasis in the left lower lobe; however, there is no clear infiltrate at this time. Clinically he does have all the symptoms of pneumonia and he has tracheobronchitis. It is not uncommon for the infiltrate to show up early on. He does have leukocytosis. He was also hypoxic when he came in with an oxygenation noted at 70 to 90%. I believe with hydration he may show an infiltrate.

PLAN: I am going to continue him on the Rocephin and Zithromax and give him his usual home medications, DVT prophylaxis, and add Nexium as well. Will also try to get sputum for culture.

ICD-10-CM Code(s) _____

CASE STUDY 4

Brian is a very pleasant but unfortunate 44-year-old male who has been battling progressive multiple sclerosis for some 14 to 16 years. He is routinely followed by the university hospital for this condition. He unfortunately has continued to have progressive decline in his motor functions. He has been on very aggressive steroid and even chemotherapy regimens with Novantrone as well as current intrathecal baclofen therapy. Over the last several months apparently Brian has been experiencing increasing dyspnea symptoms. He has no prior history of any known pulmonary disease and has only minimal tobacco abuse history. He denies any productive cough, although freely relates his cough reflex is very ineffective at best. He denies any purulent phlegm or any fevers, chills, or sweats.

FAMILY HISTORY: Father is deceased from emphysema. Mother is living with a history of atrial fibrillation and emphysema. He has five brothers reportedly in good health.

SOCIAL HISTORY: The patient is married. He previously was employed as a blacksmith. He has a minimal tobacco abuse history. No history of alcohol or drugs. He does have some occupational exposure to pulmonary irritants having worked as a blacksmith for a number of years.

PAST MEDICAL HISTORY: Only notable for that of his progressive multiple sclerosis.

SURGICAL HISTORY: Includes previous intrathecal pump for baclofen therapy.

MEDICATIONS: Intrathecal baclofen; Provigil 200 mg qd; Temazepam; Effexor

ALLERGIES: He is allergic to IVP dye, which causes hives, rash, and dyspnea.

REVIEW OF SYSTEMS: A comprehensive review of systems was performed, as per history of personal illness described previously. He denies any fevers, chills, or sweats. No history of seizures. No odynophagia or dysphagia. Cardiovascular is negative. Pulmonary history as above, including increased dyspnea. Gastrointestinal review is negative for abdominal pain, melena, or hematochezia. Genitourinary is negative for any burning, dysuria, or frequency. Hematologic/oncologic is negative for any bleeding, diatheses, or malignancy. Endocrine is negative for diabetes and thyroid disease. Remaining systems are negative.

PHYSICAL EXAMINATION:

VITAL SIGNS: Blood pressure 140/82; pulse 90s; respiration 16; afebrile.

GENERAL: A pleasant, well-developed gentleman. He is in a wheelchair. He is in no overt distress. He is awake and oriented.

NEUROLOGIC: Normocephalic, atraumatic. Pupils were reactive. There are some sluggish extraocular eye movements. His facial muscles are symmetric. He has bilateral upper motor weakness of the hands and forearms. His deep tendon reflexes appear to be +3 out of 3 bilaterally. He had marked diminished motor strength in the lower extremities.

HEENT: Unremarkable. Nares are patent. Pharynx is clear. No icterus.

NECK: Supple. No masses or bruits. No jugular venous distention. Trachea is midline.

CARDIAC: Heart tones are distant and regular. No murmur, gallop, or rub.

CHEST: Respirations were moderately labored. He was using obvious accessory, neck, chest, and shoulder muscles for his inspiratory effort. Despite this, there was markedly diminished air excursion. I did not appreciate any wheezes, rales, or rhonchi. He had a very ineffective and weak cough.

ABDOMEN: Soft, nontender.

EXTREMITIES: No clubbing, cyanosis, or edema.

STUDIES: There is no chest X ray today.

IMPRESSION:

1. Progressive multiple sclerosis with resulting neuro-muscular respiratory insufficiency.

2. Progressive dyspnea likely secondary to his primary respiratory muscle weakness, although I cannot rule out a concomitant occult infection and retained secretions and/or lobar collapse. Additionally, he may have an occult component of underlying reactive airways disease as well.

PLAN:

1. Unfortunately, Brian clearly is deteriorating and I think we are beginning to see end-stage development of respiratory insufficiency as a consequence of neuromuscular involvement of his multiple sclerosis in terms of respiratory muscles. Our options, unfortunately, are extremely limited in this regard. Obviously, he will continue his primary treatment for his multiple sclerosis including continued intrathecal baclofen, steroids, and Novantrone as his cardiac status will tolerate.

2. We will get a PA and lateral chest X ray to exclude an occult pneumonia as a cause for the acute worsening of his dyspnea.

3. I will give him a trial of bronchodilators with Albuterol and Atrovent nebulizers q4h.

4. I do think he may benefit from some non-invasive ventilatory support mechanisms. There are a few different mechanisms available, and I will get in touch with one of my physiatrist colleagues to see what is currently available in the way of nocturnal oxygen supplementation requirements.

5. We will check a NOS for nocturnal oxygen supplementation requirements.

6. I also discussed with the patient and his wife the fact that at some point, given his progressive neuromuscular weakness, we may need to consider a tracheotomy and possible ventilatory support devices as well. Fortunately, we are not at that point yet but certainly bears discussion over time.

7. I will plan on seeing him back in approximately two weeks here in the pulmonary office for re-evaluation and follow-up regarding my research on noninvasive ventilatory support mechanisms. Obviously, I will see him back sooner if there should be any interval change in his clinical condition.

ICD-10-CM Code(s) _____

CASE STUDY 5

William is a pleasant 55-year-old gentleman who presented to you for the evaluation of hypersomnia. He had undergone a sleep study that showed that he had very severe reductions in his sleep latency of 1.7 minutes. His clinical history dates all the way back to childhood. During adolescence, high school, and college, he had great difficulties in staying awake during classes and fell asleep easily. Throughout his early adulthood, from 198x to 199x, he attributed some of his sleepiness to the fact that in addition to what he calls a "regular" job, he had aspirations of being a musician and frequently played gigs at night that resulted in his obtaining very little nocturnal sleep. In 199x, this stopped.

Initially, he had some problems with sleep fragmentation and some psychophysiologic insomnia-type symptoms but has had increasing problems with hypersomnia. He can easily fall asleep while driving and falls asleep during conversation. Previously, his sleepiness was predictable. However, over the last few months, he has been having increasing degrees of sleep attacks. He states that even on the way over for his office appointment this afternoon he almost fell asleep behind the wheel of the car and crossed the center line. The employees who work for him also have noted this.

He has frequent episodes of hypnagogic hallucinations, as well as occasional sleep paralysis. He also has episodes of automatic behavior. There also has been the development of some symptoms that are suspicious for depression, and he has been given a trial of both Trazodone and Lexapro. He took the Trazodone for six months, and the Lexapro for three to four months, but discontinued both medications about two and a half weeks ago because he didn't feel they provided him with any significant benefit. He was on the medications when he had the nocturnal polysomnogram.

He is unaware of any significant snoring, but his wife told him about some occasional irregular breathing pattern during his sleep at night. He denies any restless leg symptomatology.

The multiple sleep latency test showed no sleep-onset REM periods. Interestingly, he stated that the day he had the multiple sleep latency test, he believes that he felt more alert than he normally does.

SOCIAL HISTORY: He works as the office director for the Welfare Department of Jamison County. He denies any recreational drug use.

REVIEW OF SYSTEMS: A complete review of systems was performed and documented. Pertinent results are as above. All other systems reviewed were negative.

PHYSICAL EXAMINATION:

VITAL SIGNS: Blood pressure 137/80; pulse 91; respiration 17; body mass index 43.

GENERAL: Does not appear to be in any distress.

NEUROLOGIC: DTRs are unremarkable.

HEENT: Moist mucous membranes; oropharynx is normal.

NECK: Supple. No masses or bruits. No jugular venous distention. Trachea is midline.

CARDIAC: Regular rate and rhythm with a systolic murmur.

RESPIRATORY: Lungs clear on auscultation. No wheezes or rales noted.

ABDOMEN: Soft, nontender.

EXTREMITIES: No clubbing, cyanosis, or edema.

IMPRESSION AND RECOMMENDATION:

1. Very severe hypersomnia dating back to adolescence. There are some features that make me suspicious that he may have a primary sleep disorder such as narcolepsy. He has had an increase in his symptom complex in the last few years, and part of this may be associated with some sleep fragmentation. Certainly it is known that certain primary sleep disorders, such as narcolepsy, actually do have a sleep fragmentation component. I have recommended to him that until this data is sorted out and we put him on some treatment that will improve matters, I don't think that it is a good idea for him to drive alone, or to perform other tasks that require vigilance, such as operating potentially dangerous equipment. I told him that I recognize the potential inconvenience of that for him, but I really think it is very important that he do this until things are sorted out. I also have recommended that we obtain a CBC, Chem-7, and some thyroid function tests, as well as HLA typing for the narcolepsy disease–associated antigens.

2. For his chronic rhinitis symptoms and the mild snoring that he has, I have given him a trial of Flonase to see if that will ameliorate matters.

3. Regarding further evaluation, I am so concerned about the issue of the primary sleep disorder that, in a way, I am glad that he has not continued on the Lexapro or Trazodone, as this will afford us the opportunity to repeat the polysomnogram and multiple sleep latency test off of agents that may potentially have REM–suppressing effects, so we can best see the full physiology. I then would like to place him on a therapeutic trial of some Provigil 200 mg po bid.

4. I would like to see him back shortly after his polysomnogram. I would like to see if we can facilitate him through the laboratory because of the magnitude of his symptom complex.

5. During his physical examination, I noted that he had a systolic murmur. He states that he has been told this before, but really doesn't know anything more about the nature of it. I think it would be prudent to see if he has any significant valvular pathology, and to begin to follow that. Also, there may be recommendations needed regarding potential subacute bacterial endocarditis prophylaxis.

ICD-10-CM Code(s) _____

CASE STUDY 6

Thomas is a very pleasant 59-year-old male who has no significant prior past medical history aside from hypertension until some three to four months ago. At that time, he was noted to have been experiencing profound fatigue and weakness and ultimately was found to have significant hypercalcemia and acute renal failure. In retrospect this apparently had been preceded by several months of some increasing fatigue as well as a history of some optic neuritis/uveitis symptoms prior to his acute decompensation.

He was hospitalized in January through the first part of February for acute renal failure. Ultimately he was also found to have evidence of diffuse adenopathy and some interstitial lung disease changes on chest X ray. Ultimately he was diagnosed with having disseminated pulmonary and disseminated sarcoidosis. Transbronchial biopsies demonstrated granulomatous disease changes. He ultimately underwent pulse dose steroid therapy for his presumed sarcoidosis and has since had marked interval improvement with nearly complete resolution of his renal failure as well as complete resolution of his systemic hypercalcemia. Currently he is on Prednisone taking 15 mg of Prednisone every day. He denies any headaches or visual acuity changes to suggest optic neuritis or uveitis. He denies any skin rashes or lesions. No cough, shortness of breath, or dyspnea.

PAST MEDICAL HISTORY:

- Notable for recently identified disseminated sarcoidosis

- Chronic renal insufficiency and acute renal failure secondary to his previous disseminated sarcoidosis

- Hypothyroidism

- Hypertension

- A previous history of optic neuritis and probable uveitis as an early manifestation of his sarcoidosis

- Anemia

- Gastroesophageal reflux disease

- History of sclerotic aortic valvular disease

- A history of previous progressive headaches and visual acuity changes likely secondary to his disseminated sarcoidosis

MEDICATIONS:

- Protonix

- Zocor

- Levothyroxine

- Prednisone

- Wellbutrin

- Hydralazine

- Aspirin

See in-chart patient medication record for exact dosages.

ALLERGIES: None.

SOCIAL HISTORY: The patient is married. He is a distribution facilities manager. No alcohol, drug abuse, or tobacco abuse history is present. He does have a previous 40 pack-year history of tobacco abuse having quit two years ago.

FAMILY HISTORY: Father died of a myocardial infarction at age 59. Mother died from a myocardial infarction at age 88. One brother with lung cancer is deceased, and one brother died from complications of coronary artery bypass grafting at age 60.

REVIEW OF SYSTEMS: A comprehensive review of systems was performed as annotated per history of personal illness described previously. All other systems were negative.

PHYSICAL EXAMINATION:

VITAL SIGNS: Blood pressure 130/96; pulse 84; respiration 16; afebrile. Weight today 181 pounds.

GENERAL: A pleasant gentleman in no distress.

SKIN: Warm and dry.

HEENT: Pharynx is clear.

NECK: Without masses, bruits, or jugular venous distention. Trachea is midline.

CARDIAC: Regular rate and rhythm.

CHEST: Respirations are easy and regular. Clear to auscultation.

ABDOMEN: Soft.

EXTREMITIES: Gait normal. No edema.

NEUROLOGIC: Alert and oriented ×3.

STUDIES: His CT demonstrated diffuse interstitial lung disease changes as well as some paratracheal and hilar adenopathy.

LABORATORY: I do not see a recent sedimentaion rate or ACE level. Previous white count was 19.9; hemoglobin of 9.9. Bronchial washings were negative. Transbronchial biopsies demonstrated reactive hyperplasia and granulomatous disease changes consistent with sarcoidosis. ACE level actually was markedly elevated on initial presentation at 176. Previous creatinine was 5.2 and is 1.5 per patient as an outpatient.

IMPRESSION:

1. Disseminated sarcoidosis, clinically improved on steroids

2. Acute renal failure secondary to disseminated sarcoidosis, improved

3. Hypertension, stable

4. Chronic anemia

5. Hypercalcemia likely secondary to above

6. Bilateral visual acuity deficits and previous headaches likely secondary to neurosarcoidosis

PLAN: I had a lengthy discussion with the patient and his wife regarding the pathophysiology of sarcoidosis. I explained to them that sarcoid is an autoimmune inflammatory process that does require a very intense initial therapy but that in most patients it is very steroid-responsive. I advised him that he needs to be on at least six months of continuous immunosuppressive therapy before we begin any significant taper. In that regard, given his marked improvement, I agreed with his further tapering of his Prednisone ultimately down to a lowest dose of 20 mg alternating every other day for an additional three months. After six months of therapy, we will reassess further tapering of his Prednisone. The nice feature is we do have an ACE level as a marker of disease activity. I suggested we get a repeat CT, pulmonary functions, ACE level, and sedimentation rate now as we begin to taper his Prednisone therapy. I will plan on seeing him back in approximately three months here in the pulmonary office or sooner if there should be any interval change in his clinical condition.

ICD-10-CM Code(s) _____

CASE STUDY 7

REASON FOR VISIT: Asthma.

HISTORY OF PRESENT ILLNESS: Matthew is a new patient in our office and is a 6-year-old boy who has been having problems with asthma since the age of 2 years. His asthma symptoms have been mild and he didn't have any admissions. This summer, Matthew started to have more problems with his asthma. He had one ER visit and was initially started on AeroBid that was eventually changed to Advair. Patient's mother is not sure of the strength, but the Advair was stopped on October 28 because of chest pain. She says that since being off the Advair, Matthew seems to have a little bit more symptoms. She thinks that he wheezes some nights. Mom said that he also has occasional night-time cough. While he was on an inhaled steroid, Mom said that Matthew would not have daytime cough, and only occasionally coughed at night. She also said that Matthew used to wheeze, but only when he was sick. Matthew also has symptoms of allergic rhinitis. He is currently on Allegra and Singulair and Mom thinks that if he misses a dose, he starts having a runny nose and teary eyes.

BIRTH HISTORY: He was born full term by vaginal delivery. Birth weight was only 4 pounds. Mom said she had toxemia during the pregnancy. He didn't have any problems after birth and didn't need oxygen or intensive care.

FEEDING HISTORY: He is on a regular diet. He does not seem to complain about vomiting or heartburn.

GROWTH AND DEVELOPMENT: He is in the first grade, doing well.

IMMUNIZATIONS: Up-to-date.

HOSPITALIZATIONS AND OPERATIONS: No hospitalizations. Matthew had a T&A when he was 4 years old.

ACCIDENTS AND INJURIES: None.

ALLERGIES: None known.

MEDICATIONS: Matthew is on Singulair, the strength of which is unknown. He is also on Allegra. He is also on Ventolin, which he takes at night.

FAMILY HISTORY: Mom has a history of asthma. Dad also has a history of asthma. There are multiple allergies in dad and the paternal uncle and aunts. There is no history of cystic fibrosis in the family.

SOCIAL HISTORY: Matthew lives with his parents. He has one half-sister. They live in an old house, but they don't seem to see mold problems. There is no smoke exposure. They have no pets.

PHYSICAL EXAMINATION:

GENERAL: He is alert, active, in no distress.

SKIN: No skin lesions.

LYMPH NODES: Cervical and axillary are not enlarged.

HEENT: Throat is clear. Nasal mucosa is not congested.

TRACHEA: Central.

BREATHING PATTERN: Regular.

CHEST SHAPE: Normal.

PERCUSSION: Resonant.

CHEST AUSCULTATION: Shows food air entry bilateral, no added sounds, wheezing.

HEART: Normal S1 and S2. No murmur.

ABDOMEN: Soft, lax.

EXTREMITIES: Well perfused; no clubbing.

CNS: Grossly intact.

CHEST X RAY: An AP and lateral chest X ray was obtained today in the office and was normal.

PULMONARY FUNCTION TESTS: PFTs were obtained today and were also within normal limits.

IMPRESSION:

1. Given Matthew's history, I do think that he has mild intermittent asthma, with acute exacerbation.

2. Possible allergies

PLAN:

1. Flovent 44 mcg, two puffs twice a day

2. Allergy referral

3. Albuterol, two puffs on an as-needed basis

4. Sweat chloride test

ICD-10-CM Code(s) _____

CASE STUDY 8

REASON FOR VISIT: Evaluation of recurrent infections

HISTORY OF PRESENT ILLNESS: The patient is a 3.5-year-old female who comes with her parents as a new patient with a history of recurrent boils and fevers that started in November. The patient has had three boils, one at the beginning of November, the second at the end of November, and the last one in January. The last episode required hospitalizations overnight because it was associated with a high fever, so the patient was treated with intravenous antibiotics. During that time, blood cultures were negative. The first boil drained spontaneously, the second one was drained surgically with the child as an outpatient, and the third one drained spontaneously as well. Every time the drainage was yellow, thick, pus. The boils were on her thigh, bottom, and vagina. In addition, she has had recurrent high fevers lasting five to seven days. She has had three episodes of high fevers that started on November 12, December 8, and January 20. The fevers went up to 104°F and were not associated with cough, runny nose, or diarrhea with the skin boils. Prior to November, the patient had been quite healthy. She had only two ear infections in the past. She had two to three episodes of thrush between 9 and 18 months of age, but they were associated with antibiotic intake. She has never had problems with diarrhea. At birth she had normal detachment and healing of the umbilical cord. She had

a urinary tract infection as a newborn and was kept in the hospital for a few days.

BIRTH HISTORY: Born full term by C-section. She had jaundice for one day and the urinary tract infection. Otherwise there were no other complications.

FEEDING HISTORY: Normal. No food allergies or reflux problems.

GROWTH AND DEVELOPMENT: Normal. She is in the 50th percentile for weight and between the 50th and 75th percentile for height.

IMMUNIZATIONS: Up-to-date. She has never received Prevnar.

HOSPITALIZATIONS AND OPERATIONS: Hospitalized once in January with the boil.

ACCIDENTS AND INJURIES: None.

ALLERGIES: Penicillin with hives and wheezing.

MEDICATIONS: None.

FAMILY HISTORY: Maternal grandmother has systemic lupus erythematosus. She has a second cousin that has recurrent boils. She has no siblings.

SOCIAL HISTORY: She lives with her parents. They don't have any pets. There is no smoking exposure. She does not use hot tubs.

PHYSICAL EXAMINATION:

GENERAL: She is in no apparent distress. Weight is 14.7 kg. Height is 99 cm. Heart rate is 104.

SKIN: Clear, except for a macular lesion on her right gluteal region.

HEENT: The nasal mucosa is normal. The throat is negative.

CHEST: Lungs are clear to auscultation.

HEART: Regular rate and rhythm, no murmur.

ABDOMEN: Soft, nontender, without hepatosplenomegaly.

EXTREMITIES: Negative, with no clubbing or cyanosis.

IMPRESSION:

1. Recurrent skin boils (furuncle) and fevers

2. Rule out immune deficiency

PLAN: I will send this patient to the lab for an immune screening with CBC and differential, lymphocyte subsets, serum immunoglobulin levels, titers for diphtheria, tetanus, and pneumococcals, NBT, markers for leukocyte adhesion deficiency, and total complement. The patient will receive a Pneumovax (7 valent) today and will return in four weeks to review results and for post-pneumococcal vaccination titers. Pneumovax was given IM to the patient today. Patient's mother was counseled prior to administration of vaccine. Prescribed prescription topical treatment for skin boils.

RETURN VISIT: Four weeks.

ICD-10-CM Code(s) _____

CASE STUDY 9

Julian was seen on October 15, 20xx, for follow-up of his persistent cough and abnormal chest X ray. He had a CT scan today, results of which are pending, but he has had improvement, both in his cough and his fever. He is on Albuterol prn; Advair 250 twice a day; Albuterol premixed four times a day; Nasonex; Singulair; Zyrtec; and he is weaning off Prednisone. He is also on Biaxin 175 mg twice a day and Tessalon Perles, which he is not requiring.

His weight is 25.3 kg. His height is 125.5 cm. His blood pressure is 123/66 and heart rate is 133. Nose and throat are clear. His neck is supple without adenopathy or thyromegaly. His chest is clear to auscultation, percussion is soft without organomegaly, masses, or tenderness. Extremities are without clubbing, cyanosis, or edema. Neurologic exam is normal with good muscle strength and tone and normal gait for age. Pulmonary function tests are about the same.

My impression is that he has mild intermittent extrinsic asthma with status asthmaticus. He has a persistent pneumonitis that seems to be improving, and we are trying to rule out bronchiectasis. I ordered a CT scan and will await the results of the scan to determine a course of treatment. I went ahead and told them to follow up and perform the bronchoscopy as scheduled. We also suggested an allergy evaluation as per Dr Mooring with a return visit here in four weeks.

ICD-10-CM Code(s) _____

CASE STUDY 10

June 13, 20xx

David Jones, MD
45xx Wellborn Street
Indianapolis, IN 46236

RE: Mitchell Walden

Dear Dr Jones:

Thank you for referring Mitchell Walden to our Pulmonology group for evaluation. Enclosed is a summary of our findings. I hope that this will be of help to you in your management of the patient.

Mitchell was seen back in our office in follow-up today, with complaints of coughing and wheezing for one week. It seems to be worse at night.

Upon examination, he does not appear to be in any acute distress. Breath sounds were bilateral, with some wheezing noted. Heart was at regular rate and rhythm. Abdomen was soft and nontender.

I reviewed the test results with his parents, which were negative for cystic fibrosis. My impression is that Mitchell does have asthma with acute exacerbation. He will be treated with anti-inflammatories. We will see him in another month for follow-up, or sooner if problems arise.

If I can be of further help to you with Mitchell or any of your other patients, please do not hesitate to contact me.

Sincerely,

Victor Corsini, MD
ABC Pulmonary Specialists

ICD-10-CM Code(s) _____

CASE STUDY 11

REASON FOR VISIT: Cough

HISTORY OF PRESENT ILLNESS: Michael is a 1-year-old with a history of coughing for several months that started in July and then seemed to get a little better and then reoccurred in the fall and was very persistent until recently. He was put on aerosols with Albuterol and then later Pulmicort. They have since stopped the Albuterol because his cough has improved so much. They report that the cough was worse at night, and that he wheezed frequently. Of significance, he recently has had myringotomy tubes placed and also had his adenoids taken out. Mom and Grandma feel that this had helped him a lot in terms of his symptomatology, because he used to have a lot of ear infections. At this point he is not coughing at night or in the day. They used to think he spit up quite a bit, although that has improved dramatically as he has gotten older. He was on Zantac for some time, but that has since been stopped. When they give him aerosols they do use a mask. Currently he is not on anything.

BIRTH HISTORY: Born one month early with a birth weight of 6 pounds, 5 ounces. He went home with Mom.

FEEDING HISTORY: No choking or gagging of significance. No chronic diarrhea or constipation.

GROWTH AND DEVELOPMENT: Normal.

IMMUNIZATIONS: Up-to-date.

HOSPITALIZATIONS AND OPERATIONS: He has never been hospitalized. His only surgery was for the myringotomy tube placement and the adenoid removal.

ALLERGIES: No known drug allergies.

MEDICATIONS: Currently none.

SOCIAL HISTORY: He lives with his mom and dad in Breakenfort. They have one cat. No one smokes. He does attend daycare with about 10 other children in his room.

PHYSICAL EXAMINATION:

GENERAL: He is a well-developed white male in no acute distress.

SKIN: Clear, without lesions.

LYMPH NODES: Cervical and axillary negative.

HEENT: Bilaterally clear TMs with myringotomy tubes and no drainage. Nasopharynx was clear without drainage. Oropharynx showed mucous membranes to be moist with no lesions.

NECK: Trachea normal.

BREATHING PATTERN: Normal.

CHEST SHAPE: Normal.

AUSCULTATION: Breath sounds bilateral, with good air exchange. No wheezing.

HEART: Regular rate without murmur. Pulses equal bilaterally.

ABDOMEN: Soft, nontender, nondistended. No hepatosplenomegaly.

EXTREMITIES: No cyanosis, clubbing, or edema.

CNS: Grossly normal.

CHEST X RAY: A chest X ray single view (frontal) was normal, without hyperexpansion.

IMPRESSION AND PLAN: My impression is that his cough is most likely due to baby asthma. Because of his age we need to also check a sweat chloride level, although I think this is very unlikely to be cystic fibrosis. Sweat test was performed today, the results of which are pending at this time. I told them that because he is not coughing anymore and his X ray is normal, that I didn't think we necessarily had to treat him with anything, but if he were to develop another cough or start having symptoms, then I think he should be treated through at least until next winter with a daily anti-inflammatory because of his significant history. We will see him back in about two months unless there are problems in the interim.

ICD-10-CM Code(s) _____

CASE STUDY 12

REASON FOR VISIT: Allergy evaluation for cough.

HISTORY OF PRESENT ILLNESS: The patient is new to the practice and is a 5-year-old male who comes with his parents complaining of a chronic cough that has been lifelong. The patient also had some wheezing during the first year of life, but now he only has cough and occasional shortness of breath. The cough is worse and persistent during the fall and winter. He usually gets much better during the summertime and only has occasional episodes of cough. He has been on Albuterol nebulizers and Singulair only until a month ago when he was started on Flovent. Since then, the cough has significantly improved. Now he is not coughing at night anymore. He has also had chronic nasal congestion in previous winters, but he has not had it this winter. The cough is worse with exertion, and Dad suspects that it might be related to exposure to cats. The cough is also worse at night. He has never been hospitalized or had any ER visits for these respiratory symptoms.

BIRTH HISTORY: Born at 36 weeks without complications.

FEEDING HISTORY: Unremarkable.

GROWTH AND DEVELOPMENT: Normal. He is between the 75th and 90th percentile for weight and height.

IMMUNIZATIONS: Up-to-date.

HOSPITALIZATIONS AND OPERATIONS: Bilateral myringotomy tubes twice in March 20xx and February 20xx. He had an adenoidectomy in April 20xx and a tonsillectomy in February 20xx.

PAST ILLNESSES: Only as described above.

ACCIDENTS AND INJURIES: None.

ALLERGIES: No known drug allergies.

MEDICATIONS: Flovent, two puffs twice a day with an AeroChamber; Albuterol, two puffs as needed; Singulair 5 mg qhs.

FAMILY HISTORY: Negative for cystic fibrosis.

SOCIAL HISTORY: He lives with his parents. He doesn't have any siblings. They have one cat indoors. There is no smoking in the house. They live in a six-year-old house with carpet. There is no basement. The patient attends childcare every day with 12 to 15 other kids.

PHYSICAL EXAMINATION:

GENERAL: He is in no apparent distress. Weight 15.3 kg; height 98 cm; pulse 112.

SKIN: Clear.

LYMPH NODES: Negative in axillary and cervical.

HEENT: Clear TMs. The nose and throat could not be examined because of patient lack of cooperation.

CHEST: Lungs are clear to auscultation.

HEART: Regular rate and rhythm, no murmur.

EXTREMITIES: Negative, with no clubbing or cyanosis.

LABORATORY: Allergy skin tests were done to 27 environmental allergens, including trees, grasses, weeds, molds, and indoor allergens. He was negative for everything, with a 3+ histamine control.

IMPRESSION/DISCUSSION: Intrinsic asthma with status asthmaticus, without evidence of any environmental allergies.

PLAN OF MANAGEMENT: Continue the same medications.

RETURN VISIT: Follow up for allergy as needed.

ICD-10-CM Code(s) _____

CASE STUDY 13

HISTORY OF PRESENT ILLNESS: This is a 58-year-old smoker who is admitted to the hospital with a chief complaint of shortness of breath, mild sharp substernal chest pain, and a cough productive of green sputum. He has developed increasing dyspnea on exertion over the last several months. Whereas previously he had been able to mow his yard without stopping, he now has to rest several times. He also complained of an increased rate of decline over the last several weeks that coincided with symptoms of post-nasal drainage, a sore throat, and feeling of fullness in his sinuses. He also admitted to a "smoker's cough," which was prevalent most mornings and produced white to tan sputum. This cough had been present for several years.

PAST MEDICAL HISTORY: He had been told that he might have coronary artery disease and he had been followed for borderline hypertension.

MEDICATIONS: His only current medication is aspirin, which he takes one a day.

SOCIAL HISTORY: Notable for tobacco (cigarette) dependence, up to two packs per day for 30 years.

REVIEW OF SYSTEMS: He denied chest pain, nausea, vomiting, diarrhea, or weakness.

PHYSICAL EXAMINATION: A normotensive man with a blood pressure of 120/78 mmHg. His pulse was regular at 69 and his respiratory rate was 20. His posterior pharynx had mild erythma and there was sinus tenderness on his right frontal sinus. Neck was supple with no thyroid enlargement. Lung exam found diffuse, bilateral, mild wheezing with basilar rhonchi. Heart exam found a regular rate and rhythm with no murmur or rub. Abdomen was soft with normal bowel sounds, no hepatosplenomegaly. The musculoskeletal exam was unremarkable; there was no edema. Skin was clear. Cranial nerves intact and DTRs normal.

LABORATORY: Chest X ray was consistent with mild chronic obstructive lung disease. A CBC had a white count of 8.6 with 80% segs. Electrolytes and renal function were within normal limits. His hemoglobin was 14. Pulmonary function tests demonstrated reduction in his forced expiratory volume over 1 second to 70% of normal. His FEV_1/FEV ratio, a marker of obstructive lung disease, was reduced to 62%.

ASSESSMENT AND PLAN: The patient was started on a course of ampicillin for COPD with acute bronchitis.

ICD-10-CM Code(s) _____

CASE STUDY 14

PREOPERATIVE DIAGNOSIS: Laryngeal stenosis.

POSTOPERATIVE DIAGNOSIS: Same.

INDICATIONS: This 1-year-old, male infant was born prematurely at a gestational age of approximately 29 weeks. The patient developed respiratory distress and was intubated for three weeks. At this time, the patient subsequently failed extubation and a tracheostomy tube was placed. The patient's respiratory failure was felt to be secondary to subglottic stenosis. Previous endoscopic evaluation with laryngeal dilation was performed. The patient presents for possible ablation of subglottic tissue. The patient was prepped and draped in the usual fashion. A laryngoscope was inserted orally and examination of the larynx and pharynx revealed no abnormalities. The glottis closed as a reflex to the laryngoscope coming in contact. The telescope was withdrawn. There appeared to be subglottic narrowing. The larynx was initially dilated. A fibrous mass was visualized just above the previously inserted tracheostomy tube, somewhat obscuring visualization. The telescope was passed through the cords and stenotic area for better visualization. On close inspection it appeared to be a thick, firm mass attached to the anterior tracheal wall, just above the level of the tracheal stoma. This represented a reactive tissue fibroma. The telescope was advanced along the left lateral tracheal wall past the level of this fibrous lesion and past the tracheostomy tube to the level of the carina. After inspection, the laryngoscope was withdrawn and the patient sent to recovery in stable condition.

ICD-10-CM Code(s) _____

CASE STUDY 15

PREOPERATIVE DIAGNOSIS: Inferior turbinate hypertrophy, nasal obstruction.

POSTOPERATIVE DIAGNOSIS: Same.

OPERATION PERFORMED: Bilateral submucous resection of inferior turbinates.

SURGEON: Mark Whittier, MD.

ANESTHESIA: General endotracheal.

ANESTHESIOLOGIST: George Abelman, MD.

ESTIMATED BLOOD LOSS: Minimal.

FLUIDS: Crystalloid.

COMPLICATIONS: None.

INDICATIONS FOR PROCEDURE: The patient is a 49-year-old male with a long history of nasal obstruction secondary to inferior turbinate hypertrophy. The patient previously underwent very conservative submucous resection of inferior turbinates and continues to have some nasal obstruction. Treatment with nasal steroids was ineffective. Treatment options including risks, benefits, and potential complications were thoroughly discussed with the patient. He indicated he understood and agreed to consent to the above procedure.

DESCRIPTION OF PROCEDURE: On 02/06/199x, the patient was taken to the operating room and placed in supine position. General anesthesia was administered via endotracheal tube without complications. The patient was prepared and draped in the usual manner. 4% cocaine saturated neurosurgical cottonoids were placed in either side of the nose. After a sufficient length of time had elapsed, the cottonoids were removed. An incision was made along the inferior border of the turbinates and the flaps were elevated. Anterior and inferior redundant mucosa was then removed. The turbinates were lateralized. The patient had improved airway. The patient tolerated the procedure well. The patient was awakened and extubated in the operating room and taken to the recovery room in stable condition.

ICD-10-CM Code(s) _____

CASE STUDY 16

PREOPERATIVE DIAGNOSIS: Chronic tonsillitis.

POSTOPERATIVE DIAGNOSIS: Same.

FINDINGS: 3+ tonsillar hypertrophy with cryptic changes evident. No evidence of adenoid remnants.

INDICATIONS: The patient is a 12-year-old with chronic Streptococcus tonsillitis and bilateral hypertrophy with chronic upper airway obstruction.

DESCRIPTION OF PROCEDURE: Following administration of general endotracheal anesthesia, the patient was prepped and draped in the usual sterile fashion. Attention was first directed to the oropharynx. A tonsillar mouth gag was placed allowing adequate visualization of the oropharynx and tonsillar areas. The right tonsil was grasped with a tenaculum and retracted to the midline. An incision was begun in the superior pole and dissection was continued along the fascial plane to the base of the tonsil. The tonsil was excised, including the plica triangularis area. Hemostasis was maintained with suction Bovie cauterization. Attention was then directed to the left tonsil. In similar fashion, the left tonsil was removed. Hemostasis was maintained with electric suction cauterization. The nasopharynx, posterior pharynx, and hypopharynx were then suctioned and lavaged with saline to remove all clots and debris. Reexamination at this time revealed no further bleeding present and the operation was concluded. The patient left the operating room in good condition and there were no complications. Estimated blood loss was less than 75 cc.

ICD-10-CM Code(s) _____

CASE STUDY 17

PREOPERATIVE DIAGNOSIS: Post-traumatic hydrocephalus.

POSTOPERATIVE DIAGNOSIS: Same.

PROCEDURE PERFORMED: Right ventriculoperitoneal shunt.

FINDINGS: Clear, colorless cerebrospinal fluid (CSF) was obtained by using high-pressure anteriorly.

ESTIMATED BLOOD LOSS: Minimal.

INDICATIONS: The patient previously underwent a craniotomy due to an industrial accident 45 days ago. She has been bothered the past several weeks by increasing headaches. A CT scan showed that the right parietal tumor was surrounding the ventricle, compressing the atrium and causing a trapped temporal horn, which was greatly expanded. There was clear CSF and there was no tumor around the temporal horn. This appeared to be a form of localized hydrocephalus with raised intracranial pressure and the best solution would be a permanent ventriculoperitoneal shunt. Accordingly, I discussed with the patient the

alternatives, benefits, and risks, including the risk of shunt malfunction, hemorrhage, sepsis, meningitis, shunt malposition, stroke, loss of vision, loss of speech, loss of other neurological functions, coma, and death. All questions were answered satisfactorily. The patient wished to proceed with the procedure.

PROCEDURE: With the patient in a supine position, she was placed under satisfactory general endotracheal anesthesia. She had just completed a round of intravenous chemotherapy. The platelet count and CNC were within normal limits. The patient received prophylactic Gentamicin and Vancomycin. The right side of the scalp was shaved, prepped, and draped in a standard fashion. Prior to surgery, a skull film was obtained which showed that the flap and the titanium burr hole were centered directly over the temporal horn. Accordingly, we planned a burr hole just posterior to the base of the previous flap in an area that had not been previously operated upon. An incision was planned to use the posterior limb of the previous incision and extend it posteriorly to form a horseshoe type of flap.

A right lateral paramedian upper quadrant abdominal incision was also used. The peritoneum was identified. A #4 Penfield catheter was passed and confirmed the free peritoneal space. The superficial fascia, the rectus abdominis sheath anterior to posterior to the preperitoneal fascia, and the peritoneum were dissected.

A single burr hole just posterior to the base of the previous flap was made and the dura was coagulated with a #4 Penfield and connected to the medium pressure Medtronic valve. We connected the distal tubing after using the shunt passer and making a tunnel in the epipericranial subgaleal space. We connected the distal catheter to the valve with a 2-0 silk tie and we took the ventricular catheter and passed approximately 4 cm of catheter to obtain clear, colorless CSF under high pressure by going a more anterior route. The catheter was passed in exactly that route and approximately 7 cm of ventricular catheter tubing was tied into the temporal horn. We obtained excellent outflow. There was no blood. We tied the ventricular catheter using a right-angle connector and a 2-0 silk tie to the intravalvular tubing.

We obtained free passage of clear, colorless CSF at the digital end. The valve reservoir was used to pump and refill the valve nicely before securing it in a final resting position using two 4-0 Neurolon ties to the pericranial tissue. We used interrupted 2-0 Vicryl to approximate the galea and used surgical staples to approximate the skin.

We used 2-0 catgut to close the peritoneum. We closed the abdominal layers using 2-0 Vicryl and surgical staples to close the abdominal incision. Tefla and Steri-Strips were used over the incision.

The patient tolerated the procedure well. She was extubated and taken to the recovery room where she was awakened and found to have baseline neurological function. An immediate CT scan was obtained to confirm localization and to rule out subdural hematomas. All sponge, needle, and instrument counts were correct. Blood loss was minimal.

ICD-10-CM Code(s) _____

CASE STUDY 18

New patient is seen today for cough. He is taking Advil Cold & Flu over the counter, but no relief. He has had a cough for two weeks; the cough is worse at night.

No sore throat, no fever, no history of asthma. Patient smokes cigarettes.

Chest X ray is normal. Follow-up in one month.

IMPRESSION: Smoker's cough.

ICD-10-CM Code(s) _____

CASE STUDY 19

A 40-year old woman comes in the office today complaining of shortness of breath. She has a five-day history of increasing shortness of breath. She does not attribute the shortness of breath to any precipitating event.

No fever or chills. The patient has mild persistent asthma. Past history of tobacco dependence. She stopped smoking 10 years ago.

A breathing treatment was given. Chest X ray was normal. Albuterol inhaler was prescribed.

IMPRESSION: Shortness of breath, mild persistent asthma, history of tobacco dependence.

ICD-10-CM Code(s) _____

CASE STUDY 20

Jack presents today for a follow-up on his pulmonary fibrosis. He states that he has not had any other symptoms that might trigger shortness of breath that he is aware of. He has been feeling a little run down and had a stuffy nose, no cough, but nothing that would cause immediate concern.

IMPRESSION: Pulmonary fibrosis.

ICD-10-CM Code(s) _____

CHAPTER 7

Diseases of the Digestive System (K00-K95)

ICD-10-CM Chapter 11 Guideline Review

In this chapter you will find case studies relating to Chapter 11 of the ICD-10-CM codebook to build ICD-10-CM diagnosis coding skills in this area. Chapter-specific guidelines for coding and reporting in the digestive system have not yet been developed pending future expansion.

Many medical specialties, including primary care, gastroenterology, and other various specialties, reference Chapter 11 of the ICD-10-CM codebook for coding diseases of the digestive system. Keep in mind that you should always reference the ICD-10-CM Official Guidelines for Coding and Reporting in its entirety, along with the instructional notes, when coding these conditions.

Diseases of the Digestive System (K00-K95)

CASE STUDY 1

PREOPERATIVE DIAGNOSIS: Hematochezia.

POSTOPERATIVE DIAGNOSIS: Incomplete negative colonoscopy.

PROCEDURE: Colonoscopy.

NARRATIVE: After bowel prep and intravenous (IV) sedation in the left lateral position with multiple repositioning, the colonoscope was advanced under direct vision, probably to the upper ascending colon. The patient had a very tight curve in the sigmoid colon. Despite all of our maneuvers, we never were able to reach the cecum. Prep was adequate and mucosal surfaces were adequately visualized and appeared entirely unremarkable. In the distance a

floppy ileocecal valve versus mass effect was seen. I will arrange for barium enema for follow-up. The patient tolerated the procedure well and there were no complications.

ICD-10-CM Code(s) _____

CASE STUDY 2

Patient returns to our office for follow-up of her abdominal pain. The pain seems to have dissipated. There is some mild soreness that persists. No fever, chills, or development of guarding or rebound.

PHYSICAL EXAMINATION: Chest: Clear to auscultation and percussion. Heart: Regular rate and rhythm. Abdomen: Soft, nontender, and without distention. There is no rebound or guarding. Extremities are negative for edema.

ASSESSMENT AND PLAN: Gastroenteritis is better, but patient needs to continue on Zantac 300 mg tid and will return for follow-up in three weeks.

ICD-10-CM Code(s) _____

CASE STUDY 3

CHIEF COMPLAINT: The patient is referred by Dr Mecher for pancreatitis.

HISTORY OF PRESENT ILLNESS: This patient is a 52-year-old male who was recently hospitalized with epigastric and right upper quadrant pain and apparently was found to have elevated amylase. A liver function test on April 23, 20xx, however, was within normal limits. Gallbladder ultrasound on April 23 shows biliary sludge with a positive Murphy sign and fatty infiltration of the liver. A CT scan on April 27 showed findings consistent with acute pancreatitis and fatty liver. He denies any dark urine, light stools, jaundice, or hepatitis. He was hospitalized for seven days at St Agnes North. He notes bloating after meals. He has had some night sweats and some weight loss.

ALLERGIES: Penicillin.

MEDICATIONS: Plavix, aspirin, Lopid, Toprol XL, and Prevacid.

ILLNESSES: Arthritis, hypercholesterolemia, coronary artery disease, and peripheral vascular disease.

SURGERIES: Coronary stents (20xx), lower extremity bypass (20xx), and stents in legs.

SOCIAL HISTORY: Quit tobacco; uses alcohol occasionally.

FAMILY HISTORY: Positive for some type of cancer in his father. Mother has heart disease.

REVIEW OF SYSTEMS: Positive for alternating weight loss and weight gain. He wears corrective lenses and dentures. He notes shortness of breath with walking. He has a frequent cough. He has noted loss of appetite with the pancreatitis. He notes back pain and joint stiffness. He notes a history of bruising easily. He has a history of anxiety. Review of systems is otherwise negative.

PHYSICAL EXAMINATION: This is an adult male who is alert and oriented ×3. Temperature 97.6°F; pulse 118/80; weight 203 pounds; height 6 feet. HEENT: Reveals no icterus. Extraocular movements are intact. PERRLA: Neck is supple. Lungs are clear to auscultation bilaterally. Heart is regular without murmur. Abdomen: Soft, nontender, nondistended. I detect no mass, organomegaly, herniae, or Murphy sign. Extremities: No cyanosis, rashes, or edema. Evidence of previous left lower extremity bypass surgery.

IMPRESSION: Acute pancreatitis, sludge on ultrasound.

PLAN: I discussed with the patient and his wife laparoscopic cholecystectomy with cholangiogram. I explained to them the alternatives, benefits, and risks of that procedure, including but not limited to infection, bleeding, and conversion to an open procedure. They understand if he has a positive cholangiogram, he may require postoperative endoscopic retrograde cholangiopancreatography (ERCP).

ICD-10-CM Code(s) _____

CASE STUDY 4

Dear Dr Silverstone:

I had the pleasure of seeing Mary Odum in consultation in the ABC Medical Center on December 19, 20xx. As you know, Mary is an almost 5-year-old female with a history of intermittent vomiting. She was first diagnosed with gastroesophageal reflux at 3 months of age. While she was hospitalized at St Agnes Hospital for cardiac surgery at that time, she underwent an upper GI barium study revealing normal anatomy but the presence of gastroesophageal reflux. She was initially treated with Cisapride for many months. She was weaned off the Cisapride and remained off medications for several years. She had an asymptomatic period during this time; however, her vomiting returned approximately one year ago. She now vomits about two days per week. The vomitus is nonbloody and nonbilious. It tends to occur more frequently in the afternoon and evening. The vomitus looks like undigested food. Her appetite has been fine and she has had good weight gain. She does complain of abdominal pain, which usually occurs just before vomiting; however, she also has abdominal pain that is not associated with the vomiting. She has also complained of chest pain in the past week. She continues to complain of sour spit, and her mother continues to hear gurgling in the child's throat. In June this year, she underwent a gastric emptying study revealing normal gastric emptying of 57%. She passes normal stool daily without blood. She has recently been treated with Reglan at 2 mg once a night, and the mother feels this has decreased the frequency of vomiting.

Mary was the product of a full-term pregnancy and spontaneous vaginal delivery. Her birth weight was 8 pounds, 14 ounces. She passed meconium in the first 24 hours of life. She was noted to have a heart murmur at 2 weeks of age. Between the ages of 2 weeks and 3 months, she was in and out of the hospital on multiple occasions and finally underwent corrective heart surgery for multiple septal defects at 3 months of age at St Agnes Hospital. She has had no other hospitalizations or surgeries. Her only medication is the Reglan. She has no known drug allergies. Her immunizations are up to date.

The family history is positive for gastroesophageal reflux in the father. There are no other GI diseases in the family. She lives at home with her 40-year-old father and 30-year-old mother. The father is a teacher at Pike Elementary while the mother is a social worker. Mary has a healthy 9-year-old sister. She attends preschool.

Review of systems is positive for a history of secondary enuresis and continued primary nocturnal enuresis.

On physical examination, her weight was 26.4 kg (greater than the 97th percentile) and her height 106 cm (50th percentile). Her blood pressure was 94/58 and her pulse 100/min. She was a very anxious child in no apparent distress. HEENT examination revealed clear conjunctiva and a clear oropharynx with moist mucous membranes. The neck was supple without lymphadenopathy or thyromegaly. The chest was clear to auscultation. The heart had a regular rate and rhythm without murmur. The skin was clear. The abdomen was soft, nontender, and nondistended. There was no hepatosplenomegaly, and no masses were palpated. I deferred perianal and digital rectal examination due to the patient's significant anxiety. She had Tanner Stage I external female genitalia. Musculoskeletal examination revealed normal tone and reflexes. This child remained very anxious throughout the interview and physical examination and actually vomited just after I left the room. My impression is that Mary is an almost 5-year-old female with a history of vomiting. My differential diagnosis includes gastro-esophageal reflux disease with potential hiatal hernia, allergic eosinophilic esophagitis, delayed gastric empty-ing (although a gastric emptying study in June this year was normal), and vomiting. I felt it was best to proceed with upper gastrointestinal endoscopy with biopsies and 24-hour esophageal pH monitoring to gather the data needed for appropriate treatment. I have asked that the Reglan be stopped one week before the proce-dures in order not to bias pH monitoring results.

I certainly wish to thank you for allowing me to share in the care of this nice young lady. Please feel free to contact me if you have any questions or concerns.

Sincerely,

Frank Forestern, MD

ICD-10-CM Code(s) _____

CASE STUDY 5

CHIEF COMPLAINT: Constipation

Mark Tucker is a 5-year-old, white male with a history of constipation and soiling for many months. The par-ents describe difficulties with constipation as early as 8 months of age. He was toilet trained without difficulty. He currently passes large, hard, painful stools about once to twice a month. There has been no blood in his stool. They have had to use enemas and suppositories to ease the passage of stool. Tucker soils his underwear on a daily basis, and this also occurs while he is sleep-ing at night. His appetite had been decreased with the constipation, and the mother is concerned that he has

lost weight during this time period. She estimated the weight loss to be three to five pounds. He has had no vomiting. He was initially treated with a concoction consisting of applesauce, Metamucil, prune juice, and mineral oil. This was given on an as-needed basis approximately every other day. This may have provided some benefit; however, he had some difficulty taking this.

Mark was the product of a full-term pregnancy and spontaneous vaginal delivery. His birth weight was 7 pounds, 11 ounces. He passed meconium on the first day of life. The delivery was complicated by maternal blood loss. He has had no other hospitalizations or surgeries. His only medication is the above concoction on an as-needed basis. He has no known drug allergies. His immunizations are up to date.

The family history is negative for constipation and Hirschsprung disease. The mother has a history of ulcers and migraine headaches.

He lives with his 36-year-old mother who works in a shipping department. The father is 38-years-old and no longer lives in the home; he is an electrician. Mark attends pre-kindergarten and enjoys school.

Review of systems is only positive for a bony protrusion on his left chest wall, which has been present for many years.

On physical examination his weight was 15.4 kg (3rd percentile) and his height 106 cm (10th to 25th percen-tiles). His BMI was 13.7 kg/M2 (3rd to 5th percentiles). He was awake, alert, and in no apparent distress. HEENT examination revealed clear conjunctiva, clear tympanic membranes, and a clear oropharynx with moist mucous membranes. The neck was supple. There was mild lymphadenopathy in the anterior and posterior cervical chain. There was no thyromegaly. The chest was clear to auscultation. The heart had a regular rate and rhythm without murmur. The skin was clear except for mild perianal erythema. There was a bony protrusion on the left chest wall at the costochondral joint. The abdomen was soft, nontender, and nondistended. There was no hepatosplenomegaly and no masses were palpated. He had Tanner Stage I male genitalia with bilaterally descended testicles and a normal cremasteric reflex. There was no active or chronic perianal disease. Digital examination revealed a significant amount of formed stool in the rectal vault that was hemoccult-negative. His affect was normal.

My impression is that Mark is a 5-year-old, white male with a history of chronic constipation and soiling. I discussed the pathophysiology of this with the parents.

We will clear his impaction with a pediatric Fleet enema every 12 hours for the next three days. I will then initiate therapy with Miralax at one capful (17 g) once daily in eight ounces of fluid. My goal is for Mark to pass one to two soft stools per day. I asked that he sit on the toilet after breakfast and dinner to utilize the gastrocolic reflex. I asked the parents to call me if his stool consistency is too loose or too firm so that we can adjust the dose of Miralax by phone. I will see Mark back in two months to evaluate his progress.

ICD-10-CM Code(s) _____

CASE STUDY 6

REASON FOR VISIT: Gastrointestinal bleeding.

HISTORY OF PRESENT ILLNESS: Thomas is a 48-year-old male who presented to the emergency room (ER) via rescue squad for severe gastrointestinal rectal bleeding for one day. He states that two days ago he had an episode of bright red blood in the rectum. Today he bled profusely. He has had severe weakness and dizziness to the point where he could not drive himself to the emergency department. He denies any abdominal pain, nausea, vomiting, or fevers. There is a history of previous gastrointestinal bleeds. He drinks two pots of coffee per day.

PAST MEDICAL HISTORY: Remarkable for non-insulin-dependent diabetes mellitus on Metformin. Hypercholesterolemia on Lipitor. Hypertension. Low back pain for six months. He has been seeing a chiropractor. No known allergies.

FAMILY HISTORY: Family history is remarkable for parents with diabetes and heart disease.

SOCIAL HISTORY: He is a truck driver. He is single. He has no children. He has a history of alcohol and tobacco use but quit a while ago.

CURRENT MEDICATIONS:

- Metformin, dose unknown
- Atenolol, dose unknown
- Lipitor, dose unknown
- Indapamide, dose unknown
- Enalapril, dose unknown
- Flexeril, dose unknown

PHYSICAL EXAMINATION: Blood pressure 111/71; pulse 100; respiration 16. Pulse oximetry is 100% on room air.

GENERAL: Patient is well developed, well nourished, alert, and oriented times three, in no apparent distress. He is pale.

HEENT: Head is normocephalic and atraumatic. Eyes: Pupils equal, round, and reactive to light; extraocular movements intact; sclerae anicteric. Ears: Tympanic membranes pearly grey bilaterally with good light reflex. Nose: Patent; mucosa nonerythematous and nonboggy. Mouth: Without lesions; mucous membranes moist; oropharynx clear without exudate. No tonsillar enlargement or erythema. Sinuses: Nontender.

NECK: Supple without adenopathy; no thyromegaly or bruits. Nontender; full range of motion.

LUNGS: Clear to auscultation and percussion bilaterally; good air movement.

BACK: Straight. No costovertebral angle tenderness or spinal tenderness.

HEART: Regular rate and rhythm without murmurs, rubs, or gallop. Normal S1 and S2.

ABDOMEN: Soft and nontender. Normal active bowel sounds. No masses or hepatosplenomegaly.

RECTAL: Per emergency room physician there is bright red blood.

EXTREMITIES: No cyanosis, clubbing, or edema. Good tone and range of motion. Pedal pulses intact bilaterally.

SKIN: Good turgor without rashes. No atypical appearing moles.

NEUROLOGIC: Cranial nerves II–XII grossly intact. Motor, sensory, and cerebellar functions intact. Deep tendon reflexes are equal bilaterally at biceps, patellar, and Achilles. Strength 5/5 bilateral upper and lower extremities.

LABORATORY AND DIAGNOSTIC DATA: Prothrombin time and partial thromboplastin time are 15.1 and 36.5, which is slightly elevated. A complete blood count showed a white count of 11.3; hemoglobin and hematocrit are 9.5 and 27.6 with 315 platelets. Sodium is 135, potassium 4.0, BUN 22, creatinine 1, glucose 220.

ASSESSMENT AND PLAN:

1. This is a 48-year-old male with an acute gastrointestinal bleed, etiology unknown. His hemoglobin and hematocrit are quite low prior to hydration. He is admitted. Dr Wallen from Gastroenterology was consulted. He will be scoped today. Monitor hemoglobin and hematocrit. Keep the patient nothing by mouth.

2. Non-insulin-dependent diabetes mellitus. Continue to monitor blood sugars. Patient will continue his home medications.

3. Benign hypertension. Continue home blood pressure medications. Hold for hypotension.

4. Hypercholesterolemia with endogenous hyperglyceridemia. Continue Lipitor. I discussed the above with the patient. He understands and agrees with the plan.

ICD-10-CM Code(s) _____

CASE STUDY 7

CHIEF COMPLAINT: Linda returns with a new complaint of epigastric pain and a foul taste in her mouth.

HISTORY OF PRESENT ILLNESS: Linda Meadows is a 67-year-old lady whom I know from diagnostic laproscopy with lysis of adhesions on July 29, 20xx, for chronic epigastric pain. Evaluation prior to that included an upper endoscopy in January, which raised the question of possible hiatal hernia. In addition, she underwent a colonoscopy.

On today's visit, she notes she has lost perhaps five pounds since the surgery in July. She notes that she is having frequent episodes of epigastric discomfort not related to meals. She often notices episodes of sour and foul taste in the back of her throat in the evening that occasionally wakes her up from sleep and is especially present upon rising in the morning. She notes no frank vomiting. She states her appetite is good and her bowels are moving normally.

PHYSICAL EXAMINATION: On examination, she appears well. She wears corrective lenses. The lungs are clear and the heart is regular. Abdomen: There are multiple scars consistent with the previous surgeries. The abdomen is soft, nontender, and nondistended, and I detect no mass, organomegaly, or herniae.

IMPRESSION: Possible reflux.

PLAN: I recommended to the patient that we put her on Nexium 40 mg daily trial, and I gave her instructions and 15 day samples of that. Also, arrangements were made for an esophagram and an upper GI, and she is to follow up here with those studies in two weeks.

ICD-10-CM Code(s) _____

CASE STUDY 8

CHIEF COMPLAINT: This is a new patient being seen for small amounts/drops of blood on toilet paper yesterday after attempting to pass stool. He is 14 years old and is accompanied by his parents. Patient states he was feeling well yesterday, ran cross country at school, and then noted lower abdominal pain and felt the urge to pass stool. Although he initially did not pass stool, he noted droplets of red blood on toilet paper with rectal pain at time of onset. He was seen in the ER last night with a heme + stool and received NS bolus ×2. Hemoglobin was 12.6; normal coagulation; normal amylase/lipase. He received an enema with a passage of a large blood clot. Pain resolved last night. He passed another very large brown stool without blood this morning.

REVIEW OF SYSTEMS: No vomiting. Positive for nausea—now resolved. No fever. No urinary tract symptoms. History of allergies. No trouble breathing. Positive for weight gain (slowly). Dry skin. Positive history of constipation.

PAST MEDICAL HISTORY: Discharged at 7 weeks with cystic fibrosis (CF) and failure to thrive. Multiple sinus surgeries.

MEDICATIONS: Miralax 1 cap/8oz BID. Other medications are on history form.

ALLERGIES: None.

SOCIAL HISTORY: Lives with Mom and Dad.

FAMILY HISTORY: Negative for CF.

PHYSICAL EXAMINATION: Constitutional: Heart rate 72; respiration 20; blood pressure 95/47; playing in game room prior to examination, NAD. HEENT: Normal. Neck: No lymphadenopathy. Respiratory: clear to auscultation. Cardiovascular: Normal, S1/S2. Abdomen: Soft, positive bowel sounds, no palpable masses, no hepatosplenomegaly. Rectal examination: No active perianal discharge, no tenderness with exam, no hemorrhoids/masses palpable, scant amount of brown stool. Skin: Dry patches. Neurologic: Normal.

ASSESSMENT AND PLAN: A 14-year-old with CF, chronic constipation, and one episode of rectal bleeding with pain on defecation. Hemodynamically stable. Continue with Miralax 1 cap/8oz fluid BID with goal of two soft stools a day. Encourage fluids, increase water intake, may try Benefiber. Follow up in one month.

ICD-10-CM Code(s) _____

CASE STUDY 9

This is a patient who comes back into the office following CT scan of the gallbladder. The patient has calculus of the gallbladder. We advised him to have surgery, but he didn't show up to any of his testing.

In conversation with him I stated that he could develop acute cholelithiasis and also pancreatitis. At this point, he does not want to undergo any surgery. We will follow up with him as needed.

ICD-10-CM Code(s) _____

CASE STUDY 10
OFFICE PROGRESS NOTE

SUBJECTIVE: The patient returns for follow-up one-month status post appendectomy. When we performed a laparoscopic appendectomy, we saw a small bilateral hernia. She never had any symptoms from the hernia. She denies symptoms right now. She just wanted that checked.

PHYSICAL EXAMINATION: She has no pain in her groin. There is no palpable bulge. The abdomen examination is normal. Her incisions all look clean and dry from the previous appendectomy.

ASSESSMENT: Small hernia found during laparoscopic procedure without any symptoms.

PLAN: I discussed with her the risks of not doing any surgery. I also discussed the risks of doing surgery. She is asymptomatic and there are no physical findings. She decided not to undergo any surgical procedure. I think that is a reasonable decision at this point. We will follow up with her in approximately one year. If she starts having symptoms, we will perform a hernia repair. I also discussed the risk of hernia incarceration. She does not have abdominal pain in her right or left lower abdomen; she will look for medical advice immediately if she does.

ICD-10-CM Code(s) _____

CASE STUDY 11

I was asked to evaluate this patient for Dr Sherman. She is an 88-year-old white female with a history of abdominal pain. The pain is mainly in the right upper quadrant. There is no radiation to the back or to the lower abdomen. The pain is moderate to severe. She had two attacks in the past three months. She does not have any other signs or symptoms. No fevers or chills. No nausea or vomiting. No diarrhea or constipation. There are no aggravating or relieving factors for this pain.

PAST MEDICAL HISTORY:

- Osteoarthritis
- Osteoporosis
- Chronic obstructive pulmonary disease
- Congestive heart failure
- Status post-pacemaker placement
- Arrhythmia

MEDICATIONS:

- Bumex
- Restoril
- Coumadin
- Zantac
- Dulcolax
- Vitamins, Ocuvite

REVIEW OF SYSTEMS: No history of fevers or weight loss, chest pain, or arrhythmias. No shortness of breath or wheezing. No history of thyroid disease, diabetes, stroke, seizures, hematuria, or dysuria. No lesions or rashes. All other systems negative.

PHYSICAL EXAMINATION:

GENERAL: She is awake, alert, and oriented ×3.

LUNGS: Clear.

HEART: Regular.

ABDOMEN: Soft and tenderness in the right upper quadrant. No palpable liver or spleen. Bowel sounds in all four quadrants. No other herniations. Well-healed incisions of the midline. Ultrasound today verified cholelithiasis with cholecystitis.

ASSESSMENT AND PLAN: Cholelithiasis with cholecystitis. I do not feel there is any obstruction. We will ask Gastroenterology to see this patient for possible ERCP. We will keep npo for now and on IV antibiotics. We will get cardiac clearance for possible surgical intervention if her coagulopathy is corrected and if the patient decides to have surgery performed.

ICD-10-CM Code(s) _____

CASE STUDY 12

I was asked by Dr McMannis to evaluate this patient. He is a 41-year-old, white male with a history of abdominal pain for approximately six months. He has on and off abdominal pain. The pain is mainly on the left side. The pain is moderate to severe, although at this point he does not have any pain. He has on and off some vomiting and diarrhea, although at this time he is just complaining of abdominal pain. He has been treated for peptic ulcer disease, although he never had an endoscopy performed. There are no other signs or symptoms.

PAST MEDICAL HISTORY: Unremarkable.

ALLERGIES: No known allergies.

MEDICATIONS:

- Cipro
- Flagyl
- Prevacid

SOCIAL HISTORY: He denies drug or alcohol abuse.

REVIEW OF SYSTEMS:

CONSTITUTIONAL: No fevers or chills.

CARDIOVASCULAR: No history of chest pain or tachyarrhythmia.

CHEST: No shortness of breath or tachypnea.

SKIN: No history of new skin lesions or rashes.

NEUROLOGIC: No history of seizure or stroke.

PSYCHIATRIC: No history of anxiety or depression.

GASTROINTESTINAL: History of peptic ulcer disease. He has been worked up for pancreatitis. Alcohol abuse. As I stated before, he has abdominal pain in the left lower quadrant.

MUSCULOSKELETAL: No history of recent fractures or dislocations.

PHYSICAL EXAMINATION:

GENERAL: He is awake, alert, and oriented ×3.

VITAL SIGNS: He is afebrile. Vital signs are stable.

CHEST: Lungs are clear.

CARDIOVASCULAR: Regular.

ABDOMEN: Soft and nondistended, nontender. No peritoneal signs. No rebound or guarding. No hepatosplenomegaly. Bowel sounds in all four quadrants. He has bilateral small inguinal hernias.

ASSESSMENT AND PLAN: The patient has bilateral inguinal hernias causing the lower abdominal pain. We will get a gastroenterology consultant to perform an upper and lower endoscopy. He also had a CT scan, which showed just diverticulosis. I will follow him after the endoscopies are performed. If endoscopy is normal and just shows diverticulosis, the option is to perform a resection of the diseased segment that could be causing him to have chronic abdominal pain.

ICD-10-CM Code(s) _____

CASE STUDY 13

PREOPERATIVE DIAGNOSIS: Ventral hernia.

POSTOPERATIVE DIAGNOSIS: Same.

PROCEDURE: Ventral hernia mesh repair.

DESCRIPTION OF PROCEDURE: The patient was prepped and draped in a supine position. The anterior abdomen was surrounded with sterile drapes and towel. A midline incision was made and the hernial defect was found. The hernial sac was transected and amputated. The defect was fully delineated. This accommodated a small circular Ventralex mesh. This was placed underneath the defect and secured in four quadrants using 2-0 Prolene suture. It was noted at this time that there appeared to be above-average bleeding that was controlled prior to final wound closure, which took an additional 45 minutes beyond the typical procedure. The patient's vital signs remained stable during the bleed. Following this, subcutaneous tissue was closed with interrupted 3-0 Vicryl and the skin was closed with 4-0 Vicryl subcuticular stitch. Sponge and needle counts were correct. There were no drains. The patient was sent to the recovery room in fair condition for monitoring and further stabilization. Postop instructions were written. Patient given Lortab 7.5 rag (dispense #30) 1-2 po q6-8 prn for pain. Follow-up arranged. Local wound care instruction given.

ICD-10-CM Code(s) _____

CASE STUDY 14

POSTOPERATIVE DIAGNOSIS: Incisional hernia.

PROCEDURES:

1. Excision of abscess, removal of foreign body.

2. Repair of incisional hernia.

ANESTHESIA: General, laryngeal mask airway.

INDICATIONS: Patient is a pleasant 37-year-old gentleman who has had multiple procedures including a laparotomy related to trauma. The patient has had a recurrently infected cyst of his mass at the superior aspect of his incision, which he says gets larger and then it drains internally, causing him to be quite ill. He presented to my office and I recommended that he undergo exploration of incisional hernia with obstruction without gangrene. The procedure, purpose, risks, expected benefits, potential complications, and alternative forms of therapy were discussed with him and he was agreeable to surgery.

ICD-10-CM Code(s) _____

CASE STUDY 15

CURRENT CONDITION: Dysphagia and hematemesis while vomiting.

HISTORY OF PATIENT ILLNESS: A 53-year-old female who has AIDS presents today with complaint of stuck food in her esophagus, bloody cough, and bloody vomiting since 4 o'clock.

She ate a meal of eggplant parmigiana. She denied fever, diarrhea, dysuria, and abdominal pain. This is the first episode of hematemesis and feeling of globus pallidus. CAT scan of the chest showed diffuse esophageal dilatation with residual food in it, no mediastinal air was identified.

PLAN: Dysphagia, oropharyngeal and hematemesis. We will put her npo, we will administer IV fluid, half normal saline D5 100 mL per hour. I discussed the case with Dr. Y, a gastroenterologist. The patient planned for esophagogastroduodenoscopy and is scheduled for next week.

ICD-10-CM Code(s) _____

CHAPTER 8

Diseases of the Skin and Subcutaneous Tissue (L00-L99) and Diseases of the Musculoskeletal System and Connective Tissue (M00-M99)

ICD-10-CM Chapters 12 and 13 Guidelines Review

In this chapter you will find a summary of the chapter-specific coding guidelines for Chapters 12 and 13 of the ICD-10-CM codebook followed by case studies to build ICD-10-CM diagnosis coding skills in these areas.

Many medical specialties, including primary care, dermatology, plastic and reconstructive surgery, and other various specialties reference Chapter 12 of the ICD-10-CM codebook for coding diseases of the skin and subcutaneous tissue. Chapter 13, Diseases of the Musculoskeletal System and Connective Tissue, includes information often referenced by specialties including primary care physicians, orthopedic surgeons, neurosurgeons, and other specialties as well. Keep in mind you should always reference the ICD-10-CM Official Guidelines for Coding and Reporting in its entirety when making a code selection.

ICD-10-CM Official Coding Guidelines for Diseases of the Skin and Subcutaneous Tissue

PRESSURE ULCERS

Codes for pressure ulcers (category L89) are combination codes that identify (1) the site of the pressure ulcer and (2) the stage of the pressure ulcer. Pressure ulcers are coded based on severity and site and are designated by stages (stage 1–4 and unspecified stage or unstageable). The user may report as many codes in category L89 to identify all pressure ulcers the patient may have.

When coding pressure ulcers, the following guidelines apply:

- An unstageable pressure ulcer is classified as L89.-0 and is based on clinical documentation. Only use a code from this category when the stage cannot be clinically determined. An unstageable ulcer is an ulcer that is:

  - covered by eschar,
  - treated with a skin or muscle graft, or
  - documented as a deep tissue injury not due to trauma.

- This code is not to be confused with codes for unspecified stage (L89.-9) whereas the documentation does not specify the stage of the ulcer.

- Assignment of the pressure ulcer stage code should be guided by clinical documentation of the stage or documentation of the terms found in the Alphabetic Index.

- For clinical terms describing the stage that are not found in the Alphabetic Index, and there is no documentation of the stage, the provider should be queried.

- No code is assigned if the documentation states that the pressure ulcer is completely healed.

- Pressure ulcers described as healed should be assigned the appropriate pressure ulcer stage code based on the documentation in the medical record.

- If the documentation does not provide information about the stage of the healing pressure ulcer, assign the appropriate code for unspecified stage.

- If the documentation is unclear as to whether the patient has a current (new) pressure ulcer or if the patient is being treated for a healing pressure ulcer, query the provider.

- For ulcers that were present on admission but healed at the time of discharge, assign the code for the site and stage of the pressure ulcer at the time of admission.

- If a patient is admitted with a pressure ulcer at one stage and it progresses to a higher stage, two separate codes should be assigned: one for the site and stage of the ulcer on admission and a second code for the same ulcer site and the highest stage reported during the stay.

It is time to build skill and knowledge by coding the following exercises relative to the skin and subcutaneous tissue. Make certain to reference the ICD-10-CM codebook and the ICD-10-CM Official Guidelines for Coding and Reporting, along with the instructional notes, when coding these exercises.

Diseases of the Skin and Subcutaneous Tissue (L00-L99)

CASE STUDY 1

CHIEF COMPLAINT: This 37-year-old, new patient has been experiencing facial breakouts, a severe itchy scalp, and spots on the lip and hand. She has been using tretinoin gel in the past. She has tried selenium sulfide shampoo in the past for the itchy scalp. She also has a bump on the inside of the lower lip that has been present for a couple of months that bleeds. She also has some mild hand eczema.

MEDICATIONS: Singulair, Loratadine, and Cimetidine, as needed.

FAMILY HISTORY: No family history of skin cancer.

REVIEW OF SYSTEMS: Negative for any eye complaints, including grittiness.

EXAMINATION: Acne today on the central face with no evidence of scaling on the scalp at this time. She has a small, cystic lesion on the inner aspect of the right lower lip, and mild, eczematous changes on the dorsum of the hands.

ASSESSMENT AND PLAN: Diagnosis: Rosacea, seborrhea, and atopic dermatitis. Prescribed tretinoin gel to spot treat qd prn, minocycline, 100 mg 1× day, and moisturizer for the hands. She is to contact the office if the treatment is not successful and will recheck in one month.

ICD-10-CM Code(s) _____

CASE STUDY 2

HISTORY: This is a follow-up visit for this 65-year-old female patient with a history of IDDM (Type 1). She was admitted to the hospital three days ago with cellulitis of the left foot. She was placed on IV therapy for her cellulitis. She is recovering well and the infection is almost gone. She denies chest pain or shortness of breath. Patient is positive for pain in the left foot that is sometimes severe in nature.

MEDICATIONS: 70/30 insulin in the morning and 20 units in the evening; Cardizem CD 180 once daily; Imdur 60 mg once a day; Lasix 80 mg one a day; Pepcid 20 mg twice a day; Paxil 10 mg three times a day; Nitrostat as needed.

EXAMINATION:

GENERAL: Well-developed, well-nourished female in no acute distress. Blood pressure 128/75; pulse 80, regular and strong; respiration: 12, unlabored and regular. Temperature is normal.

HEIGHT: 5 feet.

MUSCULOSKELETAL: Left foot shows slight reddening on the upper surface. Infection had decreased significantly. All other areas are normal.

ASSESSMENT AND PLAN: Patient is doing well and will be taken off IV Vancomycin. She will be discharged home tomorrow and will be given a prescription for penicillin. She is to follow up in my office in one week.

ICD-10-CM Code(s) _____

CASE STUDY 3

HISTORY OF PRESENT ILLNESS: This 47-year-old white male is a new patient seen in the office with history of lesions on his right elbow, wrist, and hairline on the neck. He thinks that the lesions on his neckline are due to his sleep apnea problems. He has just recently noticed some ulceration in that area. He does not have any other complaints.

CURRENT MEDICATIONS:

- Lotrel
- Lopressor
- Zoloft

PAST MEDICAL HISTORY:

- Hypertension
- Increased cholesterol

PAST SURGICAL HISTORY: Appendectomy.

SOCIAL HISTORY: Does not smoke, drink, or use drugs.

REVIEW OF SYSTEMS:

CONSTITUTIONAL: No fevers and no weight loss.

CARDIOVASCULAR: No heart attack but history of high blood pressure.

RESPIRATORY: No asthma or cancer.

GASTROINTESTINAL: No gastric ulcer or gastro-esophageal reflux disease.

GENITOURINARY: No kidney stones or urinary tract infections.

MUSCULOSKELETAL: No arthritis or fractures.

DERMATOLOGIC: Obviously has multiple skin eruptions.

NEUROLOGIC: No seizures or strokes.

PSYCHIATRIC: No depression.

ENDOCRINE: No diabetes or thyroid disease.

PHYSICAL EXAMINATION:

He has multiple lesions on his right upper extremity including a 2 × 2-cm lesion on his elbow, a 2 × 2-cm lesion on the right wrist, and a 3 × 3-cm lesion on the hairline of his back. They are all raised lesions, well-circumscribed with skin discoloration.

ASSESSMENT: Senile dermatosis

PLAN: Prescribed medication. We will see him in approximately one to two weeks in follow-up.

ICD-10-CM Code(s) _____

CASE STUDY 4

HISTORY OF PRESENT ILLNESS: This 77-year-old Type I diabetes patient who is brought to the hospital emergency room (ER) by paramedics after she had been confused, weak, having diarrhea, having fallen, unable to stand, and poor appetite. The patient is unable to give a decent history at this time because she is very slow to respond and not accurate in her responses. She is unsure when the symptoms started. Most of the history has been obtained from the paramedics, ER notes, and currently there is no old chart available to me. She has also been noticed to have leg redness and swelling bilaterally. The patient also says that she is on chronic oxygen therapy.

PAST MEDICAL HISTORY: Includes multiple medical problems: hypertension, coronary artery disease, status post CABG, congestive heart failure, osteoarthritis, depression, chronic renal insufficiency, baseline creatinine unknown, acute inflammatory arthritis history, pseudogout, and protein malnutrition.

CURRENT MEDICATIONS:

- Allopurinol 50 mg daily
- Alphagan eye drops, 1 drop twice daily each eye
- Aspirin 81 mg daily
- Colchicine 0.6 mg daily
- Lantus insulin 55 units subq daily
- Lexapro 20 mg in the morning
- Insulin sliding scale with NovoLog
- Prednisone 5 mg daily
- Senna tablets 2 tablets daily
- Torasemide 50 mg twice daily
- Zocor 20 mg daily

FAMILY HISTORY: Mother and father deceased. Has one sibling with diabetes.

SOCIAL HISTORY: She has a sister and a brother.

REVIEW OF SYSTEMS: Unreliable secondary to current status. However, her extended care facility knows she has had fever and chills, positive cough, nausea, and diarrhea. The patient has no allergies. Other systems are negative.

PHYSICAL EXAMINATION:

GENERAL: She is awake, alert, confused, oriented ×2. Not in distress and mildly short of breath.

HEENT: Her extraocular movements are intact. No jaundice. Throat is clear.

NECK: No JVD, lymphadenopathy, or masses.

LUNGS: Clear.

HEART: Regular rate and rhythm. Normal S1 and S2, no S3. No murmur. There is central scar of old surgery on the chest.

ABDOMEN: Obese, nontender. Umbilicus is everted. I cannot appreciate any distinct fluid thrill. There are no bruits.

EXTREMITIES: Shows erythema and redness of the left lower extremity and swelling 2+, and there are open erosions at three or four spaces on the left lower extremity, which are superficial. It is warm and tender.

NEUROLOGIC: She is moving her extremities. She does seem to have a tremor of upper extremities and periodically gets mild spasm of the upper extremity muscles, too. Cranial nerves seem to be intact. Facial movements are slow. There is flattening of her expressions. Gait was not tested due to her current status. She is moving lower extremities. There is no focal deficit.

LABORATORY: Her lab data upon admission shows a white count of 16.99 and hemoglobin 11.9. Platelets are normal. Electrolytes: Sodium 136; calcium 9.6; BUN 154; creatinine 3.6; glucose 133. Urinalysis shows three to four WBCs. She does seem to be making urine. There is urine in the bag.

ASSESSMENT AND PLAN: The patient comes in with infection, cellulitis, severely exacerbating. I will have to check her baseline creatinine. However, the BUN seems like she does have acute component of renal failure on her chronic renal insufficiency. Will check renal ultrasounds. I am going to put her on Primaxin IV for cellulitis of her extremities. Blood cultures are pending. Will use fall precautions. I am going to hold her diuretics. She needs fluids intravenously for rehydration. Will check stool for *Clostridium difficile*. Will hold her Lexapro and Allopurinol. Will continue her Prednisone. The reason for her Prednisone is not clear to me. Most likely it has been given secondary to her chronic arthritis, inflammatory variety. However, it probably is contributing to worsening of her sugars. She is not hypotensive. I do not feel we need to give her IV steroids at this time unless and until blood pressure becomes an issue. We will also take a BNP, liver panel, calcium, magnesium, phosphorus next draw. Also will check 24-hour urine for protein and creatinine clearance. I will place her on remote telemetry. Check serum protein electrophoresis and urine amino electrophoresis. Continue her eye drops. Hopefully with treatment for her infection, the delirium will clear. Will

continue her insulin. Reduce the dose of Lantus to 40 units and put her on sliding scale and give her DVT prophylaxis with Heparin subq. Will watch patient for signs of toxicity. Will contact Nephrology and have them follow the patient as well.

ICD-10-CM Code(s) _____

CASE STUDY 5

HISTORY OF PRESENT ILLNESS: New basal cell carcinoma (BCC) right nose treated with Mohs surgery in Florida two months ago. The patient now has a scaly spot on the right ear, which is irritating.

REVIEW OF SYSTEMS:

GENERAL: Denies fatigue, malaise, weight loss, fever.

HEENT: Denies visual problems, sinus symptoms, headache, glaucoma.

CARDIOVASCULAR: Denies chest pain, SOB with exertion, palpitations, murmur, leg swelling.

RESPIRATORY: Denies cough, SOB, hemoptysis.

GI: Denies nausea, vomiting, diarrhea, change in bowel habit, melena.

GU: Denies kidney problems, problems urinating, UTI.

MUSCULOSKELETAL: Denies joint pain or muscle weakness.

NEUROPSYCHIATRIC: Denies seizures, memory problems, depression.

ENDOCRINE: Denies cold or heat intolerance, polyuria, polydipsia.

ALLERGY/IMMUNOLOGY: Denies unusual allergic reactions, asthma, hay fever.

HEMATOLOGIC: Denies unusual bleeding, bruising, anemia, lymph node enlargement.

INTEGUMENT: See History of Present Illness.

PHYSICAL EXAMINATION: General appearance: Well developed, well nourished, no acute distress. Eyes: Normal conjunctiva and eyelids. Extremities: Digits normal; joints with full range of motion; nails normal. Skin: Scalp and body hair: Male pattern alopecia. Head and face: BCC right ear.

ASSESSMENT: BCC right ear. Removed lesion and sent to Pathology. The patient was counseled concerning skin cancer, monthly self-exams, and the significant risk of developing new skin cancers because the patient has already had skin cancer. The patient should call if he identifies any new or unusual spots or moles and return sooner than his scheduled appointment.

ICD-10-CM Code(s) _____

ICD-10-CM Official Coding Guidelines for the Musculoskeletal System and Connective Tissue

The following chapter-specific guidelines apply to Chapter 13 of the ICD-10-CM codebook (Diseases of the Musculoskeletal System and Connective Tissue). Most codes in Chapter 13 have site and laterality designation. The site can represent the bone, joint, or muscle. Site designations for the limbs are:

- Upper arm
- Lower arm
- Upper and lower leg
  - Humerus
  - Ulna
  - Femur
  - Tibia
  - Fibula

When coding diseases of the musculoskeletal system and connective tissue, the following guidelines apply:

- For conditions where more than one bone, joint, or muscle are involved, the multiple sites are reported.
- If the category does not have a multiple site code and more than one bone, joint, or muscle is involved, each is reported separately.
- When a condition is described as arm or leg without further elaboration as to whether the site is upper or lower, the code for the upper arm or lower leg should be used.
- When the condition identifies more than one bone, joint, or muscle, a code for multiple sites is selected.

- If a multiple site code is not available and multiple sites are involved, each site is coded separately.

Many musculoskeletal conditions are a result of previous injury or trauma to a site or are recurrent conditions. Bone, joint, or muscle conditions that are the result of a healed injury; recurrent bone, joint, or muscle conditions; and chronic conditions are usually located in Chapter 13. Any current, acute injury should be coded to the appropriate injury code from Chapter 19, Injury, Poisoning, and Certain Other Consequences of External Causes. If it is difficult to determine from the documentation in the record which code is best to describe a condition, query the provider.

CODING OF PATHOLOGIC FRACTURES

If the patient is receiving care for an active treatment of the fracture, the seventh character "A" is used. Examples of *active* treatment include:

- surgical treatment,
- an emergency department encounter, and
- evaluation and treatment by a new physician.

The seventh character "A" is to be used as long as the patient is receiving active treatment for a fracture.

The seventh character "D" (*subsequent*) is to be reported for encounters after the patient has completed active treatment (healing phase).

The other seventh characters, listed under each subcategory in the Tabular List, are to be used for subsequent encounters for treatment of problems associated with healing, such as malunions, nonunions, and sequelae. Care for complications of surgical treatment for fracture repairs during the healing or recovery phase should be coded with the appropriate complication codes. Traumatic fractures are coded in Chapter 19 of ICD-10-CM.

OSTEOPOROSIS

Osteoporosis is a systemic condition, meaning that all bones of the musculoskeletal system are affected. When coding osteoporosis, the following guidelines apply:

- Codes in category M80, Osteoporosis with current pathological fracture, are for patients who have a current pathologic fracture at the time of an encounter.
- Codes in category M80 identify the site of the fracture.

- A code from category M80, not a traumatic fracture code, should be used for any patient with known osteoporosis who suffers a fracture, even if the patient had a minor fall or trauma and that fall or trauma would not usually break a normal, healthy bone.

- For codes in category M81, Osteoporosis without current pathological fracture, site is not a specified component.

- The site codes under category M81 identify the site of the fracture, not the osteoporosis.

- Category M81 codes are used for patients with osteoporosis who do not currently have a pathologic fracture due to the osteoporosis, even if they have had a fracture in the past.

- For patients with a history of osteoporosis fractures, status code Z87.310, Personal history of (healed) osteoporosis fracture, should be reported as a secondary diagnosis with a code from category M81.

- In certain conditions, the bone may be affected at the upper or lower end (eg, avascular necrosis of bone). Although the portion of the bone affected may be at the joint, the site designation will be the bone, not the joint.

It is time to build skill and knowledge by coding the following exercises relative to the musculoskeletal system and connective tissue. Make certain to reference the ICD-10-CM codebook and the ICD-10-CM Official Guidelines for Coding and Reporting, along with the instructional notes, when coding these conditions.

Diseases of the Musculoskeletal System and Connective Tissue (M00-M99)

CASE STUDY 6

HISTORY OF PRESENT ILLNESS: This established patient presents with right shoulder pain. Her pain on the 0-10 pain scale is 8. The pain radiates from the bicep to the right scapula and sometimes the pain goes down her arm. The pain has been bothering her for about four months but over the last few days has worsened and she cannot sleep. The patient denies recent trauma, no pain in other extremities. She has been taking aspirin for the pain.

PHYSICAL EXAMINATION:

GENERAL: Well-developed, well-nourished, 34-year-old female who appears in distress.

MUSCULOSKELETAL: Grip strength equal bilaterally. Reflexes equal bilaterally. She has some tenderness on the right shoulder at the head of the biceps. Also she was tender over the subscapular bursa right scapula. Minimal positive impingement sign. Pulses and sensation good.

CARDIOVASCULAR: Regular heart rate and rhythm.

PULMONARY: Clear to auscultation and percussion.

ABDOMEN: Soft, nontender; no splenomegaly.

ASSESSMENT: Rheumatoid bursitis right shoulder.

PLAN: Gave injection of Depo-Medrol 80 mg intramuscularly. Prescribed Oxycodone for pain. If patient not feeling better in a week, will send her to outpatient physical therapy. She is to use heating pad twice a day to help with pain relief.

ICD-10-CM Code(s) _____

CASE STUDY 7

SUBJECTIVE: This normally active, healthy 57-year-old female patient presents to the office today for evaluation of hip pain after falling at home out of her bed. She reports her right hip became immediately sore and painful with difficulty bearing weight on her right side. No other complaints or injuries reported. Patient took three Advil after the fall this morning with limited relief.

OBJECTIVE: Patient appears to be in mild distress. She ambulated to the exam room slowly favoring her right hip/leg. Blood pressure is 145/82. HEENT within normal limits. Lungs clear. Abdomen soft, normal bowel sounds. Patient is not taking any medication. Musculoskeletal exam revealed right hip tender to touch with bruising. Walking is painful. Patient did drive herself to the office with some discomfort. X rays taken in office today ruled out fracture.

ASSESSMENT: Superficial injury to right hip.

PLAN: Patient to limit physical activity for two weeks, apply alternative heat/cold during the next 72 hours, and continue with over-the-counter medications as directed by the manufacturer. Patient instructed to call office if pain worsens. Patient declines pain medication at this time. I anticipate a full recovery. No fractures noted on X ray.

ICD-10-CM Code(s) _____

CASE STUDY 8

A 35-year-old patient presents with right shoulder joint pain.

HISTORY OF PRESENT ILLNESS: Shoulder pain present for five months. Occurred suddenly and noticed when wearing new shoes. Reports burning pain. Rated as 6/10 in severity right now and 8/10 in severity all the time. Occurs constantly.

REVIEW OF SYSTEMS: Constitutional: Denies shaking chills, fever, night sweats, and weight change. General health stated as good. Cardiovascular: Denies angina, cardiac arrhythmia, and hypertension. Respiratory: Denies productive cough and dyspnea. Gastrointestinal: Denies hepatitis, reflux, and ulcer disease. Genitourinary: Denies dysuria, incontinence, and kidney disease. Musculoskeletal: Denies poor balance, herniated disc, and limitations of movement. Skin: Denies rash and ulcers. Neurologic: Denies seizures and stroke. Endocrine: Denies diabetes and thyroid disease. Hematology/Lymph: Denies bleeding/clotting disorder and neoplasms.

MEDICATIONS: Darvocet N 50 mg.

ALLERGIES: Seafood (makes him cry); Amoxicillin (gives him a rash).

PHYSICAL EXAMINATION: Constitutional: Appears healthy and well developed. Speech is appropriate. Head/Face: Normal on inspection. Facial strength normal. CV: Extremities: No cyanosis, edema, or mottling. Head/Neck: Inspection/Palpation: Head is erect; symmetric. No hypertrophy. Spine: Inspection/Palpation: Spinal contour is normal. Increased pelvic tilt. Stability: No obvious instability. Range of Motion: Full ROM left and right shoulders. Skin: No rashes, lesions, or ecchymosis. Neurological: Alert and oriented ×3. Displays distrustfulness during encounter. Psychological: Patient's attitude is cooperative. Judgment is realistic. Insight is appropriate.

ASSESSMENT: Joint pain, right shoulder.

PLAN: X ray: shoulder, one view, RT.

ICD-10-CM Code(s) _____

CASE STUDY 9

PREOPERATIVE DIAGNOSIS: Multilevel degenerative disc disease of lumbar spine, severe spinal stenosis of L4-5 and L5-S1.

POSTOPERATIVE DIAGNOSIS: Same.

INDICATIONS: This patient is a 64-year-old female who has osteoporosis unresolved with conservative treatment. She had a hysterectomy at age 40 and was not diligent about taking calcium supplements.

PROCEDURE: Intravenous access was established in the preoperative holding area. Preoperative intravenous antibiotics were given. The patient was placed in the prone position on the fluoroscopy table. The back was prepped and draped in the usual sterile manner. The exact spinal level was identified by fluoroscopy and the needle was passed to the transverse process. The depth was noted and the needle was redirected to pass inferior and approximately 1 cm anterior to the transverse process. Following this, 1 cc of Omnipaque was injected to verify positioning in the epidural and paravertebral space and outline the course of the spinal nerve into the epidural space. After this, 80 mg Depo-Medrol, 2 cc 2% Xylocaine, and 2 cc normal saline with 100 mcg fentanyl was slowly injected at the left L4-5 and L5-S1 with reproduction and relief of the patient's symptoms being recorded. After this, 80 mg Depo-Medrol, 2 cc 2% Xylocaine, and 2 cc normal saline were slowly injected at the right L4-5 and L5-S1 with reproduction and relief of the patient's symptoms being recorded. The patient was returned to the recovery room in satisfactory condition, discharged after being stable, and will follow up in an outpatient setting.

ICD-10-CM Code(s) _____

CASE STUDY 10

This well-groomed, established patient presents to renew her blood pressure medication and have blood work done. The patient has bilateral knee pain, tender and swollen. The patient was doing yard work and states she was on her knees too long. Patient denies shortness of breath or chest pain.

PHYSICAL EXAMINATION: Height 5 feet, 2 inches; weight 125 lbs; blood pressure 140/70; heart rate 72. Head and neck are within normal limits. Chest is clear. CVS is normal. Knee pain bilaterally, and knees appear swollen.

ASSESSMENT AND PLAN: Hypertension; benign, bilateral knee pain. Hydrochlorothiazide, 50 mg, once a day, #100; and Calan SR 240 mg, once a day, sample was given. The patient will return for electrocardiogram (EKG) next week. Also Voltaren, 75 mg once bid, sample given. The patient is non-compliant. She is not exercising and not dieting. Advised patient to continue low-fat diet.

ICD-10-CM Code(s) _____

CASE STUDY 11

REASON FOR CONSULT: The patient is a very pleasant 59-year-old female whom I have been asked to consult by Dr Haywood for multiple medical conditions, signs, and symptoms as outlined below. Dr Haywood specifically requested information regarding the perioperative management of these conditions.

HISTORY OF PRESENT ILLNESS:

1. Acute fracture of right hip. The history, examination, and diagnosis are well documented in Dr Haywood's note of today, which I have reviewed. In brief, the patient injured her right hip in 198x when she fell through a ceiling. She notes a slow deterioration since then. On 08/28/20xx she saw a chiropractor and while he was manipulating her right hip, she heard a pop. The pain has been severely worse since that time. She was admitted to Duncan Memorial Hospital earlier this week after Orthopedics diagnosed a fracture of the hip.

2. Hypertension. Currently taking Zestril 5 mg po daily and Coreg 12.5 mg po bid. Blood pressure has been well controlled recently per patient. She is tolerating these medications well. She denies any history of myocardial infarction, congestive heart failure, cerebrovascular disease, or known renal insufficiency.

3. Fibromyalgia. I have no records supporting the details of the diagnosis; however, patient reports chronic pain that has been reasonably controlled through exercise and diet.

4. History of hyponatremia with a sodium to 129. She was on hydrochlorothiazide and this was discontinued with an improvement in her hyponatremia upon admission to Duncan Memorial this week; however, she was noted to be hypoatremic again. At that time her Paxil was discontinued as hyponatremia is a potential side effect of this medication.

5. Hypothyroid. Well-controlled with Synthroid.

6. History of severe depression for which the patient sees a psychiatrist. Most recently on Paxil, Remeron, Zyprexa, and Ambien.

7. Insomnia. Ambien and Trazodone have allowed her to have generally good sleep up until she fractured her hip as described above.

8. Allergic rhinitis. The patient reports allergies to mold, as well as other seasonal allergies for which Flonase has worked reasonably well.

9. Dyspepsia. Nexium has been added empirically recently.

ALLERGIES: Codeine, Prednisone, hydrochlorothia.

MEDICATIONS:

- Synthroid 1.233 mg po q am
- Wellbutrin SR 150 mg po tid at 7 am, 11 am, and 3 pm
- Valium 2 mg po bid
- Zestril 5 mg po daily
- Coreg 12.5 mg po bid
- Nexium 40 mg po bid
- Remeron 60 mg po qhs
- Trazodone 100 mg po qhs
- Ambien 10 mg po qhs
- Zyprexa 2.5 mg po qhs
- Flonase one spray each nostril qhs
- Colace 100 mg po bid

INJURIES/ACCIDENTS: The patient fell through ceiling as noted above in 198x.

FAMILY HISTORY: No history of untoward reaction to anesthesia in her family.

SOCIAL HISTORY: The patient is a nun with the Sisters of St. Francis. She is unmarried and lives in Miami. No tobacco or alcohol use.

REVIEW OF SYSTEMS:

GENERAL: Negative for recent weight change or fatigue. No fever or chills.

SKIN: Complains of itching since starting on morphine yesterday. No rashes.

HEAD: Denies headache or head pain.

EYES: No recent change in vision, blurred vision, or eye pain.

EARS: No recent change in hearing, ear pain, or ear drainage.

SINUSES: Sensitivity to mold as listed above.

MOUTH/THROAT: No sores in mouth or throat or difficulty swallowing.

NECK: No fullness or tenderness in her neck.

RESPIRATORY: Denies shortness of breath, cough, or productive cough.

CARDIAC: Denies chest pain, heaviness, or tightness with exercise or climbing stairs. No syncope, presyncope, orthopnea, or paroxysmal, nocturnal dyspnea.

GI: Denies nausea, vomiting, abdominal pain, abdominal tenderness, diarrhea, or blood in her stool. She had had constipation and states that she has been immobilized with her hip. She has had no bowel movement in the past four days.

GU: Denies urgency or dysuria.

PERIPHERAL VASCULAR: Negative for claudication.

MUSCULOSKELETAL: As above in history of present illness.

NEUROLOGIC: Negative for stroke, transient ischemic attack, fainting, blackouts, seizures.

ENDOCRINE: Thyroid disease as above. No known diabetes.

PSYCHIATRIC: As above. The patient reports she has been well controlled and that her mood has been fabulous recently.

PHYSICAL EXAMINATION:

GENERAL: Well-developed, well-nourished female in no acute distress. Weight: 159 pounds. BP: 148/81. Respirations: 16 and unlabored.

HEENT: Normocephalic, atraumatic. Oropharynx is clear with good dentition; PERRL.

NECK: Supple. No lymphadenopathy or thyromegaly noted. No bruits over the carotid arteries.

CHEST: Clear to auscultation, bilaterally, with good air movement. No focal wheezes or rales.

CARDIAC: Regular rate and rhythm with normal S1, S2. No murmur, gallop, or rub. Nondisplaced PMI.

ABDOMEN: Obese, soft, nontender, and nondistended with good bowel movements. No hepatosplenomegaly, masses, or bruits were noted.

EXTREMITIES: Without clubbing, cyanosis, or edema.

MENTAL STATUS: The patient is awake, alert, oriented, pleasant, and answers questions appropriately. Normal mood and affect.

SKIN: Warm and dry.

ASSESSMENT AND PLAN:

1. Acute right hip fracture. Anticipate need for total hip replacement tomorrow.

2. Hypertension. Adequate control with above medications. These will be continued and patient will be monitored closely during her hospitalization. Adjust accordingly during hemodynamic status and perioperative time frame.

3. Hypothyroid. Continue Synthroid daily.

4. Dyspepsia. Continue empiric Nexium 40 mg daily.

5. Fibromyalgia. Comfort measures only during her hospitalization. No specific intervention.

6. Severe debilitating depression now well controlled. Continue Zyprexa, Trazodone, Remeron, and Wellbutrin. I agreed with holding the Paxil. Watch for changes in patient's mental status around the time of surgery.

7. Acute constipation with no bowel movement times four days. Add glycerin suppository now.

8. Allergic rhinitis. Continue Flonase.

9. Insomnia. Continue Ambien and Trazodone.

10. Generalized anxiety. Continue Valium 2 mg bid.

11. Hyponatremia. Monitor closely during her hospitalization. Overall, this patient has relatively mild to moderate risk factors for significant perioperative morbidity and/or mortality. She is clinically stable and I did not identify any condition that would prohibit her from proceeding with surgery.

ICD-10-CM Code(s) _____

CASE STUDY 12

Ms Warren is an 83-year-old female who has had a previous right total knee replacement and who now complains of right shoulder pain that she has had for quite some time now. She states that her shoulder pain started approximately six to seven years ago after a fall on the ice, and since that time, the pain has been progressive. She did have a full evaluation at that time, and there was no evidence of any fractures or dislocations. Her main complaint right now is both decrease in motion especially with cross arm adduction and also pain about the shoulder. She has had no other conservative measurement including injections. She does state that she has pain in the shoulder almost constantly and that she does have pain when sleeping on that shoulder at night. She does find that she is starting to be limited by the pain and also loss of range of motion of that shoulder.

CURRENT MEDICATIONS: Premarin, potassium, and Maxzide.

ALLERGIES: Sulfa.

PAST MEDICAL HISTORY: High blood pressure and arthritis.

PAST SURGICAL HISTORY: Right total knee replacement done on June 22, 20xx, in addition to a hysterectomy.

FAMILY HISTORY: She has a history of diabetes on her mother's side and also a family history of arthritis.

SOCIAL HISTORY: Patient denies smoking. She states an alcohol history of approximately one to two drinks per week, and she does not exercise regularly. She does not need assistance with daily activities and does not use any type of assistance device for walking.

REVIEW OF SYSTEMS: Negative for fever, weight gain, chills. Negative for nausea and vomiting. No other musculoskeletal problems.

PHYSICAL EXAMINATION: Patient is 5 feet, 2 inches tall. She weighs 165 pounds. There was no tenderness to palpation of her cervical spine, and she had painless range of motion of her cervical spine with a negative Spurling maneuver. There were no rashes, erythema, or ecchymosis about the right shoulder. She also had 2+ pulses distally in her radial artery. She did have mild tenderness to palpation over the acromioclavicular joint, and mild tenderness to palpation over the biceps tendon and also laterally over the greater tuberosity. Her active forward flexion was to 150 degrees,

external rotation with the arm at the side was to 45 degrees, and internal rotation was only to the sacrum. Her strength, she had 4+/5 strength throughout her rotator cuff musculature. She had full and painless range of motion of her right elbow.

IMAGING STUDIES: Three views of the right shoulder were obtained. AP, scapular Y, and axillary lateral view of the right shoulder show joint space narrowing of the glenohumeral joint with osteophyte formation off of the inferior aspect of the humerus. The humeral head appears to be well located on the glenoid and the axillary lateral view with no significant posterior erosion of the glenoid itself.

ASSESSMENT: Primary localized osteoarthritis, right shoulder

PLAN: The nature and etiology of the diagnosis was explained to Ms Warren. We stated at this time that she does have arthritis of the shoulder and whether this was hastened after the fall she had on that side, it is difficult to say. From her clinical examination today, she still has fairly decent range of motion except that she has lost a significant amount of internal rotation. The X rays also show clear-cut evidence of joint space narrowing and osteophyte formation on the humeral head. Treatment plans would include conservative measures with a shoulder injection and also physical therapy for some strengthening exercises versus a total hemiarthroplasty replacement. At this time, she would like to proceed with some of the conservative measures first, and she was given a cortisone injection of her shoulder through an anterior approach with which she had relief of 75% of her pain. She was given a prescription for physical therapy, and we will see her back in the office in six weeks for a repeat clinical evaluation.

ICD-10-CM Code(s) _____

CASE STUDY 13

This is a 53-year-old, male aircraft mechanic who has had increasing pain in his left knee since January of 20xx. He has been working as an aircraft mechanic for some time. He is working security as a second job. He has had difficulty with knee pain, which came on slowly. He had been on Relafen for one week, which has helped. He has a history of knee arthroscopy back in September of 20xx. His pain is currently occasional but not serious. He stands on his feet all day which aggravates the knee. It gets puffy on the sides and stiff. He has had arthroscopy with meniscectomy in the past. He has unlimited walking activity. He has difficulty with squatting and twisting activities.

PAST MEDICAL HISTORY: Past medical history is otherwise negative.

MEDICATIONS: Current medications include Nembutone and Relafen.

ALLERGIES: He has no known allergies.

PHYSICAL EXAMINATION: Patient is 6 feet, 0 inches tall and weighs 190 pounds. Heart rate is 56 and regular. He ambulates with an antalgic gait mildly to the left. He is tender over the medial compartment. He has mild synovitis and trace effusion. There is no motor loss. He has normal pulses. He has no ligamentous instability. There is no patellofemoral crepitus. There is no lag. There is no motor loss. There is no atrophy. Skin is intact.

X RAYS: Radiographs show early degenerative changes throughout with preservation of the joint space. I see no fracture or dislocation.

ASSESSMENT: Left knee early degenerative changes

PLAN: I have recommended lateral heel wedges, activity modifications, intermittent corticosteroid injections, and continue on Relafen. Should his symptoms persist, we will consider repeat imaging.

ICD-10-CM Code(s) _____

CASE STUDY 14

Michael is a 58-year-old man who presents to our office today for evaluation of right knee pain. Michael dates his problems back to 196x when he suffered a football injury. At that time, he had an open medial meniscectomy. Over the years, he has developed progressive pain and a progressive varus deformity associated with his right knee. The problem has now reached a point where it is a significant one for him, interfering with significant elements of his day-to-day life and quality of life.

He categorizes his problem as marked and continuous with serious limitations. He experiences moderate pain each day while walking. He does not require any ambulatory aids for walking and can walk short distances without stopping due to pain. He climbs stairs normally with a rail. He has difficulty reaching his feet, shoes, and socks. He has moderate pain at rest. He reports a severe limp without support. No assistance is required for getting out of bed and he is unable to sit one hour on any chair. He is able to use public transportation.

PAST SURGICAL HISTORY: Arthroscopic surgery of left knee.

CURRENT MEDICATIONS: None.

FAMILY HISTORY: None listed. His mother is alive and his father died at the age of 32 from an accident.

SOCIAL HISTORY: He is married. He admits to consuming 6 to 12 alcoholic beverages per week and denies tobacco use. He has an office job.

REVIEW OF SYSTEMS: Positive for lungs: Asthma and wheezing. Negative for fever, weight loss, fatigue, weakness, eyes, ear, nose, throat, heart, circulation, digestive tract, kidney, urinary, skin, endocrine, neurologic, psychiatric, blood, lymph, and musculoskeletal.

PHYSICAL EXAMINATION: Height 70.5 inches. Weight 232 pounds. Michael is well developed, well nourished, and alert. Oriented and appropriate. He walks with evidence of a varus deformity of the right knee with a mild varus thrust. His skin condition is normal. He has no gross neurologic deficits. He has easily palpable pulses in his feet. Passive range of motion of his knee, 5-degree flexion deformity with further flexion to 120. Ligamentous examination is normal. His hip examination is normal.

RADIOGRAPHS: Weight-bearing radiographs of his right knee were obtained and reviewed. These show evidence of advanced medial compartment osteoarthritis. On the weight-bearing AP radiographs he has bone-on-bone articulation, subchondral sclerosis, and irregularity of articular surfaces.

ASSESSMENT: Advanced osteoarthritis, right knee with varus deformity as described above.

RECOMMENDATION: Right total knee arthroplasty.

PLAN: Michael's right knee has reached a point where he finds it unacceptable from the pain, function, and quality-of-life standpoint and he wishes to proceed with a right total knee arthroplasty. I have described to him the nature of total knee replacement surgery, the risks, benefits, rehab, and expected outcome as well as answering all of his questions. We have provided him with our written educational materials regarding total knee replacement surgery and we will begin making plans for his surgery.

ICD-10-CM Code(s) _____

CASE STUDY 15

Mr James is a 54-year-old sales executive here in Mount Randall who presents to us with posterior ankle pain that he has had for approximately a year. The patient has been fairly active in that he walks on a treadmill and walks outside fairly extensively, although has been recently limited by his posterior heel pain. The right Achilles tendon became symptomatic approximately a year ago and has been intermittent and persistent and somewhat limiting in activity. However, it resolved until the left side became symptomatic approximately four to five weeks ago and has prohibited him from doing any activity over the last three weeks due to the severe pain in the left Achilles. He states that the pain can be worse in the morning then loosens up, and then after some activity or ambulation, the tendon begins to ache. He states that the pain is localized just above the tendon insertion on his heel, again, bilaterally but most recently along the left side. The patient has taken Aleve and ibuprofen on a prn basis somewhat sporadically although he did take some for a two-week time frame without much alleviation of symptoms.

PAST MEDICAL HISTORY: Negative with the exception of some mildly elevated blood pressure that was diagnosed by his primary physician approximately two and half months ago, which is not currently being treated.

PAST SURGICAL HISTORY: The patient has had three prior right knee surgeries in 196x, 198x, and 198x. The first two surgeries involved torn meniscal cartilage and the third surgery in 198x was an open reduction, internal fixation of a patella fracture.

CURRENT MEDICATIONS: None.

ALLERGIES: No known allergies.

FAMILY HISTORY: Grandmother has history of diabetes, mother had colon cancer, and father has rheumatoid arthritis. Mother and father are both still living.

SOCIAL HISTORY: He is married with two children. Does not smoke tobacco and occasionally drinks alcohol. He is a sales executive for local insurance company.

REVIEW OF SYSTEMS: The patient has a prior history of pulmonary embolism with his second knee surgery requiring six weeks of anticoagulation but does not currently take any anticoagulation medication. Otherwise, review of systems is negative.

PHYSICAL EXAMINATION: The patient is a well-developed and well-nourished man who has a normal gait. On examination of his right foot and ankle, he has minimal tenderness to palpation along the Achilles tendon. However, he does have a fusiform enlargement of the Achilles tendon approximately 2 cm proximal to the insertion on the calcaneus. The length of the fusiform swelling is approximately 2 to 3 cm long and is mildly tender to palpation. The Achilles tendon is intact throughout its length all the way to the insertion without any palpable defect. There is no tenderness anterior to the tendon in the retrocalcaneal bursal area. He has normal strength in the right lower extremity with dorsiflexion and plantar flexion, 5/5. He has no pain with plantar flexion against resistance, and no pain with active plantar flexion against resistance. He has a small fusiform enlargement of the Achilles tendon, again, at approximately 2 cm proximal to insertion. However, the left Achilles tendinous enlargement is tender to palpation more significantly on passive stretching and during passive dorsiflexion. Again, there is no retrocalcaneal bursal tenderness to palpation. The patient does not have any bony tenderness along the calcaneus or either malleoli.

RADIOGRAPHS: Bilateral AP, lateral, and Mortise view of the ankle X rays were obtained for the diagnosis of chronic Achilles tendonitis. The right ankle showed some mild ossification along the interosseous membrane between the tibia and fibula distally consistent with an old ankle injury. Mortise was well maintained. On the lateral view of the right ankle, there was a small osteophyte at the posterior talocalcaneal joint but there was no evidence of any significant spur or osteophyte formation along the Achilles tendon. Radiographs of the left ankle demonstrated again a normal mortise without any significant osteophyte formation along the Achilles tendon on the lateral view and there does not appear to be any significant tibiotalar to talocalcaneal arthritis on the lateral view or the AP and mortise views of the ankles bilaterally.

ASSESSMENT AND PLAN: Chronic bilateral Achilles tendonitis/tendinosis, left greater than right. My impression is that Mr James has bilateral Achilles tendonitis and tendinosis, certainly a combination of degenerative changes that is exacerbated with activity. His physical examination corresponds to the watershed area of decreased vascularity approximately 2 cm proximal to insertion of the calcaneus. Recommendations for treatment include rest with an ankle-foot orthosis (AFO) for the most symptomatic left side. I have encouraged him to wear the AFO for approximately two weeks to rest the Achilles tendon, and in addition he will take anti-inflammatory medication. He has been taking Aleve currently, and I recommended he take that daily for two weeks' time. Finally, the patient will have physical therapy for instruction on heel cords stretching exercises and any further modalities recommended by the therapist to decrease the inflammation of the Achilles tendon. With this combination of conservative care, we will see how he progresses and we will see him back in six weeks' time for further follow-up. If he gets no relief from these conservative measures, we will consider an MRI of his more symptomatic side at that time. We discussed at length the physiologies involved in this process and its chronic nature related to degenerative changes. We also discussed that this is certainly not a condition which we prefer to operate on, but we will consider that should all conservative measures fail.

ICD-10-CM Code(s) _____

CASE STUDY 16

The patient is a 70-year-old retired physician who continues to work part-time, who presents today with complaints of intermittent bilateral knee pain, left worse than right. This is a new patient to our office. The patient states that she has a 15- to 20-year history of bilateral knee pain and osteoarthritis that she treats with intermittent nonsteroidal anti-inflammatories and activity modification. She states that she has had a recent flare of pain on the medial side of the left knee that has been present for the past three to four weeks. She has not had any injections to the left knee. She currently takes one Naprosyn 500 mg a day and when the pain occurs intermittently she takes glucosamine sulphate as well. She denies any mechanical symptoms. She states it is worse when she bends or flexes the knee. The pain is isolated in the medial side. She also states that she has been diagnosed with degenerative joint disease of the spine and she does have some occasional back pain.

PAST MEDICAL HISTORY: Significant for diabetes, osteoarthritis, and hepatitis B from a blood transfusion she received from a C-section in 197x.

PAST SURGICAL HISTORY: She had a C-section in 197x and an additional C-section in 197x, otherwise negative.

CURRENT MEDICATIONS: Theo-Dur, Loratadine, Synthroid, Naprosyn, glucosamine sulfate, Metformin, and calcium carbonate.

ALLERGIES: The patient has no known drug allergies.

SOCIAL HISTORY: She is married and her husband is a pediatric neurologist at Valley Hospital. She does not smoke or drink.

FAMILY HISTORY: Mother died at age 39 from unknown causes. Father died at age 53 from heart disease.

REVIEW OF SYSTEMS: Significant for the musculoskeletal abnormalities listed above and also positive for asthma and otherwise review of systems is negative.

PHYSICAL EXAMINATION: She is 59 inches tall. She weighs 174 pounds. The patient is a slightly obese female who walks with a normal gait without any evidence of antalgia. On physical examination of her knees, her right knee has no tenderness to palpation. She has excellent range of motion from full extension to 140 degrees of flexion. She has no ligamentous laxity with varus or valgus or anterior and posterior stressing. She has no patellofemoral crepitus and no effusion or warmth to the right knee.

Examination of the left knee demonstrates no effusion, no warmth. She has a mild tenderness to palpation along the medial joint line but only in significant flexion past 90 degrees. She has range of motion from full extension to 140 degrees. She has no ligamentous instability to varus or valgus stressing. She has no pain with McMurray compression meniscus signs. She is also stable to anterior and posterior testing of the knee. She has no tenderness about the pes anserine bursa bilaterally to palpation and again she has no patellar crepitus on the left side as well.

Examination of her hips with internal and external rotation does not demonstrate any groin pain or knee pain with those maneuvers and also with full flexion of the hips.

X RAYS: X rays taken in the office today were bilateral standing AP, 45-degree flexion views, bilateral lateral X rays, and Merchant views of the patella. X rays demonstrate mild early degenerative changes in the medial compartment of both knees, left worse than right. There is subchondral sclerosis and decreased joint space, again more pronounced in the left and small osteophytes along the medial proximal tibia. There is no evidence of any vascular necrosis and no other abnormalities noted.

ASSESSMENT: Medial side knee pain with early localized osteoarthritis of the medial compartment, left knee.

PLAN: I discussed with the patient that the conservative treatment at this point should be the mainstay treatment. She has not been taking anti-inflammatory dosage of her Naprosyn, so I encouraged to bump up her dose of Naprosyn to two tablets a day for the next two weeks to gain the anti-inflammatory effect of the medication. In addition, I emphasized quadriceps-strengthening exercises and reiterated her to do that on a regular basis. After discussion of intra-articular corticosteroid injection, she did not feel that that was appropriate at this time, but we will keep that as an alternative should she fail to gain relief from the knee exercises and the anti-inflammatory medication. Her X-ray changes and her symptoms do not warrant any surgical intervention at this point. She is instructed to call with any other concerns or questions.

ICD-10-CM Code(s) _____

CASE STUDY 17

The patient has a loose body in the superior medial aspect of the left knee. This was somewhat mobile and tender. It has been causing constant pain. It seems to be increasing in size according to the patient. X rays indicate a large, partially calcified mass. Options were discussed with the patient and she elected surgical removal. The operation, including risks and complications, were discussed. Consent for surgery was obtained.

SURGICAL PROCEDURE: The patient was brought to the operating room and placed on the table in supine position. After a satisfactory anesthetic, a pneumatic tourniquet was placed around the uppermost aspect of her leg. The leg was placed in a leg holder. The leg was prepared from toes to leg holder with Hibiclens and draped sterilely. The patient was given a gram of Kefzol preoperatively. The leg was elevated and exsanguinated using an Esmarch, and the tourniquet was inflated to 300 mmHg. Superolateral and anterolateral portals were created and the knee was infused with lactated Ringer's solution to the superolateral portal because the mass was superomedial. The arthroscope was introduced through the anterolateral portal and the knee was examined. The suprapatellar pouch was noted to be normal except for what appeared to be a somewhat encapsulated mass on the medial aspect of the femur superiorly. The mediolateral and intercondylar regions were normal. Attention was then redirected to the area of the mass. A medial portal was created using the needle as a guide. A hook probe was introduced and the mass was palpated. It was felt to be a somewhat encapsulated bony mass. A knife was introduced, and the soft tissue overlying it was incised. Using several instruments,

the mass was dissected free and the soft tissue overlying it was debrided using the shaver. Using the shaver, punches, and the scissors, the mass was mobilized. Using a grasping device, the mass was firmly grasped and advanced toward the medial portal. The medial portal was much too small to accommodate the mass, and the incision was enlarged to approximately an inch plus in length allowing removal of the mass with a moderate amount of difficulty. The knee was irrigated through the wound with lactated Ringer's solution. The wound was closed by approximating the capsule of the joint with interrupted figure-of-eight sutures of 0 Vicryl. The knee was reexamined. No area causing generation of this mass could be identified on either of the femoral condyles, tibial plateau, or patellar surface. The knee was thoroughly irrigated through the arthroscopic sleeve. The wounds were injected with 0.5% Marcaine plus epinephrine. The larger anteromedial wound was closed with a running horizontal mattress suture of 3-0 nylon. The other wounds were closed with interrupted simple and vertical mattress sutures of 3-0 nylon. The knee was injected with 0.5% Marcaine plus epinephrine. Xeroform and a bulky dressing were applied and held in place with a Kerlix roll. An ace wrap was applied for gentle compression. The tourniquet was released and the drapes removed. After transfer to a gurney, the patient was awakened, the elevator removed, and she was transferred to the recovery room in satisfactory condition.

ICD-10-CM Code(s) _____

CASE STUDY 18

PREOPERATIVE DIAGNOSIS: Ganglion of dorsum, right wrist.

POSTOPERATIVE DIAGNOSIS: Same (2 cm diameter).

OPERATION PERFORMED: Excision of ganglion.

SURGEON: Stephanie Morrison, MD.

ANESTHESIA: Local.

DESCRIPTION OF OPERATION: The patient was taken to the operating room suite. The hand was prepped and draped in the usual manner and then anesthetized with Xylocaine infiltration. An incision was made overlying this large ganglion cyst and dissection was carried down until the cyst was encountered. There were no major structures covering this. Small vessels were ligated. The cyst was opened, drained of its contents, and then the cyst wall was dissected away from surrounding structures through the areolar tissue.

Dissection was carried down into the joint space where a small neck was found and it was excised. There was good hemostasis. The subcutis was closed with PDS sutures and the skin closed with dermal Vicryl. A splint was then applied, and it will be worn for about ten days. He will be seen in the office at that time.

ICD-10-CM Code(s) _____

CASE STUDY 19

CHIEF COMPLAINT: A 73-year-old white female is admitted to the hospital with a right hip fracture.

HISTORY OF PRESENT ILLNESS: The patient states she leaned over to pick up some trash in the courtyard of her condo where she resides, lost her balance, and fell over. She never lost consciousness and had severe hip pain. She called for help. She was able to move her hip somewhat and the nursing staff at her residence felt that most likely there was not a fracture, but just to be certain, called me and I ordered an X ray of the right hip. This indeed did show a right hip fracture. It is subcapital in location. The patient has pain of the right hip, but no other complaints at present. It is much better after IV medication was used in the ER.

MEDICATIONS:

Her medication list is extensive and consists of the following:

- Actonel
- Lasix
- Synthroid
- Nexium
- Bentyl
- K-Dur
- Neurontin
- Voltaren

ALLERGIES: None.

SOCIAL HISTORY: She does not smoke or drink. She usually performs ADLs fairly well and is fairly sharp for her age. She is a retired nun.

REVIEW OF SYSTEMS: Head, eye, ENT, neck, pulmonary, cardiac, GI, GU, skin: No complaints. Positive right hip pain. No other musculoskeletal complaints except for chronic arthritis pains here and there that respond to Tylenol she states. Inability to ambulate correctly without pain. All other systems reviewed and negative.

PHYSICAL EXAMINATION:

VITAL SIGNS: She is afebrile. Blood pressure 122/75. Respirations 22 per minute when she was in pain. Oxygen saturation on room air apparently was 87% at one point in the ER. At present, the oxygen saturation has gotten as low as 78%. I am not sure if this was after Dilaudid was administered or not. We will put her on an oxygen protocol, keeping saturations at 90 or above.

HEENT: Normocephalic and atraumatic. Pupils equal, round, and react to light and accommodation. Extraocular muscles are intact. The discs were not visualized. Eyelids: Some droop on the right eyelid. She says this is chronic. No masses on the eyelids. Conjunctivae pink. Sclerae white. No otic or nasal discharge. The oropharynx is clear. Tongue is midline.

NECK: Supple. No JVD, bruits, thyromegaly, or lymphadenopathy.

LUNGS: Clear on auscultation and percussion. No rales, rhonchi, wheezes, dullness, or tympanism on percussion.

HEART: Distant S1 and S2. No audible murmur, gallop, or rub. The PMI is nondisplaced. Extremities, no edema.

ABDOMEN: Nontender. Bowel sounds positive. No organomegaly or masses noted. No rebound, rigidity, or guarding.

EXTREMITIES: Negative Homans sign. Negative cyanosis or clubbing.

NEUROLOGIC: Alert and oriented ×3. Cranial nerves II–XII intact. No obvious motor or sensory deficits, but a full exam could not be done secondary to the right hip fracture.

LABORATORY: EKG shows normal sinus rhythm, no acute ischemic changes, no signs of old MI, positive for poor R-wave progression, otherwise only some nonspecific ST-T changes. X ray of right hip shows a right hip fracture.

BLOOD WORK: BMP shows a blood sugar of 102; BUN and creatinine 13/0.9; sodium 130; potassium 3.6; chloride 94; bicarb 27; and calcium 8.7. CBC shows a slightly elevated white count of 12.61 with no left shift, platelet count 197,000, hemoglobin normal at 12.4. GFR is 63% estimated.

ASSESSMENT:

1. Pathological right hip fracture

2. Osteoarthritis

3. Hypothyroidism

4. Idiopathic peripheral neuropathy

PLAN: I feel that she is medically clear for surgery. Dr Williams has already seen the patient and is planning surgery in two days. We will continue some of her old medications and treat her with IV narcotics for pain (Dilaudid being the drug of choice for this patient). We will continue same medications that are necessary.

ICD-10-CM Code(s) _____

CASE STUDY 20

PREOPERATIVE DIAGNOSIS: Painful plantar fasciitis with heel spur, left foot.

POSTOPERATIVE DIAGNOSIS: Same.

PROCEDURE PERFORMED: Plantar fasciotomy, left foot.

ANESTHESIA: IV sedation with local anesthetic that consisted of 15 cc of a 50/50 mixture of 0.5% plain Marcaine and 2% plain Xylocaine, posterior tibial sural nerve block, and local infiltration into the left heel.

DESCRIPTION OF PROCEDURE: The patient was taken into the operating room and placed on the table in the regular supine position. Once adequate IV sedation had been obtained, a pneumatic tourniquet was placed on the left ankle. Local anesthetic was injected into the left surgical site. The left foot was prepped and draped in the usual sterile manner. The left foot was elevated and exsanguinated with an Esmarch bandage and the left ankle pneumatic tourniquet was inflated to 250 mmHg. Attention was directed to the medial aspect of the left heel where a predetermined site for the incision was planned at 45 mm anterior to the posterior surface of the heel and 21 mm superior to the inferior border of the heel, which was the identified location of the plantar fascial attachment to the infracalcaneal medial tubercle of the calcaneus. Once through the skin layer, hemostats were used to bluntly separate the subcuticular tissue away from the adipose layer below. At this time, a straight Kelly hemostat was used to identify the superior and inferior borders of the plantar fascia as it inserted into the medial tubercle of the calcaneus. Once these are defined, a soft tissue elevator was inserted plantarly and it was advanced until tinting was seen on the lateral surface. At this

time, the tissue elevator was removed and replaced with the obturator and cannula to exit the skin laterally, and the obturator was removed. The cannula was held in place and two swipes of a cotton-tipped applicator were performed. The endoscope was then inserted from medial to lateral identifying a thick plantar fascial band that was fully intact preoperatively. At this time, a blunt probe was marked with a skin marker and inserted from lateral to medial identifying the lateral extent of the plantar fascial release. This was noted to be approximately the medial two-thirds of the plantar fascial band. Once this was marked, a hook blade followed by a right angle blade was advanced across the plantar fascia from medial to lateral with the hallux dorsiflexed. Several swipes of the cutting blade were performed with good release noted. The endoscope and the hook blade were repositioned to opposite ends of the cannula and complete plantar fascial release was noted medially through the cannula. Intraoperative photos were taken prior to plantar fascial release and post plantar fascial release with release noted in the flexor belly noted dorsally. The wound was copiously irrigated with normal saline solution. Adequate release was noted intraoperatively. The scope and cannula were removed at this time. The skin was repaired with 3-0 nylon in a simple suture technique. Following the procedure, a sterile and compressive dressing was applied. The left ankle pneumatic tourniquet was released. The patient tolerated the anesthesia and procedure well without complications and was transferred from the OR to the recovery room with vital signs stable. Normal vascular return was noted to all five digits of the left foot upon tourniquet release. The patient will follow up with Dr Miller in five to seven days. Postoperative care instructions and pain medications have been dispensed to the patient.

ICD-10-CM Code(s) _____

CASE STUDY 21

Michele is here for initial evaluation of her right thumb. Approximately one year ago, she was bitten by a dog and had to have stitches that she received in the ER. Today she comes in and states she has a bone spur that feels like it is going to pop out of her hand.

ASSESSMENT AND PLAN:

Right thumb pain and acquired trigger finger, thumb; discussed the option of a cortisone injection today versus applying a split to the thumb. Overall, patient is doing well, and she refuses the injection at this time.

ICD-10-CM Code(s) _____

CASE STUDY 22

Ms Johnson has been experiencing significant right shoulder muscle spasms for months. The muscle spasms come and go. It is worse when she is lying flat on her back. Muscle relaxers don't always help. She also has left knee pain. She has had trigger point injections on her knee, which brings some relief. She just had an injection two weeks ago. She is on Oxycodone and Methadone.

PLAN: Continue current medications. Follow-up in three months for shoulder muscle spasm and left knee pain.

ICD-10-CM Code(s) _____

CHAPTER 9

Diseases of the Genitourinary System (N00-N99)

Pregnancy, Childbirth, and the Puerperium (O00-O9A); Certain Conditions Originating in the Perinatal Period (P00-P96); and Congenital Malformations, Deformations, and Chromosomal Abnormalities (Q00-Q99)

ICD-10-CM Chapters 14–17 Guidelines Review

In this chapter you will find a summary of the chapter-specific coding guidelines for Chapters 14 through 17 of the ICD-10-CM codebook followed by case studies to build ICD-10-CM diagnosis coding skills in these areas.

Many medical specialties reference Chapters 14–17 of the ICD-10-CM codebook, which include diseases of the genitourinary system; pregnancy, childbirth, and the puerperium; certain conditions originating in the perinatal period; and congenital malformations, deformations, and chromosomal abnormalities. Keep in mind that you should always reference the ICD-10-CM Official Guidelines for Coding and Reporting in its entirety when making a code selection.

ICD-10-CM Official Coding Guidelines for the Genitourinary System

Many of the conditions in the genitourinary system follow the general coding guidelines as well as any instructional notes. Chapter-specific guidelines for the system involve chronic kidney disease (CKD).

STAGES OF CHRONIC KIDNEY DISEASE (CKD)

CKD is classified by the severity of the disease, which is designated in six stages: stages 1–5 and end-stage renal disease (ESRD). The following codes apply:

- N18.1 (stage 1)
- N18.2 (stage 2, mild CKD)
- N18.3 (stage 3, moderate CKD)
- N18.4 (stage 4, severe CKD)
- N18.5 (stage 5)
- N18.6 (ESRD requiring dialysis)
- N18.9 (Chronic kidney disease, unspecified)

CODING TIP When both a stage of CKD and ESRD are documented in the medical record, only code N18.6 is reported.

CHRONIC KIDNEY DISEASE AND KIDNEY TRANSPLANT STATUS

Patients who have undergone kidney transplant may still have some form of CKD because the kidney transplant may not fully restore kidney function. The presence of CKD alone does not constitute a transplant complication. When coding CKD and kidney transplant status, the following rules apply:

- Report code N18 for the patient's stage of CKD and code Z94.0, Kidney transplant status.

- If a transplant complication such as failure or rejection or other complication is documented, see section I.C.19.g of the ICD-10-CM Official Guidelines for Coding and Reporting for information on coding complications of a kidney transplant.

- If the documentation is unclear as to whether the patient has a complication of the transplant, query the provider.

CHRONIC KIDNEY DISEASE WITH OTHER CONDITIONS

Patients with CKD may also suffer from other serious conditions, most commonly diabetes mellitus and hypertension. Sequencing of CKD in relationship to codes for other contributing conditions is based on the conventions in the Tabular List. For guidance in coding, refer to the following sections of the ICD-10-CM Official Guidelines for Coding and Reporting:

- Section I.C.9 (Hypertensive chronic kidney disease).
- Section I.C.19 (Chronic kidney disease and kidney transplant complications).

It is time to build skill and knowledge by coding the following exercises relative to the genitourinary system. Be sure to reference the ICD-10-CM codebook and the ICD-10-CM Official Guidelines for Coding and Reporting, along with the instructional notes, when coding these conditions.

Diseases of the Genitourinary System (N00-N99)

CASE STUDY 1

PROCEDURE: Ablation of seroma cavity using Doxycycline.

ADMITTING DIAGNOSIS: Persistent seroma drainage.

INDICATION: Persistent seroma of the broad ligament.

PROCEDURE: The seroma cavity was ablated using 500 mg of Doxycycline, which was instilled into the seroma cavity following local anesthetic instillation. The patient tolerated the procedure well. No complications were encountered. Appropriate catheter care instructions have been given to the patient.

ASSESSMENT: See above.

ICD-10-CM Code(s) _____

CASE STUDY 2

HISTORY: A 29-year-old white female presents to the hospital emergency department with a chief complaint of vomiting for the last four days, abdominal pain, back pain, urinary frequency, and dysuria.

HISTORY OF PRESENT ILLNESS: The patient states that four days ago she started off Thursday with stomach pressure. She promptly vomited and could not hold much food or liquid down. The abdominal pain at first was moderate and became severe over the last several days. She also developed a headache and experienced muscle aches as well as bilateral back pain. She states that she had some dysuria on Thursday but it was mild to moderate, but now it has worsened gradually over the last four days.

PAST MEDICAL HISTORY: Fairly unimpressive. She has had two cesarean sections for twins and one child, so she has three children. They are all healthy. She got hit by a car when she was 12 and had open reduction, apparently, of her left radius and right ankle. Other than that, she states she really is fairly boring as far as past medical history.

FAMILY HISTORY: Positive in two female relatives for diabetes mellitus, her grandmothers on both sides of the family.

SOCIAL HISTORY: She does not smoke, drink alcohol, or take recreational drugs.

MEDICATIONS: She has no current medications, including over-the-counter health food–type medications, etc. No allergies.

EXAMINATION:

LUNGS: Clear on auscultation and percussion. No riles, rhonchi, or wheezing. No dullness or tympanism.

HEART: S1 and S2 regular. No audible murmur, gallop, or rub. The point of maximal impulse is nondisplaced.

BREASTS/PELVIC/RECTAL: Not performed at present. This will be left in follow-up as outpatient, either with me or someone else.

ABDOMEN: Positive tenderness, most pronounced in the hypogastric area. No rebound, rigidity, or guarding. Bowel sounds positive in all four quadrants. No organomegaly or masses. Positive bilateral costovertebral angle tenderness on mild to moderate percussion.

EXTREMITIES: Negative Homans' sign, negative edema, cyanosis, or clubbing of the upper and lower extremities. Pedal pulses are palpable, as are popliteals, radials, ulnars, and brachials.

SKIN: No plaque, scaling, vesicular eruptions, or rashes. Turgor appears somewhat decreased.

NEUROLOGIC: Alert and oriented ×3. Cranial nerves II–XII intact. No motor deficits found. No pathological reflexes on examination.

MUSCULOSKELETAL: Mild tenderness on palpation with the paravertebral muscles, deltoids, quadriceps, and calf muscles but nothing severe.

ENDOCRINE: Negative central obesity. Negative buffalo hump, moon facies, exophthalmus, or thyromegaly.

HEMATOLOGIC/LYMPHATIC: Negative petechiae, purpura, or ecchymoses. Negative cervical or axillary or inguinal lymphadenopathy. Negative splenomegaly.

PSYCHIATRIC: No undue signs of anxiety, depression, suicidal ideation, or psychotic behavior on interview.

LABORATORY: An electrocardiogram (EKG) shows sinus tachycardia, nonspecific ST-T changes throughout. Her basic metabolic panel: Blood sugar 88; BUN 12; creatinine 0.8; sodium 135; potassium 3.5; chloride 96; bicarb slightly low at 20; calcium 9.4. Her CBC shows a white count of 23,000; hemoglobin normal at 15; platelets 241. There is a left shift in the differential. Magnesium normal. Pregnancy test is negative. Urinalysis is significant for positive nitrites, moderate blood, large leukocyte esterase, many WBCs, 2+ bacteria.

ASSESSMENT:

1. Acute pyelonephritis

2. Nausea and vomiting, which was intractable on admission

3. Hypokalemia secondary to nausea and vomiting

PLAN: Admit as inpatient. Replace her potassium. Replace her IV fluids as I believe she is also clinically dehydrated. Give her IV Cipro. We have cultures cooking, both of blood and urine. Hopefully these will give us some answers so we can be specific in our treatment, but Cipro is a good choice. I will give her anti-emetics and narcotics for pain control, mostly in the muscular areas, with oral medication.

ICD-10-CM Code(s) _____

CASE STUDY 3

A 59-year-old white female presents to an OB/GYN on the advice of her primary care doctor. Based on her medical records, her hemoglobin was 6.3. He had wanted her to go to the hospital for transfusion. She refused and presents here today for evaluation. This patient had a D&C four months ago in another state. Pathology was suggestive of perimenopause. She had been amenorrheic for the first two months following the D&C, then had a normal period menses last month. This month she has had an extremely heavy menses for 10 days. Her previous doctor started her on Climara .025 and Provera and she has not had a withdrawal period since. The plan was to have her stop the Provera, and expect a period, but he had doubled the dose up to 20 a day to try and keep her amenorrheic.

She has had some fatigue, occasional headache, and dizziness. She states her heart feels like it's beating fast. All other systems are negative by review with the patient.

Her past medical history is notable for anemia, and her social history does not include alcohol, tobacco, or social drug use. She has previously had three vaginal deliveries, G3, P3. She is a well-developed, well-nourished pale white female in no acute distress. Her pulse is 92; blood pressure 130/80; and weight 190 lbs. A & O ×3, affect normal. Her neck and thyroid are normal. Her heart has regular rhythm with no murmur. Lungs clear. The abdomen is soft, non-tender, no masses, and the liver and spleen are non-palpable. No inguinal or axillary adenopathy. The vulva, vagina, periurethral, perirectal, and periclitoral areas are normal. The cervix and uterus are normal and adnexa negative. Skin warm and dry. Hurricane spray and a single-tooth tenaculum to the cervix result in its coming down moderately. Her uterus and vagina are well-supported. Her diagnosis is menorrhagia with severe anemia. We discussed the complexity of the problem. She has tried a hormonal regimen in the past and it did not work. She tried a D&C and it did not work. There has been no anatomical problem found. I suggest a hysterectomy as the only viable option. She understands this will make her infertile. We need to build up her hemoglobin and stop her period. The Hemocyte Plus bothers her stomach and she will be switched to a slow iron. She is also taking Biaxin for upper respiratory problems and her chronic cough.

We need to keep her amenorrheic. We'll continue the Provera 20 mg per day. We'll give her Lupron 3.75 IM today. We discussed the risks and benefits of this. She will get a surge of estrogen in about 10 to 14 days. That is when she is likely to get a period. If the bleeding gets heavy, we can try switching her to Aygestin at that point. We will plan for surgery in about seven weeks. She should return in two weeks for a hemoglobin check. She will report any further bleeding in the meantime. We also discussed Depo-Provera, but I am concerned that in about six weeks the lining may get too thin and she could bleed from that between the Depo-Provera and the Depo-Lupron. If there is any more significant bleeding she will need to be transfused. If this occurs in the next few days for any reason, we will proceed with the hysterectomy much sooner to prevent another bleeding episode. Thirty to thirty-five minutes of the hour-long session were spent discussing our options.

ICD-10-CM Code(s) _____

CASE STUDY 4

This 35-year-old established female patient comes in today with some concerns about irritability and vaginal dryness on intercourse over the past three months. She has no other concerns. There has been no increase in weight since her previous yearly examination last year. There has been no change in her menstruation cycle.

PHYSICAL EXAMINATION:

Patient is a well-developed, well-nourished female. Blood pressure is 100/65; pulse 76; weight 150 pounds.

HEENT: Negative.

NECK: Supple. Trachea is midline.

CHEST: Lungs clear.

HEART: Normal rhythm. No murmurs appreciated.

ABDOMEN: Soft. No tenderness, masses, or organomegaly.

GENITOURINARY: Vagina dry with poor lubrication. External genitalia are negative. No cystocele or rectocele appreciated. Rectovaginal examination reveals no nodules or tenderness but a bit of inflammation. No CVA tenderness.

ASSESSMENT: Acute vaginitis, cause unknown.

TREATMENT: Prescribed Naprosyn to help with redness and inflammation. Patient will return in six weeks or sooner if needed.

ICD-10-CM Code(s) _____

CASE STUDY 5

A 67-year-old female reports symptoms of stress urinary incontinence. Examination revealed a large cystocele with loss of urethro-vesicle support. Formal cystometric evaluation revealed stress urinary incontinence, a

normal bladder volume, and no evidence of detrusor instability.

The patient undergoes a Pereyra procedure with anterior colporrhaphy. The vaginal mucosa overlying the bladder is incised and dissected off of the bladder. Through two small lower abdominal incisions, a suture is placed retropubically and looped around the neck of the bladder where it joins the urethra. This suture is anchored to the abdominal wall fascia, thus suspending the urethrovesicle angle (Pereyra procedure). The perivesicle fascia is then plicated in the midline and the previously incised vaginal mucosa is re-approximated thus completing the anterior colporrhaphy. A Foley catheter is placed for gravity drainage and a vaginal pack is also placed. The small abdominal incisions are closed.

She does well postoperatively and is discharged on the third post-op day. She is unable to void adequately at the time of the discharge; therefore, she is instructed in self-catheterization. She is seen weekly in the office until she voids adequately, approximately 14 days after surgery. She is seen six weeks' post-op to assess her healing and recovery and is allowed to resume her usual activities.

ICD-10-CM Code(s) _____

CASE STUDY 6

A 63-year-old, sexually active, gravida five, para five underwent abdominal hysterectomy 20 years ago for leiomyomata. She developed a symptomatic cystocele and rectocele and was treated with anterior and posterior repair three years ago. Now she is being evaluated for discomfort and tissue prolapsing through the introitus. Examination documents prolapse of the vaginal vault through the introitus and good anterior and posterior support.

At surgery an abdominal incision is made through all layers. After the abdominal cavity is explored, the vagina is identified. The bladder is dissected off the anterior vaginal wall and the posterior wall is freed. The peritoneum overlying the sacrum is incised and the periosteum cleared. Using a variety of techniques, the vagina is secured to the periosteum of the sacral promontory.

ICD-10-CM Code(s) _____

CASE STUDY 7

The patient is a 29-year-old female who presents for follow-up of left-sided renal calculi. The patient was originally seen in the emergency room (ER) down state for left-sided flank pain. She was found to have an obstructing renal calculi with CT stone protocol per the patient. We do not have those records available here. The patient was seen here in the office on 7/31/20xx. The attending physician refilled her Vicodin, Flomax, and prescribed a 14-day prescription of Cipro 500 mg to prevent pyelonephritis. A culture was also done at that time and grew beta hemolytic strep greater than 100,000 organisms. In the office today the patient continues to have colicky left-sided flank pain, continued chills, nausea, and loss of appetite. She has no documented fevers and no vomiting. She has one day left of Flomax and eight days left of Ciprofloxacin. The patient is out of Vicodin.

The patient has been increasing her smoking use; she is up to a half-pack per day. She is waking up with chest discomfort, tightness, and shortness of breath. She has recently found herself smoking in front of one of her children and she has decided that she needs to quit smoking.

Blood pressure is 140/70; weight 224 lbs. Heart regular rate and rhythm, no murmurs. Lungs are clear to auscultation bilaterally. Abdomen has positive bowel sounds times four quadrants. There is CVA tenderness and left lower quadrant pain on palpation. There is no guarding and no rebound tenderness. Skin is clean without rashes, erythema, or jaundice.

1. Left nephrolithiasis

2. Urinary tract infection with beta hemolytic strep (group B)

3. Tobacco use, uncontrolled

4. Elevated blood pressure secondary to pain

5. Patient will stop her Ciprofloxacin

6. A prescription for amoxicillin 850 mg po bid times seven days

7. Vicodin 5/500 1 to 2 po every four hours prn for pain, #60 were given with no refills

8. Chantix prescription. The side effects were discussed with the patient, as well as instructions for taking this medication with food. The patient was also encouraged to start this medication after she passes the kidney stone.

9. The patient was encouraged to continue to strain her stone. She was also given encouragement to drink two liters of Coke.

ICD-10-CM Code(s) _____

CASE STUDY 8

PREOPERATIVE DIAGNOSIS: High-grade moderate dysplasia, grade II, with two-stage difference between Pap smear and colposcopy results.

POSTOPERATIVE DIAGNOSIS: High-grade moderate dysplasia with two-stage difference between Pap smear and colposcopy results.

OPERATION: Cervical loop electrosurgical excision procedure.

ESTIMATED BLOOD LOSS: 10 cc.

FLUIDS: 500 cc lactated Ringer's solution.

ANESTHESIA: General endotracheal anesthesia.

SPECIMENS: Cervical LEEP, a separate posterior ectocervical specimen, endocervical specimen.

PROCEDURE: Prior to surgery, the patient was counseled extensively regarding the risks and benefits of the planned procedure including the risk of bleeding, the risk of infection, and the risk of damage to adjacent organs. After extensive discussion, the patient expressed understanding and strongly desired to proceed.

At this point the patient was transferred to the operating room (OR) where adequate endotracheal tube anesthesia was administered. The patient was then prepped and draped in the usual sterile fashion for vaginal surgery. The vagina and cervix were not prepped, however. The bladder was straight cathed prior to beginning the procedure. At this point a plastic-coated speculum was placed in the vagina for visualization of the cervix. A sidewall retractor was placed. The cervix was coated with Lugol's solution noting a normal appearance. Because of the angle of the cervix, we were able to get primarily anterior cervix and a very small sliver of posterior cervix in the initial LEEP pass. We then made a second pass to get a little more of the posterior cervix. A final narrow LEEP was then performed of the endocervical canal yielding three specimens. The bed of the biopsy site was then cauterized with the Bovie for excellent hemostasis. The surrounding cervical tissue was also cauterized outward about 3 to 4 millimeters circumferentially to make sure that we did not miss any dysplasia that we were otherwise unable to see. At this point, because of the normal findings, I went ahead and coated the remainder of the vaginal canal with Lugol's solution noting no other non-highlighting regions. At this point Monsel's solution was placed on the bed of the biopsy site again noting excellent hemostasis. The procedure was concluded. The patient tolerated the procedure well. All sponge, lap, and needle counts were correct at the end of the procedure. The patient was then taken to the recovery room in stable condition where she will be discharged home per protocol. She was given a prescription for Lortab 5 #24 with no refills. She is to follow up with me in one week for discussion of results and further therapy if needed.

ICD-10-CM Code(s) _____

CASE STUDY 9

INDICATIONS: An 11-year-old male with phimosis, which is symptomatic and requires circumcision.

FINDINGS: Phimosis.

PROCEDURE: The patient was taken to the operating room. After the induction of general anesthesia, the patient was placed in the supine position and prepped and draped in the usual sterile fashion. The foreskin was able to be retracted after the patient was asleep, and the glans was also prepped. After draping, the foreskin was retracted and the frenulum was found to be tethering the glans. We dissected out the frenulum, and divided and cauterized this very carefully, straightening out the penis. We then made a circumferential incision approximately 1 cm proximal to the glans with the foreskin retracted; we took this through the skin. We then replaced the foreskin in its normal position and made a mirror-image circumferential incision around the coronal sulcus. We connected both incisions sharply and sharply removed the foreskin. We then achieved meticulous hemostasis with electrocautery. We took great care to avoid injury to the deep structures of the urethra.

After satisfactory hemostasis, we approximated the skin with 4-0 chromic interrupted sutures with a U-stitch ventrally. At the termination of the procedure, there was excellent hemostasis. The glans was healthy. There was a good cosmetic result. We placed 3 cc of 0.25% Marcaine without epinephrine circumferentially around the base of the penis for a ring block. We sterilely dressed the wound.

The patient tolerated the procedure well and was transferred to recovery in good condition.

ICD-10-CM Code(s) _____

CASE STUDY 10

Patient comes in the office today to follow-up on his recent ER visit and labs. He was diagnosed with acute kidney failure with tubular necrosis. His urine decreased dramatically and his creatinine and BUN increased. He could not produce adequate urine. He was given IV fluids. His BP readings are in normal range. BP today was 130/80.

PLAN: Continue current medications; follow-up in two months.

IMPRESSION: Acute kidney failure w/tubular necrosis, essential hypertension.

ICD-10-CM Code(s) _____

CASE STUDY 11

A 55-year-old female patient is seen today who has type 2 diabetes and chronic kidney disease (CKD), stage 3. Her blood sugar is slightly elevated. She has been on insulin for the past seven months. According to the patient her blood sugars are always elevated during lunch time. In the morning, sugars run between 100 and 120.

No headaches, blood sugar 180. Patient has been compliant with medication and exercising two days a week.

PLAN: Follow-up in two months.

IMPRESSION: Type 2 diabetes with CKD, stage 3.

ICD-10-CM Code(s) _____

ICD-10-CM Official Coding Guidelines for Pregnancy, Childbirth, and the Puerperium

The postpartum period begins immediately after delivery and continues six weeks following delivery. The peripartum period is the last month of pregnancy to five months postpartum. A postpartum complication can occur within the six weeks following delivery. When the provider documents the complication is related to the pregnancy, codes from Chapter 15 of the ICD-10-CM codebook may be used to report complications after the postpartum or peripartum period.

The following guidelines apply to Chapter 15 of the ICD-10-CM codebook, Pregnancy, Childbirth, and the Puerperium:

- Codes for pregnancy, childbirth, and the puerperium have sequencing priority over codes in other chapters. Additional codes from other chapters may be reported in conjunction with these codes to further clarify the patient's condition, if applicable.

- When pregnancy is incidental (ie, the patient is being treated for another condition but is also pregnant), code Z33.1 is reported secondarily to the condition being treated.

- Codes in Chapter 15 may only be used on the maternal record, not the newborn record.

- For the majority of the codes in Chapter 15, the final character identifies the trimester of the pregnancy. Time frames for trimester selection are located in the beginning of the chapter.

- Certain codes have characters for only certain trimesters because the particular condition may not occur in all trimesters, but may occur in more than one trimester.

- For some codes, the trimester is not applicable.

- The provider's documentation of the trimester or number of weeks should be documented in the patient encounter including assignment of pre-existing condition and conditions developed during or due to the pregnancy.

- When delivery occurs during the patient admission or encounter and there is a childbirth option for the OB complication, the childbirth code should be assigned.

- When the patient is admitted to the hospital during one trimester and remains into a subsequent trimester, the character for the antepartum complication code should be reported based on the trimester when the complication developed. If the condition is pre-existing, the trimester character should be based on the admission or date of patient encounter.

- There are codes in each category for unspecified trimester that should only be used when the documentation is not sufficient to assign the appropriate trimester and the provider cannot be queried due to circumstance.

- For certain complications, a seventh character is required for reporting the fetus for which the complication code applies (eg, O31, O32, O33.3-O33.6, O35, O36, O40, O41, O60, O60.1, O60.2, O64, and

O69). The seventh character "0" is assigned for the following:

- Single gestations.

- When documentation in the medical record is not sufficient to determine the affected fetus and it is not possible to query the provider.

- When clinically it is not possible to determine which fetus is affected.

SELECTION OF FIRST-LISTED DIAGNOSIS FOR OB CASES

To report routine outpatient prenatal visits when no complications are documented, follow these guidelines:

- Select a code from category Z34, Encounter for supervision of normal pregnancy, as the first-listed diagnosis.

- A code from Chapter 15 should not be used if there are no complications.

- When the patient is high-risk and is receiving routine outpatient prenatal care, a code from category O09, Supervision of high-risk pregnancy, is reported as the first-listed diagnosis. Additional codes from Chapter 15 may be listed as secondary diagnoses if applicable. If there are no complications during the labor or delivery episode, assign code O80, Encounter for full-term uncomplicated delivery.

- When no delivery occurs, the first-listed diagnosis should be reported based on the complication of the pregnancy. When more than one complication is documented and all are treated, any of the complication codes may be sequenced first.

- When a delivery occurs during the admission, the condition that prompted the admission should be sequences as the principal (first-listed) diagnosis. A code for any complication of the delivery should be assigned as an additional diagnosis.

- For cesarean deliveries, the first-listed diagnosis should be the condition responsible for the patient admission. When the complication results in the reason for the cesarean delivery, that condition is reported as the first-listed diagnosis. If the reason is unrelated to the determination to perform the cesarean procedure, the condition for the reason for the admission should be reported as the first-listed diagnosis.

- When a delivery occurs, the outcome of delivery is reported on the mother's record with a code from category Z37, Outcome of delivery. Never report a code in this category on the newborn record.

PRE-EXISTING CONDITIONS VERSUS CONDITIONS DUE TO PREGNANCY

To correctly report codes from Chapter 15, it is important to determine whether a condition is pre-existing or a direct result of the pregnancy. For example, for a patient who has diabetes mellitus and who is now pregnant, the diabetes mellitus is considered a pre-existing condition. However, some conditions are considered due to the pregnancy, such as gestational diabetes.

To report patients who have pre-existing hypertension complicating the pregnancy, follow this guideline:

- A code from category O10, Pre-existing hypertension complication pregnancy, childbirth, and the puerperium, is reported as the first-listed diagnosis, followed by a secondary diagnosis to identify the appropriate type of heart failure or chronic kidney disease if these conditions are present.

FETAL CONDITIONS AFFECTING MANAGEMENT OF MOTHER

When reporting codes from category O35, Maternal care for known or suspected fetal abnormality and damage, and category O36, Maternal care for other fetal problems, follow these guidelines:

- The fetal condition does not justify a code from these two categories when the fetal condition is responsible for modifying the management of the mother including:

  - Diagnostic studies

  - Additional observation

  - Special care

  - Termination of pregnancy

- When surgery is performed on the fetus, a diagnosis code from category O35 is reported as the first-listed diagnosis to report the fetal condition.

- A code from Chapter 16, Certain Conditions Originating in the Perinatal Period, should not be reported on the mother's record to report the fetal condition. Surgery performed in utero is coded as an OB encounter.

HIV INFECTION IN PREGNANCY, CHILDBIRTH, AND THE PUERPERIUM

To report a patient who is treated for an HIV-related illness during pregnancy, childbirth, or the puerperium, follow these guidelines:

- Report code O98.7-, Human immunodeficiency (HIV) disease complicating pregnancy, childbirth, and the puerperium, as the first-listed diagnosis, with a secondary code to report the HIV-related illness.

- A patient who is HIV positive but asymptomatic during pregnancy, childbirth, or the puerperium should be reported with code O98.7- as the first-listed diagnosis followed by Z21, Asymptomatic human immunodeficiency virus (HIV) infection status.

DIABETES MELLITUS AND GESTATIONAL DIABETES IN PREGNANCY

A patient who has diabetes mellitus and is pregnant is assigned the following codes:

- A code from category O24 is selected to report the diabetes mellitus in pregnancy, childbirth, or the puerperium.

- A second code is selected from category E08-E13 to report the type of diabetes, which is located in Chapter 4 of the ICD-10-CM codebook.

- A patient who is a type 2 diabetic and on long-term (current) use of insulin should also be reported with code Z79.4 in addition to the diabetes complication code and the type of diabetes mellitus. If the patient is on oral hypoglycemic drugs, an additional diagnosis code should be reported as Z79.84 for the long-term (current) use of oral hypoglycemic drugs. If the patient is treated with both oral medications and insulin, only the code for the use of insulin (Z79.4) should be reported.

- A patient who develops gestational diabetes (pregnancy induced) should be reported with a code from subcategory O24.4, Gestational diabetes mellitus. No other code from category O24 is reported.

- Codes in subcategory O24.4 include treatment of a patient with diet, insulin, and/or oral hypoglycemic drugs. Codes Z79.4 and Z79.84 should not be reported with code O24.4.

- Abnormal glucose tolerance in pregnancy is reported with a code from subcategory O99.81, Abnormal glucose complicating pregnancy, childbirth, and the puerperium.

SEPSIS AND SEPTIC SHOCK COMPLICATING ABORTION, PREGNANCY, CHILDBIRTH, AND THE PUERPERIUM

When severe sepsis is present and documented, a code from category R65.2, Severe sepsis, and codes for an associated organ dysfunction(s) should be assigned as additional diagnoses. When reporting sepsis and septic shock complicating abortion, pregnancy, childbirth, and the puerperium, follow these guidelines:

- For puerperal sepsis, code O85 is assigned with a secondary diagnosis code to identify the causal organism. For example, if the patient has a bacterial infection, a code from category B95 or B96, Bacterial infections in diseases classified elsewhere, is reported as the secondary diagnosis.

- Do **not** report a code from category A40, Streptococcal sepsis, or category A41, Other sepsis. These two categories are not to be used to report puerperal sepsis.

- An additional code for severe sepsis (R65.2-) may be reported along with any associated acute organ dysfunction.

USE OF ALCOHOL AND TOBACCO DURING PREGNANCY, CHILDBIRTH, AND THE PUERPERIUM

Following are the guidelines to report alcohol use complicating pregnancy, childbirth, and the puerperium with subcategory O99.31:

- Report a code from subcategory O99.31 when a mother uses alcohol during the pregnancy or postpartum.

- A secondary diagnosis from category F10, Alcohol-related disorders, should be also reported to identify the manifestation of the alcohol use.

The following guideline should be followed to report tobacco use complicating pregnancy, childbirth, and the puerperium when a mother uses a tobacco product during pregnancy or postpartum with subcategory O99.33:

- Report O99.33 as the first-listed diagnosis followed by a code from category F17, Nicotine dependence, to identify the type of nicotine dependence.

POISONING, TOXIC EFFECTS, ADVERSE EFFECTS, AND UNDERDOSING IN A PREGNANT PATIENT

To report poisoning, toxic effects, adverse effects, and underdosing in a pregnant patient, three codes are required:

- The first-listed diagnosis code is a code from subcategory O9A.2, Injury, poisoning, and certain other consequences of external causes complicating pregnancy, childbirth, and the puerperium.

- The second-listed diagnosis is the appropriate injury, poisoning, toxic effect, adverse effect, or underdosing code.

- The third-listed diagnosis is the condition caused by the poisoning, toxic effect, adverse effect, or underdosing.

NORMAL DELIVERY

Code O80 is always the first-listed diagnosis when a woman is admitted for a full-term normal delivery and delivers a single, healthy, liveborn infant without any complications and/or:

- The complication is not present during the delivery.

- An outcome of delivery code for the single live birth (Z37.0) is reported as a secondary diagnosis.

CODING TIP Do not report code O80 when a complication code is necessary to describe the patient's condition.

CODING TIP Additional codes from other chapters in the ICD-10-CM codebook may be reported when not related to or complicating the pregnancy.

When a patient is admitted for routine postpartum care following delivery outside the hospital and no complications are documented, follow this guideline:

- Report code Z39.0, Encounter for care and examination of mother immediately after delivery, as the first-listed diagnosis code.

Report code O90.3 only when cardiomyopathy develops as a result of pregnancy in a woman who did not have pre-existing heart disease. This condition can be diagnosed in the third trimester of pregnancy but may progress months after delivery and is referred to as *peripartum cardiomyopathy*.

SEQUELAE OF COMPLICATION OF PREGNANCY, CHILDBIRTH, AND THE PUERPERIUM

Use code O94, Sequelae of complication of pregnancy, childbirth, and the puerperium, in cases when an initial complication of a pregnancy develops sequelae requiring care or treatment at a later date. The code may be used any time after the initial postpartum period (six weeks following delivery). Sequence code O94 after the code describing the sequelae of the complication.

ABORTIONS

The following guidelines should be used when reporting abortions:

- Report Z33.2, Encounter for elective termination of pregnancy, and a code from category Z37.-, Outcome of delivery, when an attempted termination of pregnancy results in a liveborn fetus.

- Report a code from category Z37, Outcome of delivery, as a secondary diagnosis.

- Retained products of conception following abortion or elected termination of pregnancy are reported with subcategory O03, Spontaneous abortion, or code O07.4, Failed attempted termination of pregnancy without complication, followed by code Z33.2, Encounter for elective termination of pregnancy. These codes are also to be used when the patient was previously discharged with the diagnosis of complete abortion. Diagnosis codes from Chapter 15 may be used as additional diagnosis codes to identify any documented complication of the pregnancy in conjunction with codes in categories O07 and O08.

ABUSE IN THE PREGNANT PATIENT

Three codes may be reported as the first-listed diagnosis to code abuse when a patient is pregnant:

- Code O9A.3, Physical abuse complicating pregnancy, childbirth, and the puerperium

- Code O9A.4, Sexual abuse complicating pregnancy, childbirth, and the puerperium

- Code O9A.5, Psychological abuse complicating pregnancy, childbirth, and the puerperium

A secondary diagnosis is reported (if applicable) to identify any associated current injury due to physical abuse, sexual abuse, and the perpetrator of abuse.

ICD-10-CM Official Coding Guidelines for Certain Conditions Originating in the Perinatal Period

Codes in Chapter 16 of the ICD-10-CM codebook (Certain Conditions Originating in the Perinatal Period) are for use in the newborn record and are never to be reported in the mother's medical record. If the condition remains present during the patient's lifetime, codes in this chapter may be reported. The perinatal guidelines are the same as the general coding guidelines for "additional diagnoses," except for the final point regarding implications for future health care needs. Codes should be assigned for conditions that

have been specified by the provider as having implications for future health care needs.

When coding the birth episode in a newborn record, follow these guidelines:

- Report a code from category Z38, Liveborn infants according to place of birth and type of delivery, as the first-listed diagnosis. Other conditions can be reported as an additional diagnosis.

- A code from category Z38 is assigned only once to a newborn at the time of birth.

- If a newborn is transferred to another institution, a code from category Z38 should not be used at the receiving hospital.

- A code from category Z38 is used only in the newborn record, not in the mother's record.

- Codes from Chapter 16 may be reported with codes from other chapters of the ICD-10-CM codebook if codes from other chapters provide more detail. If a definitive diagnosis cannot be supported, codes for signs and/or symptoms may be reported from Chapter 18 of the codebook. When the reason for the encounter is the perinatal condition, the perinatal condition is sequenced first.

- When a condition originated in the perinatal period and continues throughout the life of the patient, the perinatal code should continue to be used regardless of the patient's age.

- If a newborn has a condition that may be either due to the birth process or community-acquired, and the documentation does not indicate which it is, the default is due to the birth process and the code from Chapter 16 should be used. If the condition is community-acquired, a code from Chapter 16 should not be assigned.

All clinically significant conditions noted on routine newborn examination should be coded. A condition is clinically significant if it requires:

- clinical evaluation,

- therapeutic treatment,

- diagnostic procedures,

- extended length of hospital stay,

- increased nursing care and/or monitoring, or

- if the condition has implications for future health care needs.

OBSERVATION AND EVALUATION OF NEWBORNS FOR SUSPECTED CONDITIONS NOT FOUND

Assign a code from category Z05, Encounter for observation and evaluation of newborn for suspected diseases and conditions ruled out, to identify those instances when a healthy newborn is evaluated for a suspected condition that is determined after study not to be present. Do not use a code from category Z05 when the patient has identified signs or symptoms of a suspected problem; in such cases code the sign or symptom.

A code from category Z05 may also be assigned as a principal or first-listed code for readmissions or encounters when the code from category Z38 code no longer applies. Codes from category Z05 are for use only for healthy newborns for which no condition after study is found to be present. A code from category Z05 is to be used as a secondary code after the code from category Z38, Liveborn infants according to place of birth and type of delivery.

CODING ADDITIONAL PERINATAL DIAGNOSES

Report codes for conditions that require treatment or further investigation, prolong the length of stay, require resource utilization, or have implications for future health care needs. Do not report these codes for adult patients.

PREMATURITY AND FETAL GROWTH RETARDATION

A code for prematurity should not be reported unless the documentation supports this diagnosis. Codes in the following categories should be based on the recorded birth weight and estimated gestational age:

- P05, Disorders of newborn related to slow fetal growth and fetal malnutrition

- P07, Disorders of newborn related to short gestation and low birth weight, not elsewhere classified

Codes from category P05 should not be assigned with codes from category P07. When both birthweight and gestational age are available, two codes from category P07 should be reported, with the code for birthweight sequenced first and the code for gestational age reported as the secondary diagnosis. Codes from category P07 are used for a child or adult who was premature or who had a low birthweight as a newborn that is affecting the patient's current health status.

BACTERIAL SEPSIS OF NEWBORN

If an infant in the perinatal period is documented as having sepsis without documentation of whether it was congenital or community-acquired, the default is congenital and a code from category P36 should be assigned. In addition, the following guidelines should be followed:

- If the code from category P36 includes the causal organism, an additional code from category B95, Streptococcus, Staphylococcus, and Enterococcus as the cause of diseases classified elsewhere, or B96, Other bacterial agents as the cause of diseases classified elsewhere, should not be assigned.

- If the code from category P36 does not include the causal organism, assign an additional code from category B96. If documented, use additional codes to identify severe sepsis (R65.2-) and any associated acute organ dysfunction.

STILLBIRTH

Diagnosis code P95, Stillbirth, is only reported in institutions that maintain separate records for stillbirths. No other code should be used with code P95. Code P95 should not be used in the mother's record.

ICD-10-CM Official Coding Guidelines for Congenital Malformations, Deformations, and Chromosomal Abnormalities

Report codes from Chapter 17, categories Q00-Q99, Congenital Malformations, Deformations, and Chromosomal Abnormalities, when a malformation/deformation or chromosomal abnormality is documented. These codes may be the first-listed or secondary diagnosis depending on the circumstance of the patient encounter. The following guidelines apply:

- If there are additional manifestations present, report the manifestations as additional diagnoses.

- When the manifestation is inherent to the anomaly, the manifestation should not be reported.

- When a manifestation is not inherent to the anomaly, it may be reported as an additional diagnosis.

- Codes from Chapter 17 may be used throughout the life of the patient.

- If a congenital malformation or deformity has been corrected, a personal history code should be used to identify the history of the malformation or deformity.

- Although present at birth, these conditions may not be diagnosed until later in life. Whenever the physician diagnoses the condition, it is appropriate to report a code from categories Q00-Q99.

For a birth admission, the appropriate code from category Z38, Liveborn infants according to place of birth and type of delivery, should be sequenced as the first listed diagnosis followed by a code from categories Q00-Q99.

It is time to build skill and knowledge by coding the following exercises. Be sure to reference the ICD-10-CM codebook and the ICD-10-CM Official Guidelines for Coding and Reporting, along with the instructional notes, when coding these conditions.

Pregnancy, Childbirth, and the Puerperium (O00-O99); Certain Conditions Originating in the Perinatal Period (P00-P96); and Congenital Malformations, Deformations, and Chromosomal Abnormalities (Q00-Q99)

CASE STUDY 12

A 20-year-old patient suffering from severe (preeclamptic) toxemia was hospitalized during the second trimester of her pregnancy. The patient was a juvenile onset diabetic. She presents to our office today in follow-up.

Examination reveals no abnormal heart sounds. I reviewed the series of blood glucose tests that had been drawn and analyzed every four hours to determine the best course of insulin therapy for the woman during her hospital course of treatment. Based on review of all the data available, it was apparent that the pregnancy is increasing the woman's insulin needs. The patient's insulin dosage will be increased. Instructions for continued monitoring have been outlined and counseling and explanations were provided to the patient.

ICD-10-CM Code(s) _____

CASE STUDY 13

The patient is a 25-year-old, gravida 1, para 0, who was admitted at 37 weeks and 4 days' gestation with intrauterine fetal demise. There was no obvious cause. She had an unremarkable prenatal history. All diabetic testing was negative. Toxoplasmosis testing was negative. HIV was negative. Hepatitis screening was negative. She presented with complaint of decreased fetal movement. No fetal heart was noted. She was induced with Cervidil, artificial rupture of membranes, and Pitocin. There was an eight-hour labor. At one point, her contractions became 240 Montevideo units, and at this point the Cervidil was removed and we had her back down to roughly 200 Montevideo units. She progressed to full dilatation. She pushed for about 40 minutes. She had a normal spontaneous vaginal delivery. It was a male infant who was nonviable and there were no obvious defects. The placenta was spontaneous. I was unable to get cord blood because there was thrombosis in the cord. She did have a third degree laceration that was repaired in layers with O-Chromic, 2-Chromic, and 3-Chromic suture. I did place 0.5% Marcaine afterwards, subcuticularly 10 mL without epinephrine, for long-term pain control and she did have an epidural in labor. We gave her IV Valium as well. She seemed to do well with the delivery. There was appropriate grieving. We did not note a knot in the cord. There was no obvious abruption. The insertion of the cord was at the center of the placenta. There was no velamentous insertion noted. There was just no obvious problem. The mother is being started on Lexapro and she will go through grieving and counseling.

ICD-10-CM Code(s) _____

CASE STUDY 14

The patient is a 21-year-old, gravida 2, para 1, with an estimated delivery date of 11/27/20xx, which puts her at 38 weeks and 6 days. She was admitted at about 4:30 this morning in spontaneous labor at 5 cm, 75%, and a -2 station with bag of water intact. She stated that her contractions started between 3:30 and 4:00 and were every two to four minutes. An IV was started per protocol and she was given an epidural per Dr Marcus with good relief. At 6:27 am, I artificially ruptured membranes with clear fluid. She was 8 to 9 cm at that time and at 0 station. She was turned on her side and allowed to labor down. Push times three contractions, and at 7:56 am we had a spontaneous delivery of the head over an intact perineum. A tight nuchal cord was noted. The baby's nose and mouth were bulb-suctioned. The posterior shoulder was live and the baby was delivered through the cord. The baby was vigorous upon delivery and placed on the mother's abdomen, at which time he was dried thoroughly and began to cry. The cord was then doubly clamped and cut. Cord blood was obtained. This was followed shortly by a spontaneous delivery of a grossly intact placenta with an eccentric insertion of a three-vessel cord. The fundus firmed with massage and 20 units Pitocin to the IV fluid. Inspection of the perineum and vaginal vault revealed no lacerations or tears. Estimated blood loss was 300 mL. This was a male infant weighing 6 pounds, 6 ounces, 19.5 inches long, with Apgar scores of 9 and 9. Mom and baby are both stable.

ICD-10-CM Code(s) _____

CASE STUDY 15

The patient presented in labor at 41 weeks and 2 days' gestation. She had a normal spontaneous vaginal delivery with delivery of a liveborn infant.

NONOPERATIVE PROCEDURES: Amniotomy.

ANESTHESIA: Epidural.

ESTIMATED BLOOD LOSS: 400 mL.

FINDINGS: A female infant, cephalic presentation, with meconium-stained fluid. Apgar scores were 8 and 9. Time of birth was 04:17 on 04/12. The fetus weighed 7 pounds, 5 ounces.

HOSPITAL COURSE: This 20-year old, G2, PO-0-1-0 presented at 41 weeks, 2 days' gestation with regular painful contractions. She was at least 5 to 6 cm upon arrival on the April 11th. Later that day an amniotomy was performed after she had made no real significant change in her cervix. The patient progressed slowly through labor and then, after getting an epidural, her labor course progressed more quickly. She pushed for at least an hour.

PAST MEDICAL HISTORY: Not significant for diabetes, hypertension, or asthma. She is healthy and Rh positive, rubella immune, and GBS negative.

DESCRIPTION OF PROCEDURE: The patient was positioned in a semi-Fowler's position. With a series of successful pushes, the fetal vertex was delivered without nuchal cord. The cord was clamped shut and cut. The infant was not stimulated initially and taken over to the warmer where deep suction was performed with wall suction. A moderate amount of meconium-stained fluid was obtained. After the fetus was delivered and transferred to the warmer, appropriate resuscitation

was begun. The fetus responded with a brisk response initially, only lacking color in its initial response.

Attention was then turned to the peritoneum. There was noted to be small, superficial periurethral lacerations on the left and right. The patient's right had more significant bleeding and therefore 3-0 Chromic was used to reapproximate vaginal and vulvar epithelium in interrupted sutures. A left-sided superficial periurethral laceration was also noted, but this was not bleeding and it was not repaired. At this point the placenta was delivered. The placenta had a central insertion and was noted to be intact. Attention was then focused on the peritoneum. The peritoneum was noted to have a second-degree midline perineal laceration that extended into a left laceration. This was repaired in a continuous fashion, locking above the hymen and then running just below the hymen without being locked with 0-Vicryl; this was repaired in the usual fashion. A superficial area of the perineum was reapproximated with 0-Vicryl. The sites were all hemostatic at the end of the procedure. The patient tolerated the procedure without complication and remained in delivery room for recovery.

ICD-10-CM Code(s) _____

CASE STUDY 16

A 21-year old female comes in the office today because she thinks she may be pregnant. She has not had a menstrual cycle in two months. She is not on any birth control and wants a pregnancy test. She has no other complaints.

Urine pregnancy test administered with a positive result. Follow-up in one month for OB care.

IMPRESSION: Positive pregnancy test.

ICD-10-CM Code(s) _____

CASE STUDY 17

This OB patient comes in for follow-up of glucose tolerance results. She is 22 weeks pregnant in her second trimester. Patient is positive for gestational diabetes and will be put on insulin to control her gestational diabetes. Patient was given a handout explaining her condition and how to control her diabetes.

IMPRESSION: Gestational diabetes, insulin controlled.

ICD-10-CM Code(s) _____

CASE STUDY 18

Patient is admitted to the hospital at 39 weeks for severe labor pains. She was dilated to 3 cm on admission.

An epidural was placed for labor pains. At approximately 0730 hours, she was 10 cm dilated. She progressed well and completely dilated, pushed approximately three times and proceeded with delivery. Normal vaginal delivery with no complications.

IMPRESSION: Normal vaginal delivery.

ICD-10-CM Code(s) _____

Symptoms, Signs, and Abnormal Clinical and Laboratory Findings, Not Elsewhere Classified (R00-R99); Injury, Poisoning, and Certain Other Consequences of External Causes (S00-T88)

ICD-10-CM Chapters 18 and 19 Guidelines Review

In this chapter you will find a summary of the chapter-specific coding guidelines for Chapters 18 and 19 of the ICD-10-CM codebook followed by case studies to build ICD-10-CM diagnosis coding skills in these areas.

Every medical specialty references Chapter 18 of the ICD-10-CM codebook for signs and symptoms and abnormal clinical findings, and Chapter 19, which includes information on injuries, poisonings, and certain other consequences of external causes. Keep in mind that you should always reference the ICD-10-CM Official Guidelines for Coding and Reporting in its entirety when making a code selection.

ICD-10-CM Official Coding Guidelines for Symptoms, Signs, and Abnormal Laboratory Findings, Not Elsewhere Classified

Codes in this category include conditions for which no diagnosis classifiable elsewhere is found. If a sign or symptom commonly occurs with a definitive diagnosis, code only the definitive diagnosis and not the sign and/or symptom, unless the instructional notes provide other guidance.

Signs and symptom codes are reported when a confirmed diagnosis is not determined by the provider and may be reported in addition to a related definitive diagnosis when the sign or symptom is not routinely associated with the particular diagnosis. The definitive diagnosis should always be reported as the first-listed diagnosis.

There are many combination codes that identify both the definitive diagnosis and common symptoms of the condition. For these codes, additional signs and/or symptoms codes are not reported.

Following are guidelines for coding specific signs and/or symptoms:

- Code R29.6, Repeated falls, is used when the patient has recently fallen or reason for the fall is under investigation.

- Code Z91.81, History of falling, is reported when the patient has fallen in the past and has a higher risk for future falls.

- Codes R29.6 and Z91.81 may be assigned together.

- Codes from category R40.2-, Coma scale, may be reported in conjunction with:

  - traumatic brain injury codes,

  - acute cerebrovascular disease codes, and

  - sequelae of cerebrovascular disease codes.

- Codes from category R40.2-, Coma scale, are typically used by trauma registries but may be used in any setting. These codes can be used in conjunction with traumatic brain injury diagnosis codes, acute cerebrovascular disease, or sequelae of cerebrovascular disease codes. The coma scale codes may also be used to assess the status of the central nervous system for other non-trauma conditions such as monitoring patients in the intensive care unit regardless of the patient's medical condition.

- Code R40.24 is assigned when only the total score is documented in the medical record and not the individual scores.

- Codes R40.2-, one from each subcategory, are needed to complete the scale. The seventh character indicates when the scale was recorded. The seventh character should match for all three codes.

- The NIH Stroke Scale (NIHSS) codes (R29.7-) can be used in conjunction with acute stroke codes (I63) to identify the patient's neurological status and the severity of the stroke. The stroke scale codes should be sequenced after the acute stroke diagnosis code(s). At a minimum, report the initial score documented. If desired, a facility may choose to capture multiple stroke scale scores.

- Code R53.2, Functional quadriplegia, should be used only if specifically documented in the medical record and is not used in cases of neurologic quadriplegia.

- SIRS (Systemic Inflammatory Response Syndrome): When SIRS is documented with a non-infectious condition, and no subsequent infection is documented, the code for the underlying condition, such as an injury, should be assigned, followed by code R65.10, Systemic inflammatory response syndrome (SIRS) of non-infectious origin without acute organ dysfunction, or code R65.11, Systemic inflammatory response syndrome (SIRS) of non-infectious origin with acute organ dysfunction.

- If an associated acute organ dysfunction is documented, the appropriate code(s) for the specific type of organ dysfunction(s) should be assigned in addition to code R65.11.

- If acute organ dysfunction is documented, but cannot be determined if the acute organ dysfunction is associated with SIRS or due to another condition, query the provider.

- Code R99, Ill-defined and unknown cause of mortality, is used when a patient has died before arrival at the healthcare facility and is pronounced dead upon arrival.

It is time to build skill and knowledge by coding the following exercises relative to symptoms, signs, and abnormal clinical and laboratory findings. Be sure to reference the ICD-10-CM codebook and the ICD-10-CM Official Guidelines for Coding and Reporting, along with the instructional notes, when coding these conditions.

Symptoms, Signs, and Abnormal Clinical and Laboratory Findings, Not Elsewhere Classified (R00-R99)

CASE STUDY 1

This patient is a 10-year-old boy who gets tonsillitis maybe two or three times a year. His mother is concerned because his tonsils remain enlarged in between attacks and also because he sometimes has a snoring problem.

EXAMINATION: The nasal airway seems to be adequate. Both tonsils are average size and not considered to be too enlarged and do not seem to be causing any obstruction of the airway. Eardrums and ear canals are normal.

The mother was reassured that T&A is not required at this stage and that the adenoid tissue will regress and the snoring problem will eventually diminish.

ICD-10-CM Code(s) _____

CASE STUDY 2

CHIEF COMPLAINT: Follow-up for hypertension.

Follow-up visit; using relaxation and Atenalol. Still experiencing severe headache pain with severe throbbing pain. Feeling steadier on his feet. No chest pain or shortness of breath. Still stating symptoms change with weather, today a particularly bad day. In hospital earlier this month with CT negative, MRI with periventriular changes with ischemia.

NECK: Carotids without bruits.

LUNGS: Clear to A&P.

HEART: RRR.

EXTREMITIES: No edema.

Blood pressure elevated but much improved, controlled compared to initial evaluation. Patient last took medications at 4 pm yesterday—elevation may be trough effect. Continue Atenalol 50 mg OD. Check blood pressure in the morning; if better controlled, will change dosage to 25 mg bid. Headaches persistent. EEG without pathological significance. Refer to specialist. Follow up in one month.

ICD-10-CM Code(s) _____

CASE STUDY 3

REASON FOR THE VISIT: Sepsis

HISTORY OF PRESENT ILLNESS: This is a 43-year-old male with a history of hepatitis C, cirrhosis, and a history of alcohol abuse currently in remission who presented in the emergency room (ER) on 04/10/20xx for a ground-level fall secondary to weak knees. He complained of bilateral knee pain but also had other symptoms including hematuria and epigastric pain for at least a month. He ran out of prescription medications one month ago. In the ER he was initially afebrile, but then spiked up to 101.3°F with a heart rate of 130 and a respiratory rate of 24. White blood cell count was slightly low at 4 and platelet count was only 22,000. Abdominal ultrasound showed mild-to-moderate ascites. He was given one dose of Zosyn and then started on Levofloxacin and Flagyl last night. Dr X was called early this morning due to hypotension and a systolic blood pressure in the 70s. He then changed antibiotic regimen to Vancomycin and Doripenem.

PAST MEDICAL HISTORY: Hepatitis C, cirrhosis, coronary artery disease, hyperlipidemia, chronic venous stasis, gastroesophageal reflux disease, history of exploratory laparotomy for stab wounds, chronic recurrent leg wounds, and hepatic encephalopathy.

SOCIAL HISTORY: The patient is a former smoker, reportedly quit in 20xx. He used cocaine in the past, reportedly quit in 20xx. He also has a history of alcohol abuse, but apparently quit more than 10 years ago.

ALLERGIES: None known.

CURRENT MEDICATIONS: Vancomycin, Doripenem, thiamine, Protonix, potassium chloride prn, magnesium prn, Zofran prn, Norepinephrine drip, and vitamin K.

REVIEW OF SYSTEMS: Not obtainable as the patient is drowsy and confused.

PHYSICAL EXAMINATION:

CONSTITUTIONAL/VITAL SIGNS: Heart rate 101; respiratory rate 17; blood pressure 92/48; temperature 97.5°F; oxygen saturation 98% on 2 L nasal cannula.

GENERAL APPEARANCE: The patient is drowsy and morbidly obese. Height: 5 feet, 8 inches; body weight: 400 pounds.

EYES: Slightly pale conjunctivae, icteric sclerae. Pupils equal, brisk reaction to light.

EARS, NOSE, MOUTH, AND THROAT: Intact gross hearing. Moist oral mucosa. No oral lesions.

NECK: No palpable neck masses. Thyroid is not enlarged on inspection.

RESPIRATORY: Regular inspiratory effort. No crackles or wheezes.

CARDIOVASCULAR: Regular cardiac rhythm. No rales or rubs. Positive bipedal edema, 2+, right worse than left.

GASTROINTESTINAL: Globular abdomen. Soft. No guarding, no rigidity. Tender on palpation of right upper quadrant and epigastric area. Mildly tender on palpation of right upper quadrant and epigastric area.

LYMPHATIC: No cervical lymphadenopathy.

SKIN: Positive diffuse jaundice. No palpable subcutaneous nodules.

PSYCHIATRIC: Poor judgment and insight.

LABORATORY: White blood cell count is 9 with 68% neutrophils, 20% bands; H&H 9.7/28.2; platelet count 24,000. INR 3.84; PTT more than 240; BUN and creatinine 26.8/1.2. AST 76; ALT 27; alkaline phosphatase 48; total bilirubin 17.85. Total CK 1198.6; LDH 873.2. Troponin 0.09, myoglobin 2792. Urinalysis shows small leucocyte esterase, positive nitrites, 1 to 3 wbc, 0 to 1 rbc 2+ bacteria. Two sets of blood cultures from 01/07/20xx still pending.

RADIOLOGY: Chest X ray did not show any pathologic abnormalities of the heart, mediastinum, lung fields, or bony or soft tissue structures. Left knee X rays showed advanced osteoarthritis. Abdominal ultrasound showed mild-to-moderate ascites and mild prominence of the gallbladder with thickened ball and pericholecystic fluid. Preliminary report of CAT scan of the abdomen showed changes consistent to liver cirrhosis and portal hypertension with mild ascites, splenomegaly, and dilated portal/splenic and superior mesenteric vein. Appendix was not clearly seen, but there was no evidence of pericecal inflammation.

ASSESSMENT:

1. Severe sepsis with septic shock

2. Urinary tract infection

3. Ascites, rule out spontaneous bacterial peritonitis

4. Cholangitis

5. Alcoholic cirrhosis of liver

6. History of alcoholism

7. Thrombocytopenia

8. Viral hepatitis C

9. Cryoglobulinemic

RECOMMENDATIONS:

1. Continue with Vancomycin and Doripenem at this point.

2. Agree with paracentesis.

3. Send ascitic fluid for cell count, differential, and cultures.

4. Follow up with result of blood cultures.

5. We will get urine culture from the specimen on admission.

6. The patient needs hepatitis A vaccination.

ICD-10-CM Code(s) _____

CASE STUDY 4

CHIEF COMPLAINT: Abdominal pain.

HISTORY OF PRESENT ILLNESS: The patient is a 64-year-old white male with a history of acute onset of abdominal pain. He came into the ER with this abdominal pain on 3/25/20xx. He was given 10 mg of morphine at that time without much improvement. He was then given 4 mg of Dilaudid and then also Fentanyl with some improvement after that. I was asked to see this patient in consultation by the ER physician. When I saw him, he was still complaining of epigastric abdominal pain. He was not complaining of any other symptoms, although he states that the acute onset of abdominal pain the previous day was after he was eating. He also had some cold sweats at that time and he threw up. He states that this pain is just epigastric without any radiation to his back or lower abdomen. He also states that he has some dysphagia to solids that gets resolved when he drinks liquids to push the solids down the gastrointestinal tract. He states that he has had this problem for approximately one month. No other associated symptoms. No fevers in the hospital. No chills. No hematuria, dysuria, or constipation. No diarrhea.

PAST MEDICAL HISTORY:

- Hypertension

- Chronic back pain

- No allergies

PAST SURGICAL HISTORY:

- Lumbar laminectomy in 20xx

- Laparoscopic cholecystectomy in 20xx

FAMILY HISTORY: It seems that his father and mother both died from cardiovascular disease.

SOCIAL HISTORY: Divorced.

MEDICATIONS:

- Methadone

- Antihypertensive drugs

REVIEW OF SYSTEMS:

CONSTITUTIONAL: He claims that he had episodes of chills and maybe fevers. He does not refer to any weight loss recently.

CARDIOVASCULAR: No history of chest pain or tachyarrhythmia.

CHEST: No history of shortness of breath or tachypnea.

GI: Abdominal pain and some nausea.

GU: No hematuria or dysuria.

SKIN: No history of skin cancers or new skin lesions. No rashes.

ORTHOPEDIC: As stated previously; just history of chronic back pain and also knee problems. There are no recent dislocations or fractures.

NEUROLOGIC: No history of stroke.

PSYCHIATRIC: No history of anxiety or depression.

ENDOCRINOLOGIC: No history of thyroid disease or diabetes.

PHYSICAL EXAMINATION:

GENERAL: He is awake, alert, and oriented ×3.

CARDIOVASCULAR: Regular.

CHEST: Lungs are clear.

ABDOMEN: Tender in the epigastrium, but soft with no peritoneal signs and no hepatosplenomegaly. Very well healed wounds from previous laparoscopic cholecystectomy. No groin hernias. No other palpable masses.

DIAGNOSTIC DATA: He has a white blood cell count of 10.9; creatinine is 1; lipase is 23; amylase is 45. Alkaline phosphatase is 31; SGPT 12; SGOT 11. Bilirubin total is 0.9. CT scan shows bilateral renal cysts as well as hepatic cysts and calcification of his prostate. No signs of bowel obstruction or any other abnormalities.

ASSESSMENT: Patient with abdominal pain in the epigastrium.

PLAN:

1. We will start him on Lansoprazole for now and also on Carafate.

2. Perform endoscopy tomorrow to evaluate his dysphagia.

ICD-10-CM Code(s) _____

CASE STUDY 5

HISTORY OF PRESENT ILLNESS: The patient is a 30-year-old white female. I was asked by Dr Warfield to see this patient. She started developing abdominal pain yesterday. The pain is diffuse and in the lower abdomen. The pain has no radiation to her sides or back. There are no other signs or symptoms. She refers to one episode of nausea and vomiting after she took pain medicine, but she has no more nausea or vomiting now. No history of fever or chills. No history of UTI symptoms.

PAST MEDICAL HISTORY: There is a history of hypothyroidism. Allergic to sulfa.

PAST SURGICAL HISTORY: Tonsillectomy.

MEDICATIONS: Levsin prn.

SOCIAL HISTORY: She smokes one pack of cigarettes a day. She is married and has two children.

FAMILY HISTORY: Mother and father are alive and healthy.

REVIEW OF SYSTEMS:

CONSTITUTIONAL: No history of weight loss or fevers.

CARDIOVASCULAR: No history of chest pain or tacharrhythmias.

CHEST: No history of shortness of breath or tachypnea.

GU: History, in the past, of UTIs, but at this point she does not have any UTI symptoms. No history of hematuria or dysuria.

GI: As stated before, abdominal pain with some nausea and vomiting.

DERMATOLOGIC: No history of rashes or lesions.

NEUROLOGIC: Negative for seizure or stroke.

PSYCHIATRIC: No history of depression or anxiety.

ORTHOPEDIC: No history of dislocations or fractures.

PHYSICAL EXAMINATION:

GENERAL: She is awake, alert, and oriented ×3. She is afebrile.

VITAL SIGNS: Stable.

CHEST: Lungs are clear.

CARDIOVASCULAR: Regular rate and rhythm.

ABDOMEN: Soft, tender in the lower quadrant. Bowel sounds are active but decreased. No palpable masses. No palpable inguinal hernias. No hepatosplenomegaly.

EXTREMITIES: No signs of edema.

DIAGNOSTIC DATA: White blood cell count is 15,000.

ASSESSMENT: Patient with abdominal pain.

PLAN: We will perform a CT scan to rule out intra-abdominal pathology, including appendicitis and diverticulitis. Treatment options will be determined based on results from CT scan.

ICD-10-CM Code(s) _____

CASE STUDY 6

HISTORY OF PRESENT ILLNESS: This is a 35-year-old female with a history of diabetes. Dr Jones requested a consultation in regard to the patient's chest pain and shortness of breath. This patient was admitted earlier this morning. The patient says that she has been having chest pain for the past few years that has become worse over the past few months. Patient described the chest pain as tightening, squeezes across the chest, occurs every couple of days, 3 of 5 on a scale of 1 to 5. Exertion related and activity related, relieved with rest, associated with shortness of breath as well as left arm numbness. Patient also says that she has gained nearly 40 pounds in three months. Apparently, she has tried Lasix and Bumex, and her weight has not changed. Patient says that her exercise capacity is all right.

PAST MEDICAL HISTORY: Significant for history of diabetes.

PAST SURGICAL HISTORY: Significant for history of dilation and curettage, surgery on the right thumb, and surgery on the right foot.

SOCIAL AND PERSONAL HISTORY: She is married and a non-smoker. No history of alcohol or substance abuse.

ALLERGIES: Penicillin and sulfa.

MEDICATIONS: Home medications are listed and I have reviewed them.

FAMILY HISTORY: Patient's father is diabetic and has many health problems. Patient's mother also has hypertension and is diabetic. Patient's younger brother has heart problems.

REVIEW OF SYSTEMS:

CONSTITUTIONAL: Complains of weight gain and mild fatigue. No fever.

CARDIOVASCULAR: Patient has chest pain, shortness of breath, weight gain. Denies any history of orthopnea. No history of palpitations, dizziness, near syncopal or syncopal episodes.

RESPIRATORY: Shortness of breath. No cough. No sputum production.

REVIEW OF OTHER SYSTEMS: Negative.

PHYSICAL EXAMINATION: Examination reveals a well-developed, slightly obese female in no apparent distress at this time. Patient's vitals are noted. HEENT: Pupils are equal, round, and reactive to light. Extraocular movements are intact. Oropharynx is clear. Neck: There is no JVD, thyromegaly, lymphadenopathy, or bruit. Lungs: Clear to auscultation bilaterally without wheeze, rhonchi, or crackle. Heart: Reveals regular rate and rhythm without murmur, rub, or gallop. Abdomen: Soft, nontender, nondistended with good bowel sounds. Extremities: Strength is 5/5 in all four extremities. Reveal no lower extremity edema. Pulses are 2+ throughout. Neurologic: Cranial nerves II–XII are grossly intact.

ASSESSMENT:

1. Chest pain/shortness of breath, strongly suspect angina

2. Hyperlipidemia

3. Diabetes

4. Weight gain, etiology uncertain; unlikely to be fluid overload

PLAN:

1. Stress Cardiolite to evaluate for any coronary ischemia as a cause for patient's chest pain and shortness of breath.

2. Echocardiogram to look for any diastolic dysfunction as well as to look for any significant valvulopathy to explain patient's weight gain.

3. Start patient on Zocor 40 mg po daily as patient is a diabetic and has elevated lipid profile.

4. I discussed the patient's coronary artery disease risk factors and modifications.

ICD-10-CM Code(s) _____

CASE STUDY 7

OPERATION PERFORMED:
Esophagogastroduodenoscopy (EGD) and Maloney dilation.

INDICATIONS FOR PROCEDURE: This is a 40-year-old female with rheumatoid arthritis who has been developing progressive dysphagia over the last week. The patient had an outpatient attempt at an esophagram in the ER that suggested she had a proximal esophageal stricture; therefore, this examination is being done to evaluate this abnormality.

DESCRIPTION OF PROCEDURE: Informed consent was obtained from the patient. Demerol 60 mg and Versed 3 mg were given intravenous slowly for sedation. The patient was placed in the left lateral position. The GIF-100 EGD scope was passed into the esophagus via the no-touch technique. The esophagus did not demonstrate a definite stricture endoscopically. Whether or not I passed it on inserting the scope, I cannot be certain. Nevertheless, there was certainly no resistance to the passage of the 9-mm scope into the proximal esophagus. The esophagogastric junction was at 40 cm. Stomach was entered and found to be within normal limits, without ulceration. The duodenal bulb and descending duodenum were both normal. The scope was then withdrawn and Maloney dilators 36, 42, 46, and 52 were passed sequentially without difficulty. The patient tolerated both procedures well and returned to the recovery room in good condition.

ASSESSMENT:

1. Possible proximal esophageal stricture

2. Status post Maloney dilation

ICD-10-CM Code(s) _____

CASE STUDY 8

HISTORY OF PRESENT ILLNESS: This 73-year-old female presents today for initial urology evaluation. She has been found to have microscopic hematuria, never gross. An intravenous pyelogram (IVP) shows no upper or lower tract abnormalities. No history of genitourinary problems.

ALLERGIES: No known medical allergies.

MEDICATIONS: Aspirin-81, Meloxicam, Prevacid.

PAST MEDICAL HISTORY: Breast cancer, colon resection, mastectomy with reconstruction.

SOCIAL HISTORY: Patient admits alcohol and tobacco use.

FAMILY HISTORY: Patient admits a family history of heart problems, hypertension, diabetes, insulin dependent, cancer, and arthritis.

REVIEW OF SYSTEMS: Genitourinary: Admits nocturia. Denies blood in urine, dysuria, frequency, urgency, thin stream. Constitutional symptoms: Denies chills, fever, nausea, vomiting, unexplained weight change. Gastrointestinal: Denies abdominal pain, bowel habit change. Musculoskeletal: Denies back pain.

PHYSICAL EXAMINATION:

CONSTITUTIONAL: Patient is a pleasant, 73-year-old female in no apparent distress who looks her given age. She is well developed and well-nourished with good attention to hygiene and body habits. Oriented to person, place, and time. Mood and affect appear appropriate to the situation.

SKIN/EXTREMITIES: No skin rash.

TEST RESULTS: Complete urinalysis results on a specimen: Voided mid-stream specimen. Blood: trace; glucose: negative; ketones: negative; leukocyte esterase: negative; nitrites: negative. pH: 5.0; protein: negative; specific gravity: 1.025.

ASSESSMENT AND PLAN: Microscopic hematuria. NMP-22 (negative), RTC for cystoscopy.

ICD-10-CM Code(s) _____

CASE STUDY 9

A 25-year-old female, who is a new patient, requests a pregnancy test because she stopped birth control pills three months ago and has not had a period since. She also has burning on urination for three days. Patient denies vaginal discharge, fever, hematuria, nocturia, nausea, or vomiting.

PHYSICAL EXAMINATION:

VITAL SIGNS: Temperature: 98.6°F; blood pressure 120/82; weight 120 pounds.

GENERAL: Well-nourished, well-developed 25-year-old female, cooperative, nervous.

BREASTS: No masses, lumps, or tenderness.

ABDOMEN: Soft, nontender; no masses palpable.

PELVIC: Normal external genitalia; erythematous urethral meatus. Vaginal vault clear, cervix normal. Fundus small, adnexa without masses or tenderness. Bladder negative for masses or tenderness.

RECTAL: Negative for hemorrhoids or masses.

LABORATORY: Urine dip negative; urine pregnancy test negative.

ASSESSMENT AND PLAN: Dysuria and primary amenorrhea. Dysuria: Begin Doxycycline 100 mg po bid ×7 days. She may have urethritis. Will send urine for culture. Encouraged to finish this medication no matter what the culture shows. Primary amenorrhea: Apparently not due to pregnancy. May be post-pill phenomenon and explained this to her. Patient is to return for re-evaluation in one month or sooner if urinary symptoms do not improve.

ICD-10-CM Code(s) _____

CASE STUDY 10

PREOPERATIVE DIAGNOSIS: Right flank mass, 3 × 3 cm, right lower quadrant.

POSTOPERATIVE DIAGNOSIS: Same, probably lipoma.

OPERATION PERFORMED: Excision of right flank mass.

ANESTHESIA: 1% Xylocaine and MAC.

PROCEDURE: With the patient on the operating table in the left lateral position, his right flank was sterilely prepared and draped. The area over the mass infiltrated with 1% Xylocaine. Incision made, the underlying mass excised. Clinically this looked like a lipoma that went through the deep structures. The lipoma was removed. Layered closure was accomplished with interrupted sutures of 3-0 Vicryl and the skin with a running subcuticular closure of 3-0 Vicryl. Steri-Strips applied and sterile dressing applied. The patient went to the recovery room in stable condition to be discharged and followed in the clinic in two to three weeks. Given Vicodin one to two every four to six hours prn for pain.

ICD-10-CM Code(s) _____

CASE STUDY 11

CHIEF COMPLAINT: This is a 78-year-old white male with a known history of coronary artery disease and a previous history of coronary artery bypass surgery times four in May 199x. He also has a history of biventricular AICD, which was performed in September 20xx. He came in to the office earlier today complaining of chest pain and shortness of breath. It has been going on for a couple of days. We had given him a shot of Lasix in the office, but it did not seem to help. He also is known to have hyperlipidemia and peripheral vascular disease. He has no leg claudication. He exercises three times a week at the outpatient cardiac rehab center.

REVIEW OF SYSTEMS: Negative for fever, weight loss; positive for occasional heart palpitations. No allergies.

PHYSICAL EXAMINATION: Upon examination, blood pressure is 116/54. Pulse rate is 64 per minute and regular. The pupils are equal and there is no icterus. Examination of the neck demonstrates no JVD, lymphadenopathy, or thyromegaly. Cardiac examination demonstrates normal heart sounds without any S3 or S4 and there are no murmurs and no bruits. Both lungs have inspiratory and expiratory wheezes and respiratory effort seems difficult. The abdomen is nondistended, nontender, and bowel sounds are normal. The lower extremity examination demonstrates no evidence of edema and there is no calf tenderness. CNS examination demonstrated cranial nerves intact and DTRs normal.

ASSESSMENT AND PLAN: This patient is being admitted to the hospital for likely pneumonia. We will order a chest X ray for confirmation. He will continue his normal medications at this time. Once we confirm whether or not he has pneumonia, we will then start him on antibiotic therapy.

ICD-10-CM Code(s) _____

ICD-10-CM Official Coding Guidelines for Injury, Poisoning, and Certain Other Consequences of External Causes (S00-T88)

Chapter 19 of the ICD-10-CM codebook consists of "S" codes and "T" codes. S codes are used to report traumatic injuries and T codes are used to report burns and corrosions, poisonings, toxic effects, adverse effects, underdosing, complications of medical care, and other such consequences of external causes.

Most blocks in Chapter 19 require a seventh-character for the applicable code. Most code categories use the following three seventh characters:

- A—initial encounter

- D—subsequent encounter

- S—sequelae

Fractures are reported with different extensions as follows:

- Seventh character "A" is used only for each patient encounter for active treatment for the injury or condition.

- Seventh character "D"—subsequent encounter—is used for encounters after the patient has **completed** active treatment of the condition and is receiving routine care for the condition during the healing or recovery phase.

- The aftercare Z codes are used for aftercare conditions such as injuries or poisonings where seventh characters are provided to identify subsequent care. The ICD-10-CM guidelines direct the user to report the injury code that precipitated the complication and the code for the sequelae, as follows:

  - Seventh character "S" is used for complications or conditions as a direct result of a condition. A good example is scar formation following a burn. The scar would be sequelae of the burn. When reporting a code with the seventh character "S," it is necessary to use both the injury code that precipitated the sequelae and the code for the sequelae.

  - The "S" is added to the injury code, not the code for the complication or sequelae. The sequelae (ie, the complication or the condition as a result of the injury) is sequenced first, and the injury code is sequenced second.

  - Do not report an aftercare Z code for aftercare of injuries if the injuries are sequelae.

INJURIES

When reporting injuries, the following guidelines apply:

- Assign separate codes for each injury unless a combination code is available to be assigned.

- The most severe injury is sequenced first. Injury codes are categorized by type of injury and site.

- Code T07, Unspecified multiple injuries, should only be assigned in the inpatient setting when a more specific code is not available.

- Traumatic injury codes (S00-T14.9) are not used for normal, healing surgical wounds or to identify a complication from a surgical wound.

- Instructional notes indicate which other codes will describe the injury fully. (For example, for open wounds, an instructional note provides guidance to the user to code any associated wound infection.)

- For normal healing surgical wounds, a wound code from Chapter 19 is not used.

- Codes in Chapter 19 are divided into body regions. Within each body section are categories for type of injury specific to the body section.

- Superficial injuries (abrasions, contusions) are not to be separately reported when associated with more severe injuries of the same site.

- When coding superficial and open wounds, assign codes based on terms documented in the medical record. For example, if a wound is classified as a bite, it would be classified as an "open bite." Superficial wounds are not coded with a more severe injury if it is associated with that injury at the same site.

FRACTURES

Traumatic fractures are coded using the appropriate seventh character for initial encounter (A, B, C) for each encounter where the patient is receiving active treatment for the fracture. The appropriate seventh character for initial encounter should also be assigned for a patient who delayed seeking treatment for the fracture or nonunion. Fractures are coded using the appropriate seventh character for subsequent care for encounters after the patient has completed active treatment of the fracture and is receiving routine care for the fracture during the healing or recovery phase.

Care for complications of surgical treatment for fracture repairs during the healing or recovery phase should be coded with the appropriate complication codes. Care of complications of fractures, such as malunion and nonunion, should be reported with the appropriate seventh character for subsequent care with nonunion (K, M, N) or subsequent care with malunion (P, Q, R). The appropriate seventh character for initial encounter should also be assigned for a patient who delayed seeking treatment for the fracture or nonunion.

The open fracture designations in the assignment of the seventh character for fractures of the forearm, femur, and lower leg, including ankle, are based on the Gustilo open fracture classification. When the Gustilo classification type is not specified for an open fracture, the seventh character for open fracture type I or II should be assigned (B, E, H, M, Q).

When reporting fractures, the following guidelines apply:

- Fractures are coded by site for each individual fracture. As many fracture codes needed to describe the fracture should be used with the most serious fracture coded first based on the medical record documentation.

- A fracture not documented as open or closed is coded as closed. For fractures, the seventh-character extension is added to the code reported in addition to other extensions to identify whether the fracture is open or closed, for routine healing, delayed healing, and nonunion and malunion.

- For open fractures of the long bone, extensions identify the degree of severity. The fracture extensions are unique to each type of bone and type of fracture. It is necessary to review the fracture extensions carefully before assigning an extension. A fracture code is reported as long as the patient is receiving treatment for the fracture.

- A code from category M80 is reported for patients with known osteoporosis who suffer a fracture even if it is a minor fall or trauma that would not normally break a healthy bone.

- The severity of the fracture dictates sequencing.

BURNS AND CORROSIONS

ICD-10-CM distinguishes between burns and corrosions. The burn codes are to report thermal burns that come from a heat source, such as a fire or hot appliance. The burn codes are also for burns resulting from electricity and radiation; corrosions are burns due to chemicals.

When coding burns and corrosions, the following guidelines apply:

- If a burn is a thermal burn, a burn code should be used.

- If a burn is a chemical burn, a corrosion code should be used.

- The guidelines for burns and corrosions are the same.

- Sunburns are not coded in this category but coded in category L55.0-.

- Code categories T20-T25 are used to report burns and corrosions.

- Burn and corrosion codes are classified by:
  - site;
  - depth; and
  - first degree (erythema), second degree (blistering), or third degree (full-thickness).

- When coding a burn of the eye (T26), these codes are classified by site, not by degree. Each burn or corrosion site is coded by sequencing the highest degree of burn or corrosion when more than one site is affected.

- Burns and corrosions internally are reported before external burns if they require more extensive treatment or are more severe. Code burns of the same site to the highest degree using one code even if the burns or corrosions are of different degrees. Sequence first the code that reflects the highest degree of burn when more than one burn is present.

  - When the reason for the admission or encounter is for treatment of external multiple burns, sequence first the code that reflects the burn of the highest degree.

  - When a patient has both internal and external burns, the circumstances of admission govern the selection of the principal diagnosis or first-listed diagnosis.

  - When a patient is admitted for burn injuries and other related conditions such as smoke inhalation and/or respiratory failure, the circumstances of admission govern the selection of the principal or first-listed diagnosis.

- Classify burns of the same local site (three-character category level, T20-T28) but of different degrees to the subcategory identifying the highest degree recorded in the diagnosis.

- Non-healing burns are coded as acute burns. Necrosis of burned skin should be coded as a non-healed burn.

- For any documented infected burn site, use an additional code for the infection. When coding burns, assign separate codes for each burn site. Category T30, Burn and corrosion, body region unspecified is extremely vague and should rarely be used.

- Assign codes from category T31, Burns classified according to extent of body surface involved, or T32, Corrosions classified according to extent of body surface involved, when the site of the burn is not specified or when there is a need for additional data. It is advisable to use category T31 as additional coding when needed to provide data for evaluating burn mortality, such as that needed by burn units. It is also advisable to use category T31 as an additional code for reporting purposes when there is mention of a third-degree burn involving 20 percent or more of the body surface.

- Encounters for the treatment of the late effects of burns or corrosions (ie, scars or joint contractures) should be coded with a burn or corrosion code with the seventh character "S" for sequela.

- When appropriate, both a code for a current burn or corrosion with seventh character "A" or "D" and a burn or corrosion code with the seventh character "S" may be assigned on the same record (when both a current burn and sequela of an old burn exist). Burns and corrosions do not heal at the same rate and a current healing wound may still exist with sequela of a healed burn or corrosion.

- An external cause code should be used with burns and corrosions to identify the source and intent of the burn, as well as the place where it occurred.

CODING TOTAL BODY SURFACE AREA FOR BURNS OR CORROSIONS

An additional code is assigned to one of the following categories:

- T31, Burns classified according to extent of body surface involved

- T32, Corrosions classified according to extent of body surface involved

These codes are used to indicate the total body surface area (TBSA) burned and should be reported when there is mention of a third-degree burn involving 20% or more TBSA. However, these codes may also be reported if the TBSA is less than 20%.

When coding burns or corrosions based on TBSA, the following guidelines apply:

- Code categories T31 and T32 are based on the classic "rule of nines" in estimating body surface involved: head and neck are assigned 9 percent, each arm 9 percent, each leg 18 percent, the anterior trunk 18 percent, posterior trunk 18 percent, and genitalia 1 percent.

- Physicians may change the TBSA percentage assignments where necessary to accommodate infants and children who have proportionately larger heads than adults and patients who have large buttocks, thighs, or abdomen that involve burns or corrosions.

- Non-healing or infected burns and corrosions are reported as acute burns or corrosions. Necrosis of burned skin is coded as a non-healed burn.

- An infection as the result of a burn (ie, an infected burn site) should be reported as an additional code.

- External cause code(s) should be used with burns and corrosions to indicate the source of the burn, the place where it occurred, and the activity of the patient at the time of the incident.

- Seventh character "S" should be assigned to a burn or corrosion code to indicate that a sequela of the burn or corrosion exists. Both a code for the current burn or corrosion with the seventh-character extension "A" or "D" is reported followed by the codes for late effect with the seventh-character "S" for sequelae.

POISONINGS, ADVERSE EFFECTS, UNDERDOSING, AND TOXIC EFFECTS

Codes in categories T36-T65 are combination codes related to adverse effects, poisonings, toxic effects, underdosing, and external causes. When reporting these codes, the following guidelines apply:

- No external cause codes are required.

- Codes in categories T36-T65 are sequenced as the first-listed diagnosis followed by the code(s) for the nature of the adverse effect, poisoning, or toxic effect.

- For underdosing, the sequencing rule does not apply.

- Do not code directly from the Table of Drugs and Chemicals. Verify the code(s) in the Tabular List.

- Use as many codes as necessary to describe completely all drugs, medicinal, or biological substances.

- If the same code would describe the causative agent for more than one adverse reaction, poisoning, toxic effect, or underdosing, assign the code only once.

- If two or more drugs, medicinal, or biological substances are reported, code each individually unless a combination code is listed in the Table of Drugs and Chemicals.

- When coding a poisoning or reaction to the improper use of a medication (eg, overdose, wrong substance given or taken in error, wrong route of administration), first assign the appropriate code from categories T36-T50. The poisoning codes have an associated intent as their fifth or sixth character (accidental, intentional self-harm, assault, and undetermined).

- If the intent of the poisoning is unknown or unspecified, code the intent as accidental intent. The undetermined intent is only for use if the documentation in the record specifies that the intent cannot be determined. Use additional code(s) for all manifestations of poisonings.

- If there is also a diagnosis of abuse or dependence of the substance, the abuse or dependence is assigned as an additional code.

The occurrence of drug toxicity is classified in ICD-10-CM as follows:

- Assign the appropriate code for adverse effect when the drug was correctly prescribed and properly administered. Assign the code for the nature of the adverse effect followed by the appropriate code for the adverse effect of the drug (T36-T50).

- The code for the drug should have a fifth or sixth character "5."

When coding a poisoning or a reaction to the improper use of a medication (eg, overdose, wrong substance given or taken in error, wrong route of administration), the following guidelines apply:

- Report a code from categories T36-T50.

- Poisoning codes have an associated intent: accidental, intentional self-harm, assault, and undetermined.

- Use additional code(s) for all manifestations of poisonings.

- If there is also a diagnosis of abuse or dependence on the substance, the abuse or dependence is reported with an additional code diagnosis.

UNDERDOSING

Underdosing refers to taking less of a medication than is prescribed by a provider or per a manufacturer's instruction. When reporting underdosing, the following guidelines apply:

- For underdosing, assign the code from categories T36-T50 (fifth or sixth character "6").

- Codes for underdosing should never be assigned as the first-listed code.

- If a patient has a relapse or exacerbation of the medical condition for which the drug is prescribed because of the reduction in dose, the medical condition itself should be coded.

- Noncompliance (Z91.12-, Z91.13-) or complication of care codes (Y63.61, Y63.8-Y63.9) are to be used with an underdosing code to indicate intent, if known.

TOXIC EFFECTS

A toxic effect occurs when a harmful substance is ingested or comes in contact with a person. The toxic effect codes are in categories T51-T65. Toxic effect codes have an associated intent: accidental, intentional self-harm, assault, and undetermined.

A code from categories T74.- or T76.- should be reported for either suspected or confirmed adult and child abuse, neglect, or other maltreatment, followed by any applicable mental health or injury code(s). When coding a toxic effect, the following guidelines apply:

- If the documentation in the medical record states abuse or neglect, the toxic effect is coded as confirmed (T74.-).

- The toxic effect is coded as suspected if it is documented as suspected (T76.-).

- For cases of confirmed abuse or neglect, an external cause code from the assault section (X92-Y09) should be reported to identify the cause of any physical injuries.

- A perpetrator code (Y07) should be reported when the perpetrator of the abuse is known.

- If the perpetrator is suspected, do not report an external cause or perpetrator code.

- If a suspected case of abuse, neglect, or mistreatment is ruled out during an encounter, code Z04.71, Encounter for examination and observation following alleged physical adult abuse, or code Z04.72, Encounter for examination and observation following alleged child physical abuse, should be used, *not* a code from T76.

- If a suspected case of alleged rape or sexual abuse is ruled out during an encounter, code Z04.41, Encounter for examination and observation following alleged adult rape, or code Z04.42, Encounter for examination and observation following alleged child rape, should be used, *not* a code from T76.

COMPLICATIONS OF CARE

Complications of care codes are reported based on the documentation in the medical record. The following guidelines apply:

- Pain associated with devices, implants, or grafts left in a surgical site is reported with a code from Chapter 19. T codes are available to report the codes for pain due to medical devices.

- An additional code from category G89 may be reported to identify the acute or chronic pain due to the presence of the device.

- Codes in category T86 are to be used for complications of transplanted organs.

- Only assign a transplant complication code if the complication affects the function of the transplanted organ. Two codes are reported: the first-listed code from category T86 and a secondary diagnosis to explain the complication.

For example, a patient who has had a kidney transplant may still have some form of chronic kidney disease (CKD). If within the documentation it is evident the CKD still exists, report code T86.1- for the complication of the kidney transplant, such as transplant failure or rejection or other transplant complication. Do not report code T86.1- when the patient has CKD unless the transplant complication indicates failure or rejection in the documentation.

As with certain other T codes, some of the complications of care codes have the external cause included in the code. The code includes the nature of the complication as well as the type of procedure that caused the complication. No external cause code indicating the type of procedure is necessary for these codes.

Intraoperative and postprocedural complication codes are found within the body system chapters with codes specific to the organs and structures of that body system (for example, a complication of a spine surgery is located in the musculoskeletal system). These codes should be sequenced first, followed by a code(s) for the specific complication, if applicable, and not reported in this category.

Now that you have a good understanding of the chapter-specific guidelines for injuries, poisonings, adverse and toxic effects, and other external causes, it is time to build skill and knowledge by coding the following exercises. Be sure to reference the ICD-10-CM codebook and the ICD-10-CM Official Guidelines for Coding and Reporting, along with the instructional notes, when coding these conditions.

Injury, Poisoning, and Certain Other Consequences of External Causes (S00-T88)

CASE STUDY 12

SUBJECTIVE: This 17-year-old patient presents to the emergency department after racing motorcycles earlier today. He had his helmet on as well as all of his racing gear. He actively races motorcycles and has done this all summer long, winning a number of times. He came over a jump and lost control of the bike, going over the handlebars. He denies hitting his head but landed on his left elbow and his left knee and has had some discomfort in these areas since. He tells me that he was not going fast, approximately 30 mph. He

denies any loss of consciousness. The main complaints center only on the left knee and the left elbow.

OBJECTIVE: The patient is in no acute distress, nontoxic appearing. During an expanded problem-focused examination, he is alert and oriented. Eyes: PERL, EOMI conjugate without nystagmus. Fundoscopic exam reveals the disks to be sharp and the TMs normal. Throat: Clear with teeth intact. Neck: Nontender. No palpable discomfort or adenopathy. He has intact clavicles. Lungs: Clear. Heart: Regular rate and rhythm. Abdomen: Soft; no hepatosplenomegaly, rebound, or guarding. He has good upper- and lower-extremity strength. His right arm is nontender to palpation. The left arm has a small amount of tenderness around the elbow joint, but there is no obvious deformity and he does have good, active motion. He has no tenderness with movement of the hips and no tenderness down the long bones of the lower extremities. There is mild tenderness at the left knee. The knee is intact with negative drawer sign and minimal tenderness along the lateral collateral ligament region. There is no real tenderness along the joint line or over the mediocollateral ligament. Both of these ligaments are intact with stress. X rays of the left knee and left elbow are negative for fracture.

ASSESSMENT: Contusion, left elbow and left knee.

PLAN: Ice, Tylenol; recheck if not improving over the next few days, otherwise on a prn basis.

ICD-10-CM Code(s) _____

CASE STUDY 13
Operative Report

PREOPERATIVE DIAGNOSIS: Displaced right olecranon fracture.

POSTOPERATIVE DIAGNOSIS: Same.

PROCEDURE: Open reduction and internal fixation of right olecranon fracture.

ANESTHESIA: General.

TOURNIQUET TIME: Approximately 1 hour, 250 mmHg.

ESTIMATED BLOOD LOSS: Minimal.

DESCRIPTION OF PROCEDURE: Patient was identified, brought to the operating room, and placed on the operating table in supine position where appropriate monitoring devices were attached and adequate general anesthesia was obtained. The right arm was prepped and draped in the usual fashion for right arm surgery. The right arm was elevated and exsanguinated with an Esmarch bandage. Tourniquet was inflated to 250 mmHg and remained inflated for approximately one hour during this procedure. Attention was directed to the posterior aspect of the right elbow where a linear incision was made overlying the proximal ulna. Appropriate skin flaps were raised. There was noted to be a displaced fracture of the right olecranon. The fracture fragments were curetted and irrigated. The fracture was then reduced with two parallel, 2-mm K-wires and the longitudinal axis of the ulna from proximal to distal direction, thereby reducing the fracture. The reduction was checked with intraoperative fluoroscopy. The reduction was further maintained by utilizing a standard technique cerclage wire. The wire was tightened and there was noted to be compression at the fracture site. After this was completed, the previously placed K-wires were bent and gently tapped further into the bone and cut and left subcutaneously. A cerclage wire was also cut and left subcutaneously. When this was completed, the elbow was put through a range of motion. The reduction was noted to be stable. The wound was irrigated with irrigation solution. Hemostasis was obtained utilizing electrocautery. The wound was closed utilizing a 4-0 Vicryl in a running subcuticular fashion. The wound was reinforced with skin staples. A bulky compressive dressing was applied to the arm, incorporating a long arm fiberglass splint. The patient was then considered ready for discharge from the operating room.

ICD-10-CM Code(s) _____

CASE STUDY 14

CHIEF COMPLAINT: Burn, right arm.

HISTORY OF PRESENT ILLNESS: This patient, a 41-year-old male, was at a coffee shop where he works as a cook when hot oil splashed onto his arm, burning him from the elbow to the wrist on the medial aspect. He has had it cooled and presents with his friend to the ER for care.

PAST MEDICAL HISTORY: Noncontributory.

MEDICATIONS: None.

ALLERGIES: None.

PHYSICAL EXAMINATION: Well-developed, well-nourished, 41-year-old adult male who is appropriate and cooperative. His only injury is to the right upper extremity. There are first- and second-degree burns on the right forearm, ranging from the elbow to the wrist. Second-degree areas with blistering are scattered through the medial aspect of the forearm. There is no circumferential burn, and I see no areas of deeper burn. The patient moves his hands well. Pulses are good. Circulation to the hand is fine.

FINAL DIAGNOSIS:

1. First-degree and second-degree burns, right arm secondary to hot oil spill.

2. Workers' compensation industrial injury.

TREATMENT: The wound is cooled and cleansed with soaking in antiseptic solution. The patient was ordered Demerol 50 mg IM for pain, but he refused and did not want pain medication. A burn dressing is applied with Neosporin ointment. The patient is given Tylenol No. 3, tabs #4, to take home with him and take one or two every four hours prn for pain. He is to return tomorrow for a dressing change. Tetanus immunization is up to date. Preprinted instructions are given. Workers' compensation first report and work status report are completed.

DISPOSITION: Home.

ICD-10-CM Code(s) _____

CASE STUDY 15

HISTORY OF PRESENT ILLNESS: Carl is a very pleasant 43-year-old, male, federal prison worker. He presents to our office today as a new patient. He injured his left knee two weeks ago at his daughter's softball game. He has never injured the knee before. The pain is bearable on nonprescription pain medicine; however, he has significant medial joint line tenderness. It does catch and lock on him. Minimal effusion, but it is affecting him significantly. He presents to our office today with an MRI scan that shows a medial meniscal tear. No other significant pathology.

PAST SURGICAL HISTORY: None.

MEDICATIONS: Protonix.

ALLERGIES: None.

FAMILY HISTORY: Mother and father alive.

SOCIAL HISTORY: He is married and doesn't smoke or drink.

REVIEW OF SYSTEMS: Denies fever, weight loss, chest pain, shortness of breath, varicosities, itching, burning, sleep disturbances, blood disorders, loss of motion, or cramps.

PHYSICAL EXAMINATION: Height: 6 feet; weight: 255 pounds; BMI: 35. In no acute distress. Normocephalic, atraumatic, full range of motion, upper extremities, nontender spine, clear chest, soft abdomen. Lower extremities have negative log roll, full range of motion in both the knee and the hip on the right side, but his left side shows significant medial joint line tenderness, positive McMurray test, positive crepitus, stable Lachman, and anterior drawer.

RADIOGRAPHS: AP, standing views of both knees were obtained today with no significant pathology.

MRI: Medial meniscal tear.

ASSESSMENT: Complex meniscal tear, medial side, left knee.

PLAN: All risks have been discussed with Carl at length and include, but not limited to, deep vein thrombosis, pulmonary embolus, death, infection, incomplete resolution of pain, chronic degenerative changes, nerve injury, and bleeding. He accepts these risks and has elected to proceed with knee arthroscopy and medial meniscal repair versus meniscectomy. This has been scheduled by Amberly. He will call sooner if there are any problems or concerns, but otherwise I will see him at that time. He understands the rehab protocol afterwards as well.

ICD-10-CM Code(s) _____

CASE STUDY 16

CHIEF COMPLAINT: Patient was on a "ripstick" and fell off and "heard a snap" in his left elbow.

HISTORY OF PRESENT ILLNESS: This is a 10-year-old male who presents to the emergency department with left elbow pain. Patient reports that he was riding a "ripstick" when he fell, sustaining an injury to his left elbow. He states that he felt and heard a pop during the incident. He has expressed no other injuries.

REVIEW OF SYSTEMS: As indicated in the HPI. All other systems were reviewed and were negative.

ALLERGIES: No known allergies.

PAST MEDICAL HISTORY: Hepatic transplant in 20xx.

SOCIAL HISTORY: Patient lives with parent(s).

PHYSICAL EXAMINATION:

GENERAL: Alert, no acute distress. Examination focused on left upper extremity.

HAND: Normal inspection; normal range of motion; nontender to palpation; no ecchymosis; no soft tissue swelling.

WRIST: Normal inspection; normal range of motion; no tenderness to palpation, including anatomic snuff box; no ecchymosis; no soft tissue swelling.

FOREARM: Normal inspection; no tenderness to palpation; no ecchymosis; no soft tissue swelling.

ELBOW: Supracondylar bony tenderness to palpation; decreased range of motion; no ecchymosis; no soft tissue swelling; positive effusion.

ARM/SHOULDER: Normal inspection; no tenderness to palpation; no AC drop off or tenderness; no anterior fullness; no ecchymosis; no soft tissue swelling; no clavicular point tenderness; no deformity to clavicle.

NEURO/VASC/TENDON: Sensation intact to light touch; motor function intact to median, radial, ulnar, and axillary nerve testing; no vascular compromise; tendon function normal.

CARDIOVASCULAR: Distal pulses in the affected extremity strong and regular.

HEAD: Normocephalic; atraumatic.

NECK: Supple; good range of motion.

RESPIRATORY: No respiratory distress.

SKIN: Intact, warm, dry.

RADIOLOGY: X ray; Elbow three views X ray; Modifier: Left; Indications: Pain.

FINDINGS: There is an F supracondylar fracture of the elbow with slight posterior angulation of the F distal portion. There is a large joint effusion.

CONCLUSION: Left elbow supracondylar F fracture.

DESCRIPTION OF PROCEDURES:

CAST/SPLINT: Ortho-glass posterior splint was applied by physician to the left elbow. Neurovascular exam after treatment: Intact. The patient tolerated the procedure well.

ORTHOPEDIC APPLIANCE: A sling was placed on the left arm in a position of function. Patient tolerated the procedure well.

MEDICATIONS: Ibuprofen Oral 400 mg tab po.

ASSESSMENT AND PLAN: My primary concern initially was for left elbow fracture. X ray of the left elbow confirmed supracondylar fracture with no significant displacement and minimal angulation. He was neurovascularly intact. I discussed the case with Dr Kevin Shea, the orthopedist on call, who recommended treatment with a posterior splint and follow-up the following morning in clinic. I independently reviewed the left elbow X rays and agree with the radiologist's interpretation of supracondylar fracture. The treatment plan, as specified under disposition documentation, was discussed with the patient and/or the patient's family. The patient and/or the patient's family have expressed understanding and comprehension of the plan.

ICD-10-CM Code(s) _____

CASE STUDY 17

CHIEF COMPLAINT: Sternal drainage and fevers.

HISTORY OF PRESENT ILLNESS: The patient is a 59-year-old male who had complaints of exertional angina in early November 20xx. The patient had a known history of previous coronary artery disease in the left anterior descending system and subsequently had cardiac catheterization revealing evidence of recurrent disease. Based on these findings, he was advised to undergo operative revascularization. The patient underwent off-pump coronary revascularization with left internal mammary artery (LIMA) to the left anterior descending coronary artery (LAD) on 11/09/20xx. He had a fairly uneventful hospital stay and was able to be discharged on 11/14/20xx. The medical record indicated during the hospitalization there was a development of some paroxysmal atrial fibrillation that was able to be cardioverted on Amiodarone therapy. The patient was doing well at home until 11/29/20xx when he noted symptoms of some fever as well as pain in the right side of his chest radiating to his shoulder. The patient presented to his primary care physician who evaluated the patient and noted no significant EKG

changes and ruled him out for myocardial infarction with enzymes. A thorough examination revealed some purulent-type drainage from the mid-aspect of the sternum, which progressed. The patient also had fevers. Based on these findings, plans were made to admit the patient to the CVCC for further management.

PAST MEDICAL HISTORY:

- Hypertension
- Hyperlipidemia
- Depression
- Gastroesophageal reflux disease
- Sleep apnea
- Chronic low back pain
- History of disc surgery

PAST SURGICAL HISTORY:

- Umbilical hernia repair
- History of disc surgery
- Recent coronary artery bypass graft ×1 off-pump procedure on 11/09/20xx

ALLERGIES: No known drug allergies.

SOCIAL HISTORY: Non-smoker; no current alcohol use.

FAMILY HISTORY: Diabetes and heart disease.

CURRENT MEDICATIONS:

- Lopressor 25 mg bid
- Aspirin 81 mg a day
- Pepcid 20 mg bid
- Prozac 40 mg a day
- Celebrex 200 mg bid
- Tricor 145 mg a day
- Pravachol 40 mg a day
- Amaryl 4 mg a day
- Allegra 180 mg a day
- Quinine 250 mg a day
- Oxycontin 20 mg bid
- Nitroglycerin 0.4 mg sublingual prn
- Ultracef prn

REVIEW OF SYSTEMS:

CONSTITUTIONAL: He does note some weakness, increased fatigue, and some fevers. No significant weight loss or weight gain.

HEENT: Denies any eye pain, diplopia, epistaxis, hearing loss, voice changes, or dysphagia.

CARDIOVASCULAR: No anginal chest pain. Some sternal incisional pain. No palpitations. No syncopal symptoms.

RESPIRATORY: No wheezing, bronchitis, hemoptysis.

GI: No nausea, vomiting, diarrhea, gastrointestinal bleeding.

GU: No frequency, dysuria. No hematuria. No nephrolithiasis.

MUSCOSKELETAL: No bony arthropathy, gout, or herniae.

SKIN: Purulent drainage from the mid aspect of the sternal incision, with some mild erythema, no tissue loss in the lower extremities. There are no rashes.

NEUROLOGIC: No CVA. No TIA. No seizure disorder.

PSYCHIATRIC: No anxiety/depression disorder.

ENDOCRINE: No diabetes mellitus or hypothyroidism.

HEMATOLOGIC: No leukemia, lymphoma, or blood dyscrasias.

PHYSICAL EXAMINATION:

VITAL SIGNS: Temperature max is 100.6°F; temperature current is 98.6°F. Pulse is 91. Blood pressure is 114/73. Room air saturation is 93%.

GENERAL: The patient is lying in bed in no apparent distress.

HEENT: Normocephalic, atraumatic. Pupils are equal. Extraocular muscles are intact.

NECK: Soft and supple. There is no JVD or lymphadenopathy. There are no carotid bruits.

CARDIOVASCULAR: Regular rate and rhythm. No murmurs, rubs, or gallops.

RESPIRATORY: Lungs are clear to auscultation bilaterally.

CHEST: The sternal incision evaluation over the mid aspect was with gross drainage of purulent. There is mild erythema surrounding the incision. No crepitans of the skin.

GU: Normal external male genitalia; no groin herniae.

ABDOMEN: Soft, nontender; no pulsatile masses.

SKIN: Warm and dry.

NEUROLOGIC: Alert, awake and oriented ×3. No focal neurologic deficits.

PSYCHIATRIC: No evidence of anxiety/depression disorder.

ASSESSMENT: Sternal drainage secondary to sternal infection, status post coronary revascularization.

PLAN: The patient is to be admitted to the hospital for IV antibiotic therapy. Due to the nature of the purulent amount of drainage from the sternum, we will need to perform an incision and drainage of his sternal incision, to evaluate the extent of the incision. If there is a significant amount of drainage leading from the substernal space, then he may require washout and debridement. The patient's sternum appears to be stable currently, and we will plan to attempt conservative therapy if tolerated. We will plan to place a PICC line for long-term antibiotic therapy, and delineate the therapy, per the wound cultures that will be sent. We will also plan to send blood cultures to rule out a source of bacteremia, and we will follow his progress and leukocytosis.

ICD-10-CM Code(s) _____

CASE STUDY 18

PREOPERATIVE DIAGNOSIS: Ventricular empyema.

POSTOPERATIVE DIAGNOSIS: Same.

PROCEDURE(S) PERFORMED: Right frontal burr hole; endoscopic exploration of ventricle; resection of fibrinous exudates using endoscopic microdissection.

FINDINGS: Extensive exudative material was located in the ventricle.

INDICATIONS: This patient developed gram-negative meningitis and ventriculitis. Initially her cultures were clear, but CT scan today showed her right ventricular system to be trapped with a high-density material suggesting ventricular empyema. She is brought to the operating room at this time for irrigating, opening the system, and reculturing it. The procedure was discussed with her husband and he requested that we proceed.

PROCEDURE(S): After induction of adequate endotracheal anesthesia, the area on the right frontal region was prepped with DuraPrep. She was given intravenous antibiotics. An incision was marked just behind the hairline based about 3.5 cm off the midline. She was draped in the usual sterile fashion. We opened the incision down through the pericranium. The pericranium was stripped back and a burr hole was made with the TPS acorn bit. We then placed a ventricular needle into the ventricle and got some purulent material. We followed that down with the 18 French peel-away sheath. Following that, we passed the 4.6-mm endoscope into the ventricle. We identified the ventricle. There was marked exudative fibrinous material in the ventricle. We used a 2.8-mm aspirating catheter down the operating tunnel in the scope and gently aspirated the material. We were able to aspirate out most of the third ventricle. We were able to get through into the other ventricle. The septum pellucidum was opened easily and we saw the shunt catheter on the other side. We irrigated back through the main body of the ventricle. Again, we could identify the walls and aspirated the fibrinous material between the walls. Following that, we placed a rubber catheter with multiple holes down the tract into the ventricle. We hooked that up to a ventricular drainage system. The catheter was secured in place and the patient was taken off anesthesia. All sponge, needle, and instrument counts were correct. The patient tolerated the procedure well and was taken to the intensive care unit in serious but stable condition.

ICD-10-CM Code(s) _____

CASE STUDY 19

The patient is a 38-year-old man admitted to our burn center after sustaining significant burns to both hands while trying put out a trash fire in his backyard that got out of control after he poured gasoline on the blaze. He has very extensive and deep burns to the right hand. Some of these appear to be fourth-degree burns with obvious exposure into tendon. He underwent burn excision earlier this week with placement of cadaver allograft skin. Quite a bit of this skin did not take, as the underlying tissue remains nonviable due to

the severe depth of his injury. He returns to our burn center today requiring a repeat operation for re-excision of the burn wounds on his right hand. We anticipate placing a split-thickness skin graft at this time. We talked to the patient about the risks of infection, bleeding, extensive scarring with significant loss of function, and the possible need for finger amputation of the right hand.

ICD-10-CM Code(s) _____

CASE STUDY 20

POSTOPERATIVE DIAGNOSIS: Right forearm radial shaft fracture with possible mild distal radioulnar joint subluxation (Galeazzi-type injury).

OPERATION: Right radius fracture open reduction and internal fixation with closed reduction distal radioulnar joint.

DESCRIPTION OF PROCEDURE: The patient was placed under axillary block in the holding area followed by general anesthesia in the operating room. Patient identification, correct procedure, and site were confirmed. Antibiotics were provided in an appropriate fashion preoperatively. A dorsal/posterior approach to the fracture was performed with a standard recommended incision, location, and technique. The interval between the extensor carpi radialis brevis and extensor digitorum communis was developed. The extensor pollicis brevis and the abductor pollicis were gently retracted one way or the other to expose the fracture site and the fracture was just beneath this area. The radial sensory nerve was identified and protected throughout the procedure. The fracture was exposed with minimal soft tissue stripping. The bone-holding forceps were placed on either side of the fracture and the overriding fracture was manipulated with gentle traction and manipulation and the fracture reduced. This effectively reduced the distal radioulnar joint.

A small fragment, Synthes DCP locking plate was utilized to fix the fracture. Eight holes were utilized. Due to the nature of the fracture and the anatomy, there were three screws distal, four screws proximal, and the last hole was at the area of the fracture. Initially to achieve satisfactory bone to plate contact, three lag screws were required and these were placed initially. This was followed by placement of the remaining screws that were utilized proximal and distal to the fracture site to be locking screws. Intraoperative X rays utilizing the C-arm were performed throughout the procedure to guide fracture reduction and hardware replacement.

Final X rays demonstrated excellent alignment of the fracture in the distal radioulnar joint. Final irrigation of the wound was performed. The wound was closed in layers in a standard fashion. Splints were applied. Total tourniquet time was approximately 60 minutes. The patient tolerated the procedure well and went to the recovery room in satisfactory condition. Sponge and needle counts were correct ×2. Estimated blood loss was minimal.

ICD-10-CM Code(s) _____

CASE STUDY 21

EXAMINATION: MRI lower extremity.

ADMITTING DIAGNOSIS: Patient states right knee pain, effusion.

CLINICAL HISTORY: Right knee pain.

RESULT: Sagittal, axial, and coronal images of the right knee were obtained on the 0.23 Tesla open magnet. The bones are in anatomic alignment. The bone marrow signal intensity is normal. The anterior and posterior cruciate ligaments are intact. There is an oblique tear through the posterior horn of the medial meniscus extending to the inferior surface. There is horizontal tear through the posterior horn of the lateral meniscus extending to the free edge. The medial collateral and lateral collateral ligament complexes are intact. The patellar and quadriceps tendons are intact. There is thinning of the articular cartilage of both the medial and lateral joint compartments, greater laterally.

There is mild para-articular spurring with subchondral cyst formation seen in the lateral tibial plateau. There is no evidence of chondromalacia. There is a small joint effusion. No evidence of a Baker's cyst.

ASSESSMENT:

1. Complex oblique tear, posterior horn of the medial meniscus extending to the inferior surface.

2. Horizontal tear, posterior horn of the lateral meniscus extending to the free edge.

3. Small joint effusion.

ICD-10-CM Code(s) _____

CASE STUDY 22

Judy is here to discuss the results of her shoulder MRI. She states her right shoulder pain is constant on the anterior lateral aspect and radiates down into the bicep area. No numbness/tingling in her fingers. Pain is increased at night time and when she applies pressure to the shoulder. She is maintaining her range of motion. She continues to work on her home exercises.

IMPRESSION/PLAN: Rotator cuff tear and shoulder impingement. After careful discussion and consideration, Judy has decided to proceed with a right shoulder arthroscopy with arthroscopic rotator cuff repair, subacromial decompression, and treatment of pathology as indicated.

ICD-10-CM Code(s) _____

External Causes of Morbidity (V00-Y99) and Factors Influencing Health Status and Contact with Health Services (Z00-Z99)

ICD-10-CM Chapters 20 and 21 Guidelines Review

In this chapter you will find a summary of the chapter-specific coding guidelines for Chapters 20 and 21 of the ICD-10-CM codebook followed by case studies to build ICD-10-CM diagnosis coding skills in these areas.

Every medical specialty references Chapter 20 of the ICD-10-CM codebook for external cause of morbidity codes and Chapter 21, which includes information on the factors that influence the health status of the patient and the patient's contact with health services. Keep in mind that you should always reference the ICD-10-CM Official Guidelines for Coding and Reporting in its entirety when making a code selection.

ICD-10-CM Official Coding Guidelines for External Causes of Morbidity

External cause codes for injuries and other health conditions provide data for research and prevention strategies. These codes capture the cause of the injury or health condition and have been further expanded in ICD-10-CM. The External Cause codes identify whether the intent of the circumstance was (1) unintentional (accidental), (2) intentional self-harm, or (3) assault. The External Cause codes also identify the place where the event occurred and the activity of the patient at the time of the event.

Note: There is no national requirement for reporting ICD-10-CM External Cause codes. Unless the provider is subject to a state-based External Cause code-reporting mandate, or a payer requires External Cause codes, they are optional. However, providers are encouraged to report External Cause codes, which provide valuable data for injury research and evaluation of injury prevention strategies and identify coverage issues with some payers.

The following guidelines apply to the use of External Cause codes:

- An External Cause code can be used with any code range or code categories (A00-T88.9 and Z00-Z99) to report an external cause. Most are used for injuries, but the codes can be used to report diseases or infections due to an external cause, source, or health condition. These codes are optional for reporting purposes.

- External Cause codes may be used with a seventh-character extension to further identify whether it is the initial, subsequent, or sequelae encounter.

- Reference the External Cause of Injuries Index and select the appropriate External Cause code from the Tabular List.

- When reporting injuries or other conditions, make certain to reference the instructional notes, as some conditions require the use of the External Cause codes.

- External Cause codes are never to be recorded as a principal/first-listed diagnosis. These codes can be used in any health care setting.

- You may assign as many External Cause codes as necessary to explain fully each cause.

- An External Cause code is not used for poisonings.

- Sequencing of multiple External Cause codes is based on the sequence of events leading to the injury. If only one External Cause code can be recorded, assign the External Cause code that relates to the principal/first-listed diagnosis.

- Certain External Cause codes are combination codes that identify sequential events that result in an injury, such as a fall that results in striking against an object. The injury may be due to either event or both.

- The combination External Cause code used should correspond to the sequence of events regardless of which event caused the most serious injury.

- External Cause codes for child and adult abuse take sequencing priority over all other External Cause codes.

PLACE OF OCCURRENCE

In ICD-10-CM, codes from category Y92-, Place of occurrence of the external cause, are secondary codes for use with other External Cause codes to identify the location of the patient at the time of injury. The following guidelines apply to the use of place of occurrence codes:

- A place of occurrence code is used only once, at the initial encounter for treatment.

- A place of occurrence code should be used in conjunction with an activity code from the Y93- code category.

- Do not use place of occurrence code Y92.9 if the place is not stated or is not applicable.

- Place of occurrence codes are not necessary with poisonings, toxic effects, adverse effects, or underdosing codes.

The place of occurrence (Y92-) and activity codes (Y93-) are sequenced after the main External Cause code. Regardless of the number of External Cause codes assigned, only one place of occurrence code and only one activity code should be assigned to a record.

ACTIVITY CODES

Codes from category Y93- are used as secondary codes to identify the activity at the time of injury. The following guidelines apply to the use of activity codes:

- Only use an activity code one time per patient encounter.

- Activity codes should only be reported for the initial encounter for treatment and not used for subsequent care.

- Activity codes are not used for poisonings, adverse effects, misadventures, or sequelae.

- Report Y93.9 when the activity is unspecified or unstated.

SEQUENCING PRIORITY

As with ICD-9-CM, External Cause codes have a specific sequencing priority in ICD-10-CM:

- Terrorism takes sequencing priority over all other External Cause codes (exception: child and adult abuse).

- Cataclysmic events take sequencing priority over all other External Cause codes (exception: child and adult abuse and terrorism).

- Transport accidents take sequencing priority over all other External Cause codes (exception: cataclysmic events, child and adult abuse, and terrorism).

The selection of the appropriate External Cause code is guided by the External Cause of Injuries Index, a separate index in the ICD-10-CM codebook, and by the instructional notes in Chapter 20. The code indicated in the External Cause of Injuries Index for the main term is verified in the Tabular List for Chapter 20. The conventions and rules for the classification also apply. There are also sections for legal interventions, operations of war, military operations, terrorism, complications of medical and surgical care, and supplemental factors related to causes of morbidity classified elsewhere.

Codes from categories V00-Y35 require an extension to indicate whether the encounter is the initial encounter for treatment, a subsequent encounter for treatment, or the sequelae of an event. The extensions for these categories are as follows:

- A—initial encounter

- D—subsequent encounter

- S—sequelae

These extensions match the extensions for the non-fracture T codes that have extensions. An External Cause code may be used for every health care encounter for the duration of treatment of an illness or injury. Late effects are reported with the extension "S" for sequelae to identify the previous injury. Late effect External Cause codes are not used for a current injury. One exception is follow-up care where no late effect of the injury is documented.

For unintentional (accidental) injuries, the default for external cause is "unintentional." If there is no documentation in the medical record as to the intent of an injury, it should be assigned an "unintentional intent" External Cause code. All transport accidents are assumed to be of accidental intent.

EXTERNAL CAUSE FOR TERRORISM

When cause of injury is identified by the federal government (eg, FBI) as terrorism, the following rules apply:

- Select the first-listed External Cause code from category Y38, Terrorism.

- Assign a code for the place of occurrence (Y92.-) as an additional diagnosis.

- More than one code from Y38 may be reported, if applicable.

- When the cause of injury is suspected terrorism, a code from category Y38 is not assigned.

- Report code Y38.9 for a secondary effect occurring subsequent to the terrorism act, but not for the initial act.

- If there is an initial terrorism act and an injury due to the subsequent result of a terrorism act, codes Y38.- and Y38.9 may be reported together as long as the documentation supports both codes reported together. Use additional code for place of occurrence (Y92.-).

EXTERNAL CAUSE STATUS

An External Cause status is reported with a code from category Y99. A code from this category is used to report the status at the time the event occurred, including whether the event occurred during a military activity or a non-military activity at work, and whether a person, including a student or volunteer, was involved in the non-work activity at the time of the event.

This code can be used only once for the initial encounter. If the status is not documented, do not use code Y99.9 for unspecified External Cause status.

ICD-10-CM Official Coding Guidelines for Factors Influencing Health Status and Contact with Health Services

Codes in Chapter 21, Factors Influencing Health Status and Contact with Health Services (the Z codes), are provided to deal with occasions when circumstances other than a disease or injury classifiable to the other chapters of the ICD-10-CM codebook are recorded as a reason for encounters with a health care provider. There are four primary circumstances for the use of Z codes:

1. When a person who is not currently sick has a health care encounter for some specific reason.

2. When a person with a resolving disease or injury or a chronic, long-term condition requiring continuous care has a health care encounter for specific aftercare of that disease or injury.

3. When circumstances or problems influence a person's health status but are not in themselves a current illness or injury.

4. For newborns, to indicate birth status.

Z codes are for use in both the inpatient and outpatient setting but are generally used more often in the outpatient setting. Z codes are used in all health care settings to identify when a patient has contact with health services and other factors that might influence patient care.

CODING TIP A diagnosis/symptom code, not a Z code, should be used whenever a current acute condition is being treated or a sign or symptom is being studied.

CONTACT EXPOSURE

Contact exposure codes may be reported as the first-listed diagnosis code to identify the encounter for testing or as a secondary code to identify risk.

- Patients who have been in contact or exposed to a communicable disease without signs or symptoms are reported with codes from category Z20.

- A patient who has contact with and suspected exposure is reported with codes from category Z77.

INOCULATIONS AND VACCINATIONS

Patient encounters for inoculations and vaccinations are reported with code Z23. When the inoculations are provided during a routine well visit, code Z23 may be reported as a secondary diagnosis code.

STATUS CODES

Status codes are reported when a patient is a carrier of the disease or has the sequelae or residual of a former condition. A status code provides information that might affect the course of treatment or outcome of treatment. A status code may not be reported with a diagnosis that includes the information about the status codes.

HISTORY CODES

History codes may be either personal history or family history Z codes. A personal history code indicates the patient no longer has the disease or condition that previously existed, such as a personal history of colon cancer, or the patient is not receiving active treatment for the disease, but the patient is at a higher risk of recurrence and requires continued monitoring.

Family history codes are reported when a disease or condition puts the patient at a higher risk, such as a family history of diabetes mellitus, which would put the patient at risk for developing the condition. The patient requires monitoring for that particular condition.

Personal and family history codes may be used together or alone and may be reported in conjunction with screening codes. History codes may be used as the reason for the visit and may be reported as first-listed or secondary diagnosis codes depending on the circumstances of the visit.

SCREENING

Screening Z codes are reported for testing to rule out or confirm a suspected or potential diagnosis or condition. For screenings, signs and symptoms codes should be reported to explain the reason for the test.

- If the reason for the test is for the screening, the test may be reported as the first-listed diagnosis code.

- Screening Z codes may also be reported as secondary diagnoses if the screening is performed during the visit when the patient presents for other reasons.

OBSERVATION

ICD-10-CM includes three observation categories:

- Z03-, Encounter for medical observation for suspected diseases and conditions ruled out

- Z04-, Encounter for examination and observation for other reasons

- Z05-, Encounter for observation and evaluation of newborn for suspected diseases and conditions ruled out

An observation encounter is an encounter in which a person without signs or symptoms is suspected of having an abnormal condition following an accident or incident that might result in a health problem, which, after examination and observation, is ruled out. Observation codes are for use in very limited circumstances when a person is being observed for a suspected

condition that is found not to exist. The fact that the patient may be scheduled for a return encounter following the initial observation encounter does not limit the use of an observation code.

The observation codes are to be used as principal diagnosis only. The only exception to this is when the principal diagnosis is required to be a code from category Z38, Liveborn infants according to place of birth and type of delivery. Then a code from category Z05, Encounter for observation and evaluation of newborn for suspected diseases and conditions ruled out, is sequenced after the Z38 code. Additional codes may be used in addition to the observation code, but only if they are unrelated to the suspected condition being observed.

AFTERCARE

Aftercare visit codes, with such category titles as "fitting and adjustment" and "attention to artificial openings," cover situations when the initial treatment of a disease or injury has been performed and the patient requires continuing care during the healing or recovery phase, or for the long-term consequences of an illness. When coding aftercare, the following guidelines apply:

- The aftercare Z codes should not be used if treatment is directed at a current disease or injury. The disease or injury code should be used in such cases.

- An aftercare code may be used as a secondary code when some type of aftercare is provided in addition to another reason for an encounter and no diagnosis code is applicable.

- Certain aftercare codes require a secondary diagnosis code to describe the resolving condition or sequelae. For others, the condition is inherent in the code title.

- Aftercare codes are not for use for mechanical complications or malfunctioning of a device.

FOLLOW-UP

The follow-up codes are used to describe encounters for a continuing patient encounter following the completed treatment of a disease, condition, or injury. Follow-up care codes should not be confused with aftercare codes, which explain current treatment for a healing or long-term condition.

Follow-up codes are used to report the repeated visits of patients who require follow-up care to monitor a condition that may have healed or otherwise resolved. For example, a patient who had cancer that has been eradicated is reported with a history code for the resolved cancer and follow-up codes for the long-term follow-up care. If the condition is still present or reoccurs, the follow-up visit code should be reported in addition to the condition diagnosed during the visit.

Codes used in the follow-up category include:

- Z08, Encounter for follow-up examination after completed treatment for malignant neoplasm

- Z09, Encounter for follow-up examination after completed treatment for conditions other than malignant neoplasm

- Z39, Encounter for maternal postpartum care and examination

When reporting code Z08, it is necessary to assign the appropriate secondary code from category Z85, Personal history of malignant neoplasm.

DONOR

Reporting donors of organs and tissues is reported with codes from category Z52 for living persons donating blood or other body tissue. Do not report these codes for cadaveric donations.

COUNSELING

Counseling codes are used to report circumstances when a patient or family member receives counseling after an illness or injury or support with coping with other problems. These codes are not used in conjunction with a diagnosis code when counseling is a component of the treatment diagnosis.

ENCOUNTER FOR OBSTETRICAL AND REPRODUCTIVE SERVICES

Z codes for pregnancy are reported when a complication included in the code from an OB chapter does not exist. Codes in category Z34, Encounter for supervision of normal pregnancy, are always first-listed codes and are not to be used with any other code in the OB chapter. Category Z3A is used to report weeks of gestation and provides additional information about the patient's condition. Codes in category Z37 are reported for outcome of delivery and reported only on the maternal record. If family planning or procreative management and counseling occur during the pregnancy or the postpartum stage, codes in this category are also reported.

ROUTINE ADMINISTRATIVE EXAMINATIONS

General and administration examinations are reported for encounters for routine examinations. The codes from these categories are the first-listed codes. They are not used if the examination is for diagnosis of a suspected condition or for treatment purposes. In such cases, a confirmed diagnosis, sign, or symptom code should be used. Codes in the category range include those from Z00-Z01, Z02, and Z32. The instructional notes in code Z00.10 indicate that if abnormal findings are discovered during a routine examination, the abnormal findings are reported as secondary codes.

Codes used in the routine administrative examinations category include:

- Category Z00, Encounter for general examination without complaint, suspected or reported diagnosis

- Category Z01, Encounter for other special examination without complaint, suspected or reported diagnosis, which includes subcategories for general medical examinations including eye, ear, and dental examinations; general laboratory and radiology examinations; routine child health examinations; as well as encounters for examinations for potential organ donors and controls for participants in clinical trials.

- Category Z02, Encounter for administrative examinations, which includes codes for such things as pre-employment physicals.

- Z32.0, Encounter for pregnancy test and childbirth and childcare instruction

The final character of the general health examination codes distinguishes between "without abnormal findings" and "with abnormal findings." For these encounters, if an abnormal condition is discovered, the code for "with abnormal findings" should be used. A secondary code for the specific abnormal finding should be used.

MISCELLANEOUS CODES

Miscellaneous Z codes are used to report other health care encounters that do not fall into another category. Miscellaneous Z codes can provide additional information about circumstances involving the patient's care.

NON-SPECIFIC Z CODES

The non-specific Z codes should be used sparingly. Only use these codes when documentation does not permit more precise coding.

It is time to build skill and knowledge by coding the following exercises relative to Chapters 20 and 21 of the ICD-10-CM codebook. Be sure to reference the ICD-10-CM codebook and the ICD-10-CM Official Guidelines for Coding and Reporting, along with the instructional notes, when reporting these conditions.

External Causes of Morbidity (V01-Y99) and Factors Influencing Health Status and Contact with Health Services (Z00-Z99)

CASE STUDY 1

PREOPERATIVE DIAGNOSIS: Left knee medial meniscal tear, displacing.

POSTOPERATIVE DIAGNOSIS: Left knee locked, bucket-handle medial meniscal tear.

OPERATION PERFORMED:

1. Exam under anesthesia

2. Video arthroscopy

3. Partial medial meniscectomy

SURGEON: Cameron Davis, MD.

ANESTHESIA: General.

ANESTHESIOLOGIST: Martin Schuster, MD.

INDICATIONS FOR PROCEDURE: The patient is a 20-year-old male who presents at this point in time for treatment of his left knee with which he has been having problems. He was injured while playing basketball in his driveway at home. He has had intermittent locking of the knee and intermittent catching of the knee. Recently he twisted his knee and locked it. He has developed swelling and medial side pain. Secondary to this he is brought to the operating room at this time for treatment.

INTERPRETIVE FINDINGS: Examination reveals a stable knee examined with patient under anesthesia. The video arthroscopy examination reveals smooth articular surfaces throughout the entire knee. He has a lateral meniscus that is normal. His medial meniscus shows a locked, bucket-handle medial meniscal tear

that underwent excision. The cruciate ligament is intact.

DESCRIPTION OF PROCEDURE: On 02/06/199x, the patient was taken to the operating room. After adequate general anesthesia, the left lower extremity was prepped with alcohol, painted with Betadine, and draped in a sterile fashion. The tourniquet was inflated to 300 mmHg of pressure. The arthroscope was introduced through the anteromedial portal with visualization of the patellofemoral joint, negative. The medial compartment was entered where the medial meniscus was visualized and probed. It was a locked, bucket-handle medial meniscal tear noted with a rim remaining with some tearing. It underwent reduction following excision. It was removed through a combination of anteromedial and anterolateral portals through a combination of biter, shaver, and punch. Once the fragment had been removed, the remaining rim was trimmed of its remaining fragments with the shaver. The medial femoral condyle was smooth as was the medial tibial plateau. Intercondylar notch area revealed intact cruciate ligament. The lateral compartment revealed a normal-appearing lateral meniscus and chondral surfaces. At this time, a final inspection of the knee revealed no additional pathology. Therefore, attention was turned toward the closure. The knee was well irrigated with overhead solution followed by the removal of arthroscopic instrumentation with tips intact. The portal sites were closed with a simple Prolene stitch followed by injection of Marcaine 0.25% with epinephrine. The patient was transferred to the recovery room cart and taken to the recovery room in satisfactory condition having tolerated the procedure well.

ICD-10-CM Code(s) _____

CASE STUDY 2

HISTORY OF PRESENT ILLNESS: This is a 30-year-old female who comes today for follow-up. The patient is HIV positive, which was confirmed six months ago and is most likely from unprotected sex. The patient denies any symptoms associated with opportunistic infection. She is experiencing no symptoms of AIDS at this point and is doing well on medications. All systems were reviewed and were negative.

PHYSICAL EXAMINATION: General: This is a WDWN female in no acute distress. Vital Signs: Temperature 98.6°F; blood pressure 120/82; pulse 78; and weight 125 pounds. Supple neck. No adenopathy. Heart: Heart sounds S1 and S2 regular. No murmur. Lungs: Clear bilaterally. Abdomen: Soft and nontender; good bowel sounds. Neurologic: She is alert and oriented ×3 with no focal neurological deficit. Extremities: She has no pitting pedal edema, clubbing, or cyanosis. GU: Examination of external genitalia is unremarkable. SKIN: No lesions or rashes.

ASSESSMENT AND PLAN: Human immunodeficiency virus, stable on Trizivir. Continue her current medications. The patient has been educated regarding her medications and plan. Her prognosis is excellent and she will follow up in three months.

ICD-10-CM Code(s) _____

CASE STUDY 3

EXAMINATION: CT with abdomen.

ADMITTING DIAGNOSIS: Gallbladder problem. The patient has right upper quadrant abdominal pain. History of colon cancer; colostomy.

COMPARISON: None.

The study was performed with oral and intravenous contrast material. The lung bases appear normal. The liver, spleen, both kidneys, and adrenal glands appear normal. There is faint calcification density in the dependent portion of the gallbladder, suspicious for a possible gallstone. Recommend ultrasound correlation. Visualized portions of the pancreas appear unremarkable. There is no retroperitoneal lymphadenopathy. Opacified bowel loops are unremarkable. Note is made of left lower quadrant colostomy. No abnormality is noted within the pelvis.

ASSESSMENT: Small calcific density in the dependent portion of the gallbladder, suspicious for gallstone. Recommend ultrasound correlation.

ICD-10-CM Code(s) _____

CASE STUDY 4

This patient is status post laparoscopic right inguinal hernia repair with mesh performed on 12/22/20xx. He does have usual postoperative discomfort. He had ecchymosis of the scrotum that is resolved. He is eating well again and had regular bowel movements.

PHYSICAL EXAMINATION:

GENERAL: Reveals a comfortable male in no acute distress.

GI: The abdomen is soft. The incisions are healing nicely. He does have resolving ecchymosis of the scrotum. No significant swelling. No evidence of hernia recurrence.

ASSESSMENT AND PLAN: Hernia repair doing well. Status post laparoscopic repair of a right inguinal hernia. The patient is instructed to avoid any heavy lifting or vigorous activity for the next several weeks. He will call me if he has any problems.

ICD-10-CM Code(s) _____

CASE STUDY 5

HISTORY OF PRESENT ILLNESS: This patient, who had undergone a lumbar fusion of L4-L5, suffers from spinal stenosis with continual back pain. She has been on Percocet, Hydrocodone, and Neurontin at home. Other past medical history positive for coronary artery disease, positive for pacemaker placement and ulcerative esophagitis.

MEDICATIONS: Coreg, aspirin, Lisinopril, Furosemide, Hydrocodone, Advair, potassium chloride, Nexium, Ativan, Percocet, Spirolactone, Digitek, Spiriva, and Neurontin.

ALLERGIES: Codeine, penicillin, and sulfa. The patient also lists morphine; however, apparently she has tolerated Hydromorphone.

REVIEW OF SYSTEMS: The patient has had no fever and no chills. Has had no dysuria. No change in bowel or bladder habit. All other systems reviewed negative.

PHYSICAL EXAMINATION: This is a 47-year-old female who is alert and does not appear in acute distress but is clearly uncomfortable.

VITAL SIGNS: Temperature 98°F; pulse 100; respirations 16; blood pressure 128/60.

HEAD: Normocephalic, atraumatic.

EYES: Pupils equal and reactive. Sclerae and conjunctivae are clear.

ENT: Mucous membranes are moist. No cyanosis, pallor, or lesion noted.

NECK: Trachea is in the midline. No masses.

AXIAL SKELETON: Full range of motion of the upper extremities. There is a healing incision of the lower lumbar region. It does not appear indurated or infected. There is pain with motion of the lower extremities. Sensation is grossly intact.

DIAGNOSTIC STUDIES: CBC, sedimentation rate, and C-reactive protein were obtained.

PLAN: We will admit the patient for observation and pain control. The patient was given Percocet in the emergency department.

ICD-10-CM Code(s) ______________________

CASE STUDY 6

This 78-year-old patient presents today for pessary cleaning and fitting. Patient has no complaints. General: Well-developed, well-nourished female in no acute distress. Vaginal speculum examination reveals no lesions. Pessary removed, scrubbed, vagina swabbed with betadine, and pessary replaced. The patient will return to the office for follow-up in three months.

ICD-10-CM Code(s) ______________________

CASE STUDY 7

PREOPERATIVE DIAGNOSIS: History of breast cancer, status post chemotherapy with a retained MediPort catheter.

POSTOPERATIVE DIAGNOSIS: Same.

OPERATION: Removal of MediPort catheter.

ANESTHESIA: Local MAC.

INDICATIONS: This is a 49-year-old, white female who was previously diagnosed with breast cancer. She has undergone treatment including chemotherapy. Her chemotherapy treatments are finished and it is felt that she no longer needs the MediPort catheter. Therefore, she would like to have the MediPort catheter removed.

FINDINGS: The MediPort catheter was removed intact without difficulty and no other abnormalities were seen.

DESCRIPTION OF PROCEDURE: The patient was taken to the operating room, identified, and placed on the operating room table. Intravenous sedation was established by the Anesthesia department and maintained by Anesthesia throughout the procedure. The patient's right anterior chest wall was prepped and draped in a sterile fashion. Local anesthesia using 1% plain lidocaine was infiltrated in the area of the MediPort catheter. A transverse incision was made directly on top of the previous incision for the insertion of the MediPort catheter and carried through the skin and subcutaneous tissues. Dissection was undertaken to identify the MediPort catheter. The MediPort catheter was identified and cleared of its attachments. The retaining sutures were identified and were cut to free up the catheter. The catheter was then removed from the pocket and pressure was held on the insertion site as the catheter was removed. The catheter was removed intact. The wound was inspected. There was no evidence of any active bleeding. The wound was irrigated with saline solution. The wound cavity was then closed by approximating the subcutaneous tissues with a series of interrupted 3-0 Vicryl sutures. The skin edges were approximated and closed with a #4 Monocryl in a running subcuticular fashion. The wound was cleaned and antibiotic ointment and a sterile dressing were applied. The patient was then awakened and taken to the recovery room in satisfactory condition. Total blood loss was less than 10 ml. The patient tolerated the procedure well. At the completion of the procedure, all sponge, needle, and instrument counts were correct.

ICD-10-CM Code(s) ______________________

CASE STUDY 8

This 30-year-old female known to me has a positive history of HIV. The patient has been seen in the emergency department for severe abdominal pain, and I have been called in to evaluate her. She states the pain is in the right lower region and that it has become increasingly worse over the last 24 hours. She has a significant history for IV drug use and prostitution. She was confirmed positive with HIV six months ago and continues to remain asymptomatic at this time. She is divorced and has no living parents or siblings. She denies any nausea, vomiting, diarrhea, or skin lesions. She has been sexually inactive for the past two weeks and denies any dysuria or discharge. Up until the past few days, she states she had been feeling fine and has been going to drug counseling to "finally move on" with her life.

PHYSICAL EXAMINATION: Fever 101.5°F; blood pressure 145/88; pulse 92; respiration 20. She is a very frail and thin-appearing female. HEENT: Negative. Lungs: Clear. Cardiovascular: RRR. GI: Negative. GU: Negative. Skin: Dry with significant scars on the inner aspects of her arms and legs. Abdomen: Liver and spleen enlarged with considerable guarding in the right lower quadrant.

DIAGNOSTICS: Abdominal ultrasound performed in the emergency department was positive for acute pelvic inflammatory disease.

PLAN: I will start the patient on Clindamycin 900 mg IV, q eight hours. If no improvement in 24 hours, I will consider surgical consult and intervention.

ICD-10-CM Code(s) _____

CASE STUDY 9

Patient returns for removal of a Hickman catheter following knee replacement today. The patient had a Hickman catheter placed due to osteomyelitis. The patient is now recovered, and the Hickman catheter is no longer needed.

REVIEW OF SYSTEMS: Constitutional: Denies anorexia, change in appetite, chills, fatigue, fever, or weight change. Skin: Denies skin changes, pruritus, or rashes. No allergies.

MEDICATIONS: Gentamycin, Vancomycin.

PHYSICAL EXAMINATION: Constitutional: Appears healthy and well developed. No signs of acute distress present. Speech is clear and appropriate. Alert and oriented. Skin: There is a single-lumen Hickman catheter on the right anterior chest wall. The site is clean and without erythema or drainage.

ASSESSMENT AND PLAN: I advised removal of the Hickman catheter. I explained the procedure in detail including the risks, benefits, and alternatives. Informed consent was obtained. The site was prepped and draped in a sterile manner. Local anesthesia using 1% plain lidocaine was administered until adequate analgesia was established. A small curved clamp was inserted at the catheter entrance to the skin and the cuff was freed of its attachments with blunt dissection. Once the cuff was freed, the catheter was removed intact. The wound was dressed with a sterile gauze dressing. The patient tolerated the procedure well.

ICD-10-CM Code(s) _____

CASE STUDY 10

A 10-month-old patient had an illness with high fever at her preventive medicine visit two weeks ago and now returns to see the nurse for her DTaP vaccine. The nurse performs an interval history, finding the symptoms from the earlier illness resolved. Next, the nurse confirms that the infant is afebrile by taking the infant's temperature and makes the observation that the infant is playful. After assessing that the patient is currently in good health, the nurse confirms that there are no contraindications to the immunization per the CDC guidelines. The nurse reviews the VIS (vaccine information statement) with the father, antipyretic dosage for weight, and obtains the father's consent for the immunization. The nurse administers the DTaP, observes for immediate reactions, and schedules the patient for her 12-month visit in two months.

ICD-10-CM Code(s) _____

CASE STUDY 11

A 90-year old woman comes in complaining of chronic pain in her left hip. She is unable to bear weight on her left leg. She fell from the left side of her bed while resting. This happened two days ago and she still is experiencing severe pain.

This happened while she was at the nursing home. This is the second time this has happened. A hip X ray was taken and no fracture was detected.

The patient was released back to the nursing home with a prescription for pain medication.

ICD-10-CM Code(s) _____

CASE STUDY 12

A 13-year-old patient suffered a hematoma of the left ear after being hit in the ear while sparring during a boxing match in the school gymnasium. The patient was taken to the emergency department at the hospital for treatment.

ICD-10-CM Code(s) _____

CASE STUDY 13

Patient presents to the emergency room with multiple lacerations resulting from a car accident in which he was a passenger in an SUV. The car he was riding in collided with a pickup truck on the interstate. The patient suffered a laceration of the nose with glass imbedded in the wound, puncture wound of the scalp, and laceration of the left cheek.

ICD-10-CM Code(s) _____

Chapter 1

CASE STUDY 1

N10	Acute pylonephritis

B96.20	Unspecified Escherichia coli (*E.coli*) as the cause of the diseases classified elsewhere

R11.2	Nausea with vomiting unspecified

Rationale: The patient's condition is pylonephritis, which is reported as N10. The instructional notes indicate an additional code is reported for the type of infection, which is *E. coli* (B96.20). It is not clear whether the nausea with vomiting is part of this condition and may be reported as the tertiary diagnosis.

CASE STUDY 2

T81.4xxA	Infection following a procedure, initial encounter

A41.01	Sepsis due to *Staphylococcus aureus*

B95.61	Methicillin susceptible *Staphylococcus aureus* infection as the cause of diseases classified elsewhere

D72.829	Elevated white blood cell count, unspecified

D64.9	Anemia, unspecified

E10.9	Type 1 diabetes mellitus without complications

Z95.1	Presence of coronary artery bypass graft

Rationale: The first-listed diagnosis should be the reason for the primary treatment, which is the post-procedural infection. The guidelines direct that an additional code is reported for the infection, which is A41.01 as the secondary diagnosis. Because the provider indicated the patient has leukocytosis, anemia, and type I diabetes, and all of the conditions can be affected by the infection, they can all be reported as additional diagnoses.

CASE STUDY 3

B37.81	Candida esophagitis

Rationale: The Candida esophagitis is confirmed by pathology and is documented as the postoperative diagnosis. The rule for coding surgical procedures is that if the postoperative diagnosis is different from the preoperative diagnosis, the postoperative diagnosis is reported.

CASE STUDY 4

B20	Human immunodeficiency virus (HIV) disease

C46.0	Kaposi's sarcoma of skin

Rationale: Based on the ICD-10-CM Official Guidelines for Coding and Reporting, when the patient is being treated for an HIV-related illness (eg, Kaposi's sarcoma), the HIV code B20 is reported as the first-listed diagnosis followed by the manifestation.

CASE STUDY 5

B20	Human immunodeficiency virus (HIV) disease

B00.1	Herpesviral vesicular dermatitis

Rationale: The patient is treated for an AIDS-related illness (B00.1). Based on the ICD-10-CM Official Guidelines for Coding and Reporting, HIV (B20) is reported as the first-listed diagnosis followed by the manifestation.

CASE STUDY 6

B34.9	Viral infection, unspecified

Z09	Encounter for follow-up examination after completed treatment for conditions other than malignant neoplasm

Rationale: The patient is being seen for follow-up for a viral infection. Because this is a follow-up examination, Z09 can be reported in addition to the condition being treated. The main term for the viral infection is referenced in the Alphabetic Index as Infection; virus.

CASE STUDY 7

A75.2   Typhus fever due to *Rickettsia typhi*

S61.258A   Bite to the index finger (Open bite of other finger without damage to nail)—Sequela

W53.01xA   Bitten by mouse, initial encounter

Rationale: The patient has Murine typhus. Reference the Alphabetic Index: Typhus; murine, which directs the user to A75.2 in the Tabular List. In addition, the bite to the finger, which is the cause of the Murine typhus should be reported as a secondary diagnosis. The bite to the index finger would be reported as the reason the patient has the condition in addition to the mouse bite. Since the laterality (left versus right index finger) is not documented, the only choice is the code for "other finger," which includes the open bite of a specified finger with unspecified laterality. It would be appropriate in this instance for the user to query the practitioner for the laterality to code to the highest level of specificity. The guidelines instruct the user to report a seventh character to identify the initial encounter (A) for the initial encounter (treatment) for the condition.

CASE STUDY 8

B47.0   Eumycetoma

S91.341S   Puncture wound with foreign body, right foot, sequela encounter

W45.8xxS Other foreign body or object entering through skin, sequela

Rationale: The puncture wound of the foot is reported as the subsequent encounter. The infection is coded in addition to treatment of the wound. Because the infection is a late effect of the wound, the seventh character S is reported for sequela. Madura of the foot, which is the infectious process, is reported with B47.0, Eumycetoma. In addition, the External Cause code, which is optional, can be reported.

CASE STUDY 9

A23.0   Brucellosis due to *Brucella melitensis*

W55.39xA Other contact with other hoof stock

Rationale: The diagnosis is a viral infection from sheep—*Brucella melitensis*—which is reported as A23.0. The External Cause code for the contact with the sheep is reported with W55.39xA.

CASE STUDY 10

A77.1   Spotted fever due to *Rickettsia conorii*

Rationale: The Alphabetic Index is referenced under the main term Fever, followed by Boutonneuse, which is code A77.1, Spotted fever due to Rickettsia conorii, which is selected from the Tabular List.

CASE STUDY 11

E86.0   Dehydration

A08.4   Viral intestinal infection, unspecified

J45.909   Asthma, unspecified

L22   Diaper dermatitis

Rationale: In the Alphabetic Index, Gastroenteritis; viral directs the user to A08.4.

Chapter 2

CASE STUDY 1

C44.229   Squamous cell carcinoma skin of left ear and external auricular canal

Rationale: Reference the Neoplasm Table under Ear—auricular canal, external, and reference C44.22 in the Tabular List. A sixth character is required to identify laterality (right versus left).

CASE STUDY 2

C44.519   Basal cell carcinoma of skin and other part of trunk

Rationale: Because there is no specific diagnosis for the basal cell carcinoma of the right chest, the Neoplasm Table directs the user to C44.519.

CASE STUDY 3

Z45.2   Encounter for adjustment and management of vascular access device

C56.9   Malignant neoplasm of ovary, unspecified side

Rationale: In this scenario it would be beneficial to clarify right versus left ovary because C56.9 is an unspecified diagnosis code and there are two codes for the right and left ovary to identify laterality. Always reference the neoplasm in the Neoplasm Table and select the code from the Tabular List.

CASE STUDY 4

C78.7   Secondary malignant neoplasm of liver and intrahepatic bile duct

C79.89   Secondary malignant neoplasm of other specified sites (for the abdominal cavity)

C18.9   Malignant neoplasm of colon, unspecified (primary site)

Z87.891   Personal history of nicotine dependence

Rationale: Because the patient has metastatic colon cancer (primary/origin), the code is referenced in the Alphabetic Index under the main term Colon and selected from the primary column and verified in the Tabular List (C18.9). The documentation also indicates the cancer metastasized to the liver and abdominal cavity, so C78.7 and C79.89 are reported. Also, because the history indicates the patient was a smoker 15 years ago, personal history (Z87.891) would be reported.

CASE STUDY 5

D66   Hereditary factor VIII deficiency

Z95.828   Presence of vascular device (Hickman catheter)

Rationale: The Alphabetic Index is referenced for hemophilia and then factor VIII, which is reported as D66.

CASE STUDY 6

D57.219   Sickle-cell/Hb-C disease with crisis, unspecified

E11.9   Type 2 diabetes mellitus without complications

Rationale: The patient has sickle-cell/Hb-C disease and is in crisis. The Alphabetic Index is referenced under Sickle-cell and the code is selected based on the type of sickle-cell disease (with a cross-reference to "*see* Disease, sickle-cell"). The Tabular List is referenced for the Hb-C sickle-cell disease in crisis, D57.219. The diabetes mellitus is documented, and because diabetes mellitus affects every chronic condition, it is reported. The Alphabetic Index is referenced under Diabetes— type 2. The code is verified in the Tabular List as E11.9.

CASE STUDY 7

D57.20   Sickle-cell/Hb-C disease without crisis

Z79.891   Long term (current) use of opiate analgesic

Rationale: Because there is no mention in the documentation, the condition is reported without crisis, referencing Disease; sickle-cell/Hb-C in the Alphabetic Index and verified in the Tabular List.

CASE STUDY 8

I82.401   Acute embolism and thrombosis of unspecified deep veins of right lower extremity

M79.A21   Nontraumatic compartment syndrome of right lower extremity

E10.9   Type 1 diabetes mellitus without complications

Z79.01   Current use of anticoagulant

Rationale: The Alphabetic Index is referenced under Thrombosis; deep (with a cross-reference to "see Embolism, vein, lower extremity"). The code is verified in the Tabular List identifying the laterality, which is the right lower extremity, which is sixth character "1." The documentation also indicates the patient has compartment syndrome. The Alphabetic Index is referenced under Syndrome—compartment, nontraumatic. The Tabular List is verified and, as with the thrombosis, the code is selected with the sixth character 1 based on laterality. The patient is also diabetic and a Type 1 patient, which is also reported. Since manifestations are not identified, the unspecified diabetes code is reported. Because the patient is on indefinite Coumadin, use of the anticoagulant should also be reported.

CASE STUDY 9

I80.03   Phlebitis and thrombophlebitis of superficial vessels of lower extremities, bilateral

E11.9   Type 2 diabetes mellitus without complications

Z79.4   Long term (current) use of insulin

Z79.01   Long term (current) use of anticoagulants

Rationale: Thrombophlebitis for the superficial vessels is referenced in the Alphabetic Index under saphaneous (greater) (lesser) (I80.0-). The Tabular List further defines the laterality as bilateral, which is reported with fifth character 3.

CASE STUDY 10

C44.319   Basal cell carcinoma of skin of other parts of face

C44.01   Basal cell carcinoma skin of lip

Rationale: Reference the Neoplasm Table and select the final codes from the Tabular List. The documentation indicates the patient has basal cell carcinoma of the chin, which is reported as C44.01, and the right lower lip, which is reported with C44.319. Verify the codes in the Tabular List.

CASE STUDY 11

D18.02   Hemangioma of intracranial structures

Rationale: Refer to Hemangioma; cavernous in the Alphabetic Index to locate the appropriate category D18.0 and verify the correct code in the Tabular List. Because the cavernoma is stuck to the dural surface, D18.02 is the most appropriate code.

CASE STUDY 12

C34.11   Malignant neoplasm of upper lobe, right bronchus or lung

C34.2   Malignant neoplasm of middle lobe, bronchus or lung

C79.31   Secondary malignant neoplasm of brain

J44.9   Chronic obstructive pulmonary disease, unspecified

M79.89   Other specified soft tissue disorders

M25.561   Pain in right knee

M25.562   Pain in left knee

F17.200   Nicotine dependence, unspecified, uncomplicated

Rationale: The patient has several conditions to report. The Neoplasm Table should be referenced for the primary malignant neoplasm of the upper lobe. The documentation indicates the cavitary lesion extends to the middle lobe, which is a primary malignancy. Documentation also states the patient has brain metastasis. Because the area of the brain cancer is unknown, the unspecified code is reported as the secondary malignancy (C79.31). Additional diagnoses that should be reported are the COPD (Disease—pulmonary, chronic obstructive) and the swollen left leg reported with M79.89. The patient also has bilateral knee pain, which is referenced in the Alphabetic Index under Pain—joint, knee. When referencing the Tabular List, there is not a specific code for bilateral, so the right and left knee pain (M25.561 and M25.562) must be reported. Documentation also indicates the patient is an 80-pack-a-year smoker, which is reported as Nicotine dependence, unspecified.

CASE STUDY 13

Z51.0   Encounter for antineoplastic radiation therapy

C53.0   Malignant neoplasm of endocervix

Rationale: The Neoplasm Table is referenced based on the site of the cancer, which is the endocervix. Because it appears this is the primary malignancy, the code is selected from the Primary malignancy column and verified in the Tabular List. The first-listed diagnosis Z51.0 is reported for the radiation therapy and is reported first because it is the reason for treatment.

CASE STUDY 14

D03.4   Melanoma in situ of scalp and neck

Rationale: The main term in the Alphabetic Index is Melanoma—in-situ, neck, which then references D03.4. In the Tabular List D03.4 is Melanoma in situ of scalp and neck.

CASE STUDY 15

C50.211   Malignant neoplasm of upper-inner quadrant of right female breast

Rationale: Reference the Neoplasm Table and make sure the quadrant and laterality are specific in both documentation and coding. Code only from the Tabular List. In referencing the Neoplasm Table, look up the malignancy by anatomic area (breast) and then identify gender (female) and the quadrant of the breast and laterality.

Chapter 3

CASE STUDY 1

E11.641   Type 2 diabetes mellitus due to underlying condition with hypoglycemia without coma

Rationale: The patient has hypoglycemia due to an insulin reaction. The Alphabetic Index is referenced under the main term Hypoglycemia—*see* diabetes hypoglycemia E11.649.

CASE STUDY 2

E10.628   Type 1 diabetes mellitus with other specified complications

L03.116   Cellulitis of left lower limb

Rationale: The patient has cellulitis of the left foot, which is referenced in the Alphabetic Index as Cellulitis—foot, which references L03.11, with a sixth-character extension required. The Tabular List indicates the laterality in the description. The type 1 diabetes mellitus (DM) is also reported with the manifestation as other skin complications with E10.628. Coding instruction identifies that the DM is reported as the first-listed diagnosis.

CASE STUDY 3

E87.6   Hypokalemia

E87.8   Other disorders of electrolyte and fluid balance, not elsewhere classified

E87.1   Hypo-osmolality and hyponatremia

C20   Malignant neoplasm of rectum

Rationale: The rectal cancer is referenced in the Neoplasm Table and verified in the Tabular List. The conditions identified in the documentation should be

reported for the Hypokalemia (E87.6); hypochloremia, which is reported as E87.8; and the hyponatremia, which is referenced in the Tabular List as E87.1. Because all conditions are treated, any of the four conditions may be reported as the first-listed diagnosis.

CASE STUDY 4

J96.00   Acute respiratory failure, unspecified whether with hypoxia or hypercapnia

E46   Unspecified protein-calorie malnutrition

Rationale: The Alphabetic Index is referenced for the acute respiratory failure under Failure—respiratory, acute, and the code is selected from the Tabular List. The malnutrition is documented and reported as a secondary diagnosis. Because the type of malnutrition is not documented, the unspecified code E46 is reported.

CASE STUDY 5

E78.0   Pure hypercholesterolemia

M25.512   Left shoulder pain

Rationale: The Alphabetic Index is referenced for Hypercholesterolemia and verified in the Tabular List as E78.0. The pain in the left shoulder is referenced in the Alphabetic Index as Pain in shoulder (M25.51-).

CASE STUDY 6

E10.610   Type 1 diabetes mellitus with diabetic neuropathic arthropathy

I10   Hypertension

L84   Corns and callosities

Rationale: The patient has type 1 diabetes mellitus with neuropathic arthropathy documented in the medical record. In the Alphabetic Index the condition is referenced as Diabetes—type 1, arthropathy.

CASE STUDY 7

O14.03   Moderate pre-eclampsia, third trimester

O24.414   Gestational diabetes mellitus in pregnancy controlled by insulin

O99.213   Obesity complicating pregnancy controlled by insulin

E66.01   Morbid (severe) obesity due to excess calories

Z68.30   Body Mass Index 30.0–30.9

Z3A30   Pregnancy single uterine, 30 weeks' gestation

Z86.32   Personal history of gestational diabetes

Z79.4   Long term (current) use of insulin

Rationale: Seven diagnosis codes are required for this encounter. The pre-eclampsia, gestational diabetes mellitus on insulin, trimester of pregnancy, the obesity (morbid), the personal history of the gestational diabetes, and based on ICD-10-CM coding guidelines, code Z79.4 for the insulin use is required.

CASE STUDY 8

E11.22   Type 2 diabetes mellitus w/diabetic chronic kidney disease

N18.6   Chronic kidney disease, stage 6 (severe)

Z79.4   Long term (current) use of insulin

Z99.2   Dependence on renal analysis

Rationale: The Alphabetic Index is referenced as Diabetes—type 2—with chronic kidney disease. There is an instructional note to use an additional code to identify the stage of the chronic kidney disease and long-term use of insulin. In addition, because the patient is on dialysis, it is appropriate to report the dependence on renal dialysis.

CASE STUDY 9

F33.1   Major depressive disorder, recurrent, moderate

G54.7   Phantom limb syndrome without pain

Z89.511   Acquired absence of right leg below knee

Z89.512   Acquired absence of left leg below knee

Rationale: In ICD-10-CM there are two codes: one for pain and one for without pain. Because pain is not documented as to whether the patient has pain, the without pain code is reported. The depression is

reported in the Alphabetic Index under Disorder—depressive—recurrent—moderate, and verified in the Tabular List.

CASE STUDY 10

F33.0   Major depressive disorder recurrent, mild

E78.0   Hypercholesterolemia

Z82.49   Family history of ischemic heart disease and other diseases of the circulatory system

Rationale: Coding in this category for major depressive disorder and family history of heart disease is similar. For the depressive disorder, documentation must indicate whether this is a single episode or a recurrence. Because this has been ongoing, it is coded as recurrence. The documentation must also indicate whether the disorder is mild, moderate, or severe. The family history for ischemic heart disease includes family history of a myocardial infarction (heart attack). Because this information is documented as the brother died of a heart attack, Z82.49 is the appropriate diagnosis code for the family history. Elevated cholesterol is reported as E78.0.

CASE STUDY 11

F33.1   Major depressive disorder, recurrent, moderate

Z63.4   Disappearance or death of family member

Rationale: The depression is reported in the Alphabetic Index under Disorder—depressive—recurrent—moderate and verified in the Tabular List. Because the depression is related to the spouse's death, Z63.4 is reported as a secondary diagnosis.

CASE STUDY 12

F32.9   Major depressive disorder, single episode, unspecified

Z63.5   Disruption of family by separation or divorce

Rationale: Because the type of depression is not documented in the medical record, it is reported as NOS (not otherwise specified) and referenced in the Alphabetic Index as Depression.

CASE STUDY 13

F90.1   Attention-deficit hyperactivity disorder, predominantly hyperactive type

Rationale: When coding ADHD with ICD-10-CM, the type of hyperactivity is important in coding the patient encounter. Many times ADHD is not well defined. The types in ICD-10-CM include: combined, hyperactive type, inattentive type, other type, and unspecified. Use caution when selecting the appropriate diagnosis code.

CASE STUDY 14

F41.0   Panic disorder (episodic paroxysmal anxiety) without agoraphobia

F32.9   Depression NOS

Rationale: The documentation indicates the patient has a panic disorder, which is referenced in the Alphabetic Index under the main term panic (attack) (state) as F41.0. Because depression is documented and treated by the practitioner, F32.9 (depression NOS) is reported as a secondary diagnosis.

CASE STUDY 15

F03.90   Unspecified dementia without behavioral disturbance

R27.0   Ataxia, unspecified

H54.7   Visual loss unspecified

Rationale: In the Alphabetic Index, Dementia—senile is referenced. Because the cause of the dementia is unknown, F03, unspecified dementia, is the most appropriate diagnosis code.

CASE STUDY 16

R44.0   Auditory hallucinations

R41.0   Disorientation unspecified (confusion)

Rationale: In ICD-10-CM, when coding hallucinations, the specificity is reported as auditory, other hallucinations, or unspecified. Because it is documented that the patient's hallucinations are auditory, R44.0 is reported. Because the documentation indication the patient is confused, R41.0 is reported as a secondary diagnosis.

CASE STUDY 17

Z72.810   Child and adolescent antisocial behavior

Rationale: The patient is being treated for antisocial behavior in group therapy, which is reported with a code from Chapter 21: Z72.810. Always verify the code in the Tabular List.

CASE STUDY 18

F41.1   Generalized anxiety disorder

N95.9   Unspecified menopausal and perimenopausal disorder

Rationale: Perimenopausal disorder is referenced under Disorder—anxiety for the generalized anxiety disorder and referenced in the Tabular List as F41.1. The menopausal symptoms are unspecified.

Chapter 4

CASE STUDY 1

G89.18   Other acute postprocedural pain

R50.9   Fever unspecified

Z98.890   Other specified postprocedural states

Rationale: Three codes are reported. One for the postoperative pain referenced in the Alphabetic Index as Pain—postprocedural (G89.18); a code for the fever: Fever (of unknown origin); and a code to identify the patient status in Chapter 21: Status—postoperative (postprocedural) NEC (Z98.890). Make certain to follow the instructional notes in the Tabular List.

CASE STUDY 2

G96.0   Cerebrospinal fluid leak

Rationale: The code is reported for the CSF as G96.0—Cerebrospinal fluid leak. In the Alphabetic Index, refer to Leak—cerebrospinal fluid.

CASE STUDY 3

G56.02   Carpal tunnel syndrome, left upper limb

Rationale: Because the documentation supports carpal tunnel of the left wrist, which is the upper limb, the appropriate code is G56.02.

CASE STUDY 4

J35.1   Hypertrophy of tonsils

L81.9   Disorders of pigmentation, unspecified

G47.33   Obstructive sleep apnea (adult) (pediatric)

Rationale: The hypertrophy is reported as the first-listed diagnosis in addition to the pigmented lesion of the right temple, and the obstructive sleep apnea is listed as an additional diagnosis. In the Alphabetic Index the main term, Apnea—sleep, obstructive, is referenced and verified in the Tabular List.

CASE STUDY 5

G56.02   Carpal tunnel syndrome, left upper limb

Rationale: Because the documentation supports carpal tunnel of the left wrist, which is the upper limb, the appropriate code is G56.02.

CASE STUDY 6

G44.1   Vascular headache, not elsewhere classified

Rationale: The Alphabetic Index is referenced as Headache, vascular, NEC and verified in the Tabular List.

CASE STUDY 7

G56.21   Lesion of ulnar nerve, right upper limb

M77.11   Lateral epicondylitis, right elbow

Rationale: In the Alphabetic Index the neuropathy is referenced as Neuropathy—ulnar nerve and Epicondylitis (elbow)—right (laterality). The codes should be verified in the Tabular List.

CASE STUDY 8

G43.109   Migraine with aura, not intractable, without status migrainosus

G93.2   Benign intracranial hypertension

Rationale: The reason for the procedure is the benign intracranial hypertension, which is reported with G93.2 and the migraine with aura. Because there is no mention of status migrainosus, the patient encounter is reported as "without status migrainosus" (G43.109). The pseudotumor cerebri is sometimes referred to as benign intracranial hypertension.

CASE STUDY 9

G56.02   Carpal tunnel syndrome, left upper limb

Rationale: It is important to note that location is very specific in ICD-10-CM and laterality is also an issue. Good documentation for specificity is required for proper code assignment. The documentation indicates the carpal tunnel affects the left wrist and the fifth character "2" identifies laterality (left).

CASE STUDY 10

G51.0   Bell's palsy

G35   Multiple sclerosis

G93.6   Cerebral edema

Rationale: The first-listed diagnosis reported is the Bell's palsy (G51.0), which is the reason for the test. Cerebral edema (G93.6) is the finding and can be coded as a tertiary diagnosis. Even though facial weakness is documented, R29.810 is not coded, as this is a symptom of Bell's palsy. The patient also has MS (multiple sclerosis), which is reported as G35.

CASE STUDY 11

G93.6   Cerebral edema

S00.03xA   Contusion of scalp, Initial encounter

W06.xxxA   Fall from bed, Initial encounter

Y93.84   Activity, sleeping

Y92.032   Bedroom in apartment as the place of occurrence of the external cause

Y99.8   Other external cause status

Rationale: There are two conditions treated: cerebral edema and the contusion of the scalp (injury). The seventh character "A" is required to identify the phase of treatment (active treatment). An external cause code (optional) can be reported for the fall from the bed. In addition, the place of occurrence (bedroom in apartment) and the External Cause code is reported. An external cause status Y99.8 is reported based on whether the injury occurred during, employment, volunteering, military, or other cause.

CASE STUDY 12

C44.102   Unspecified malignant neoplasm of skin of right eyelid, including canthus

Rationale: The patient encounter is reported as a malignant neoplasm referenced first in the Neoplasm Table under Skin—eyelid, primary malignant. When referencing the Tabular List, laterality is important and the fifth character "1" identifies the right eyelid.

CASE STUDY 13

H25.9   Unspecified age-related cataract

Rationale: The diagnosis is referenced in the Alphabetic Index as Cataract—senile. Because no other specific information is available in the documentation, the unspecified age-related cataract is reported with H25.9.

CASE STUDY 14

H25.041   Posterior subcapsular polar age-related cataract, right eye

Rationale: In the Alphabetic Index reference Cataract—senile, subcapsular, polar. The Tabular List identifies the laterality as the right eye with sixth character "1."

CASE STUDY 15

H04.553   Acquired stenosis of nasolacrimal duct bilateral

Rationale: In the Alphabetic Index the main term is Stenosis—nasolacrimal duct (see stenosis lacrimal duct—lacrimal duct H04.44-) Reference the code in the Tabular List. The sixth character "3" is used to report the condition bilaterally.

CASE STUDY 16

H02.402   Unspecified ptosis of left eyelid

Rationale: The main term in the Alphabetic Index is Blepharoptosis and verified in the Tabular List. Report the left eyelid with the sixth character "2."

CASE STUDY 17

H40.11x0   Primary open-angle glaucoma, stage unspecified

Rationale: The main term in the Alphabetic Index is Glaucoma—open angle—primary and verified in the Tabular List. The seventh character identifies the stage of the glaucoma. Because a seventh character is required and the category subdivides into five

characters, the placeholder "x" must be added as the sixth character to code the required seven characters.

CASE STUDY 18

H04.551   Acquired stenosis of right nasolacrimal duct

H02.132   Senile ectropion of right lower eyelid

H02.135   Senile ectropion of left lower eyelid

Rationale: There is no bilateral code for senile ectropion in ICD-10-CM so the right and left lower eyelids are reported separately.

CASE STUDY 19

H05.811   Cyst of right orbit

Rationale: Laterality is key in code selection: Cyst—orbit—laterality right.

CASE STUDY 20

D23.11   Other benign neoplasm of skin of right eyelid, including canthus

Rationale: The patient encounter is reported as a malignant neoplasm referenced first in the Neoplasm Table under the Skin—Eyelid, benign column. When referencing the Tabular List, laterality is important. The fifth character "1" identifies the right eyelid.

CASE STUDY 21

H02.831   Dermatochalasis of right upper eyelid

H02.834   Dermatochalasis of left upper eyelid

Rationale: The Alphabetic Index is referenced with the main term Dermatochalasis and referenced in the Tabular List. Laterality is reported with the sixth character. Because there is not a code for upper eyelids bilateral, each is reported.

CASE STUDY 22

H05.012   Cellulitis of left orbit

H00.024   Hordeolum internum, left upper eyelid

Rationale: The Alphabetic Index is referenced with the main term Cellulitis. Remember that laterality is important when selecting a diagnosis code in this chapter.

CASE STUDY 23

H00.11   Chalazion right upper eyelid

Rationale: The main term Chalazion is referenced in the Alphabetic Index and coded in the Tabular List. Location and laterality are important when selecting a code in this category.

Chapter 5

CASE STUDY 1

J30.9   Allergic rhinitis, unspecified

J33.0   Polyp nasal cavity

Rationale: The patient has allergic rhinitis, which is referenced in the Alphabetic Index under Rhinitis—allergic and referenced in the Tabular List. Because the documentation is not more specific, report J30.9 for unspecified allergic rhinitis. The polyp is referenced as polyp—nasal—cavity and reported as J33.0.

CASE STUDY 2

H90.42   Sensorineural hearing loss, unilateral, left ear, with unrestricted hearing on the contralateral side

Rationale: The Alphabetic Index is referenced under the main term Loss—hearing—sensorineural. The Tabular List identifies the fifth-character "2" for the left ear.

CASE STUDY 3

H65.23   Chronic serous otitis media, bilateral

Rationale: In the Alphabetic Index reference Otitis—media, serous (see otitis media nonsuppurative)—Otitis media nonsuppurative—chronic. In the Tabular List the fifth-character "3" identifies the condition is bilateral.

CASE STUDY 4

H72.92   Unspecified perforation of tympanic membrane, left ear

H90.3   Sensorineural hearing loss, bilateral

B36.9   Superficial mycosis, unspecified

H62.42   Otitis externa in other diseases classified elsewhere, left ear

Rationale: The instructional note directs the user to report H72.92, Unspecified perforation of tympanic membrane, left ear. Otomycosis is reported as B36.9, Superficial mycosis, unspecified.

CASE STUDY 5

H95.89   Other postprocedural complications and disorders of the ear and mastoid process, not elsewhere classified

H93.8x1   Other specified disorders of right ear

Rationale: Because the documentation does not state whether there is an infection and just identifies the condition as straw-colored fluid, the patient encounter cannot be coded as an infection. The only other choice is Other specified disorder of the right ear. The sixth character "1" is to report the right side (laterality). Also the post-procedural complication should be reported for the ear and mastoid process with H95.89 as the first-listed diagnosis. Because the instructional note in the Tabular List indicates to "use an additional code if applicable to further specify disorder," the other post-procedural complication is listed first.

CASE STUDY 6

R20.2   Paresthesia of skin

J01.40   Acute pansinusitis

J33.0   Polyp of nasal cavity

J34.89   Other specified disorders of nose and nasal sinuses

Rationale: The documentation indicates the patient has pansinusitis with left-sided nasal polyp and synechia right nasal cavity. These three codes do not identify laterality in the description. In the Alphabetic Index the main term for the nasal polyp is polyp—nasal—cavity.

CASE STUDY 7

H65.33   Chronic mucoid otitis media, bilateral

J35.2   Hypertrophy of adenoids

Rationale: In the Alphabetic Index the main term is referenced as Otitis media—mucoid (see otitis media—nonsuppurative) then reference otitis media—nonsuppurative—chronic—mucoid (H65.3-). Hypertrophy of the adenoids is referenced under the main term hypertrophy—adenoids (infective) (J35.2).

CASE STUDY 8

I87.2   Venous insufficiency (chronic) (peripheral)

I83.219   Varicose veins of right lower extremity with both ulcer of unspecified site and inflammation

Rationale: The ICD-10-CM codes for varicose veins of the lower extremity with inflammation are selected based on laterality (right, left, or unspecified site).

CASE STUDY 9

I83.211   Varicose veins of right lower extremity with ulcer and inflammation of thigh

L95.9   Vasculitis limited to the skin, unspecified

Rationale: The ICD-10-CM code for leg varicosity of the lower extremity with ulcer is selected based on laterality (right, left, or unspecified site).

CASE STUDY 10

I83.11   Varicose veins of right lower extremity with inflammation

I83.12   Varicose veins of left lower extremity with inflammation

I87.2   Venous insufficiency (chronic) (peripheral)

G25.81   Restless legs syndrome

Rationale: Laterality is crucial in selecting diagnosis code I83.11, Varicose veins of right lower extremity with inflammation, which differs from ICD-9-CM. There is not a bilateral code in category I83.1, so both left and right must be reported with I83.11 (right) and I83.12 (left).

CASE STUDY 11

I69.051   Hemiplegia and hemiparesis following nontraumatic subarachnoid hemorrhage affecting right dominant side

E64.0   Sequelae of protein-calorie malnutrition

I69.391   Dysphagia following cerebral infarction

R13.10   Dysphagia, unspecified

F01.50   Vascular dementia without behavioral disturbance

R63.4   Abnormal weight loss

Rationale: The documentation for hemiplegia and hemiparesis indicates the right dominant side is affected, so the sixth character is "1" for code I69.051. The malnutrition is sequelae to the paralysis. Because the patient is having difficulty swallowing, the dysphagia is reported following the cerebral infarction. An instructional note instructs to report R13.1- if the type of dysphagia is known. R13.10 is reported for difficulty in swallowing.

CASE STUDY 12

I25.111   Atherosclerotic heart disease of native coronary artery with angina pectoris with documented spasm

Rationale: The atherosclerotic heart disease in category I25 must indicate with or without angina pectoris, with or without spasm, or if the patient has angina pectoris. The code range is I25.10 to I25.119.

CASE STUDY 13

K64.8   Internal hemorrhoids without mention of degree

Rationale: In the Alphabetic Index the main term is Hemorrhoids—internal and verified in the Tabular List without complication as K64.8.

CASE STUDY 14

I21.3   ST elevation (STEMI) myocardial infarction of unspecified site

Z87.891   Personal history of nicotine dependence

Rationale: The patient suffered an acute MI STEMI based on the documentation. Infarction—myocardial (acute) is referenced in the Alphabetic Index and the code is selected in the Tabular List as ST Elevation acute MI (I21.3). The personal history should be reported for the nicotine dependence as documented in the social history portion of the case: History—personal—nicotine dependence (Z87.891).

CASE STUDY 15

I21.19   ST elevation (STEMI) myocardial infarction involving other coronary artery of inferior wall

I10   Hypertension

Rationale: The documentation indicates the patient suffered an ST elevation of the coronary artery of the inferior wall that is acute. Infarction—myocardial (acute) is referenced in the Alphabetic Index and the code is selected in the Tabular List as ST Elevation acute MI of the inferior wall (I21.19). Hypertension is reported as I10, is documented in the medical record, and is reported even if not treated because the acute MI may affect the patient's blood pressure.

CASE STUDY 16

I50.23   Acute on chronic systolic (congestive) heart failure

J44.9   Chronic obstructive pulmonary disease, unspecified

I49.9   Cardiac arrhythmia, unspecified

I25.10   Atherosclerotic heart disease of native coronary artery without angina pectoris

Z95.0   Presence of cardiac pacemaker

Z87.891   History of nicotine dependence

Rationale: The documentation indicates the patient has acute on chronic systolic congestive heart failure. Failure—heart—congestive—systolic is referenced in the Alphabetic Index. The cardiac dysrhythmia is referenced under the main term Dysrhythmia. The atherosclerotic heart disease is referenced under the main term Disease—heart—ischemic—atherosclerotic (of) (I25.10).

CASE STUDY 17

I48.0   Paroxysmal atrial fibrillation

R41.82   Altered mental status, unspecified

Rationale: In the Alphabetic Index reference the main term Fibrillation—atrial—paroxysmal and verify the code in the Tabular List. Because the documentation indicates the atrial fibrillation is paroxysmal, the patient encounter is coded I48.0. In addition, in the history, because there is a mention of altered medical

state and the patient was unresponsive, R41.82 is reported as a secondary diagnosis.

CASE STUDY 18

I48.91   Unspecified Atrial fibrillation

R06.02   Shortness of breath

R07.9   Chest pain unspecified

Z82.49   Family history of ischemic heart disease and other diseases of the circulatory system

Z72.0   Tobacco use

Rationale: The atrial fibrillation may have a relationship with the shortness of breath and the chest pain, but this is not clear in the documentation so they both may be reported. The patient's family history of the ischemic heart disease is documented and is important in the treatment of the patient and should be reported. Z72.0 should be reported for tobacco use. In order to code F17.21-, we need to know what the patient smokes (cigarettes, cigars, etc) and whether the patient is dependent. In this case study, there is no documented evidence of dependence or what the patient smokes, so tobacco use (Z72.0) is the more appropriate choice.

CASE STUDY 19

I25.110   Atherosclerotic heart disease of native coronary artery with unstable angina pectoris

I25.710   Atherosclerosis of autologous vein coronary artery bypass graft(s) with unstable angina pectoris

I51.7   Cardiomegaly

Rationale: All three conditions are documented in the medical record and should be reported. Because the documentation also indicates the patient has unstable angina, the specificity of the code indicates this (combination code) in the code descriptor.

CASE STUDY 20

I50.9   Congestive heart failure, unspecified

F01.50   Vascular dementia without behavioral disturbance

Rationale: Because the type of congestive heart failure is not documented or known, the only choice in this classification is Heart failure—unspecified. The documentation for vascular dementia does not indicate there is any behavioral disturbance, so F01.50, Without behavioral disturbance, is reported.

CASE STUDY 21

I82.401	Acute embolism and thrombosis of unspecified deep veins of right lower extremity
I69.320	Aphasia following cerebral infarction
J18.9	Pneumonia, unspecified organism
R73.9	Hyperglycemia, unspecified

Rationale: The patient had a stroke two months ago, which validates reporting the sequelae of the cerebrovascular disease. The reason for the visit is due to the right-sided weakness, which is documented as an acute thrombosis of the right lower extremity. Laterality right versus left is imperative in selection of the code. The patient also has pneumonia, but the organism is not specified, so it is coded as J18.9, Pneumonia, unspecified organism. The provider is also managing the hyperglycemia, which is reported as unspecified (R73.9).

CASE STUDY 22

| I49.5 | Sick sinus syndrome |

Rationale: The diagnosis is referenced in the Alphabetic Index under the main term: Syndrome—sick—sinus and verified in the Tabular List.

CASE STUDY 23

| I73.00 | Raynaud's syndrome without gangrene |
| I73.81 | Erythromelalgia |

Rationale: The diagnosis is referenced in the Alphabetic Index under the main term: Syndrome—Raynaud's and verified in the Tabular List. Two codes are necessary: one for the Raynaud's Syndrome and one for the erythromelalgia.

CASE STUDY 24

| R07.2 | Precordial pain |

Rationale: The diagnosis is referenced in the Alphabetic Index under the main term Pain—precordial and verified in the Tabular List.

Chapter 6

CASE STUDY 1

J69.0	Aspiration pneumonia
J44.1	Chronic obstructive pulmonary disease with (acute) exacerbation
E11.9	Type 2 diabetes mellitus without complications
C34.31	Malignant neoplasm of lower lobe, right bronchus, or lung
I10	Hypertension (benign)
I26.99	Other pulmonary embolism without acute cor pulmonale
Z79.4	Long term insulin use
Z87.891	Personal history of nicotine dependence

Rationale: The first-listed diagnosis, Aspiration pneumonia, is referenced under the main term Pneumonia in the Alphabetic Index. Because there is not specificity as the manifestation of type 2 diabetes mellitus, E11.9, Unspecified, is reported. The patient is on insulin, so Z79.4 should be reported. The malignant neoplasm of the right lung lower lobe is referenced in the Neoplasm Table under Lung—lower lobe in the primary malignancy column and verified in the Tabular List. Hypertension is reported with I10, and the personal history of the nicotine dependence is reported as Z87.891. In addition, the pulmonary embolism NOS is reported with I26.99.

CASE STUDY 2

| J38.02 | Paralysis of vocal cords and larynx, bilateral |

Rationale: The documentation indicates the patient has vocal code paralysis and is referenced in the Alphabetic Index under the main term Paralysis—vocal cords—bilateral. The fifth character "2" indicates the laterality.

CASE STUDY 3

| J98.11 | Atelectasis |
| J40 | Bronchitis not specified as acute or chronic |

D72.829   Elevated white blood cell count, unspecified

R09.02   Hypoxemia

Rationale: Documentation in the impression portion of the case indicates the patient has atelectasis in the left lower lobe. The Alphabetic Index is referenced under the main term Atelectasis, J98.11. The patient has tracheobronchitis, which is reported as J40 because the documentation does not indicate it is acute or chronic. The leukocytosis is reported with D72.829.

CASE STUDY 4

G35   Multiple sclerosis

R06.00   Dyspnea, unspecified

Rationale: The diagnoses in the impression portion of the case specify the patient has multiple sclerosis and is referenced in the Alphabetic Index under Sclerosis—multiple. G35 is verified in the Tabular List. The patient also has dyspnea, which is unspecified because more information is not available in the documentation.

CASE STUDY 5

G47.10   Hypersomnia, unspecified

J31.0   Chronic rhinitis

R01.1   Cardiac murmur, unspecified

Rationale: The documentation indicates the patient has very severe hypersomnia, which is reported with G47.10. Chronic rhinitis is referenced in the Alphabetic Index under Rhinitis—chronic and is verified in the Tabular List as J31.0. The documentation indicates the patient also has a systolic murmur, which is referenced in the Alphabetic Index under the main term Murmur.

CASE STUDY 6

D86.0   Sarcoidosis of lung

N17.9   Acute kidney failure, unspecified

N18.9   Chronic kidney disease, unspecified

D63.1   Anemia in chronic kidney disease

I10   Hypertension

E83.52   Hypercalcemia

H54.7   Unspecified visual loss

Rationale: The sarcoidosis of the lung can be found in the Alphabetic Index under main term Sarcoidosis—lung. The acute kidney failure is referenced as Failure—kidney—acute and the anemia can be associated with the chronic kidney disease and is referenced under the main term Disease—kidney—chronic. All codes must be verified in the Tabular List. H54.7 should be reported for the bilateral visual acuity deficits.

CASE STUDY 7

J45.21   Mild intermittent asthma with (acute) exacerbation

Rationale: The Alphabetic Index is referenced under the main term Asthma—intermittent—with acute exacerbation. The code should be verified in the Tabular List. Even though the documentation in the assessment and plan does not indicate intermittent, it is inferred in the history portion of the case study.

CASE STUDY 8

L02.32   Furuncle of buttock

R50.9   Fever, unspecified

Z23   Encounter for immunization

Rationale: Reference the Alphabetic Index for the main term Furuncle—buttock (L02.32) and verify the code in the Tabular List. There is no indication the fever is a symptom of the boils, so it is reported as Fever, unspecified because no further documentation indicates the type of fever. The documentation in the plan is that the patient will receive a pneumovax vaccination, and the vaccination is referenced in the Alphabetic Index under Immunization—Encounter (Z23).

CASE STUDY 9

J45.22   Mild intermittent asthma with status asthmaticus

J18.9   Pneumonia, unspecified organism

Rationale: When coding for extrinsic asthma, documentation must indicate whether the condition is mild, moderate, or severe and whether the asthma is intermittent or persistent.

CASE STUDY 10

J45.901   Unspecified asthma with (acute) exacerbation

Rationale: Because the documentation does not indicate or infer intermittent or persistent asthma, Unspecified with acute exacerbation should be reported. Reference the Alphabetic Index for the main term Asthma—exacerbation (acute) (J45.90-) and verify it as unspecified in the Tabular List.

CASE STUDY 11

R05   Cough

Rationale: Because the provider did not specify a definitive diagnosis and cough is the only sign or symptom, cough is reported as R05.

CASE STUDY 12

J45.902   Unspecified asthma with status asthmaticus

Rationale: In ICD-10-CM, documentation must indicate type of asthma, whether it is mild, moderate, or severe, and whether it is intermittent or persistent. Because the type is not classified as mildly persistent, the Alphabetic Index directs the user to: Asthma; nonallergic (intrinsic), with status asthmaticus.

CASE STUDY 13

J44.0   Chronic obstructive pulmonary disease with acute lower respiratory infection

F17.218   Nicotine dependence with other nicotine-induced disorders

Rationale: The Alphabetic Index is referenced with the main term Disease—pulmonary—chronic obstructive with lower respiratory infection (acute) (J44.0) and verified in the Tabular List. The documentation also indicates in the history of present illness that the patient is a smoker, and nicotine dependence is reported as a secondary diagnosis.

CASE STUDY 14

J38.6   Stenosis of larynx

Rationale: Reference the Alphabetic Index for the main term Stenosis—larynx and verify the code in the Tabular List as J38.6.

CASE STUDY 15

J34.3   Hypertrophy of nasal turbinates

Rationale: The main term in the Alphabetic Index is Hypertrophy—nasal turbinate (J34.3) and verified in the Tabular List. The obstruction is not reported, as it results from the hypertrophy.

CASE STUDY 16

J35.01   Chronic tonsillitis

Rationale: Reference the main term Tonsillitis—chronic in the Alphabetic Index and verify the code in the Tabular List.

CASE STUDY 17

G91.3   Post-traumatic hydrocephalus, unspecified

Rationale: The postoperative diagnosis is post-traumatic hydrocephalus and is referenced in the Alphabetic Index as Hydrocephalus—post-traumatic and verified in the Tabular List.

CASE STUDY 18

J41.0   Simple chronic bronchitis

F17.210   Nicotine dependence, cigarettes, uncomplicated

Rationale: The Alphabetic Index main term is Cough—smokers' (J41.0). Because the nicotine dependence does not indicate any associated nicotine-induced disorders except the cough, the uncomplicated code F17.210 is accurate.

CASE STUDY 19

R06.02   Shortness of breath

J45.30   Mild persistent asthma, uncomplicated

Z87.891   Personal history of nicotine dependence

Rationale: Three codes are reported: shortness of breath, the asthma that is mildly persistent, and the history of nicotine dependence.

CASE STUDY 20

J84.10   Pulmonary fibrosis, unspecified

Rationale: The main term in the Alphabetic Index is Fibrosis—pulmonary and verified in the Tabular List. Because the specific type is not documented, the condition is coded as unspecified.

Chapter 7

CASE STUDY 1

K92.1   Melena

Rationale: The postoperative diagnosis cannot be reported because the documentation indicates incomplete colonoscopy, so the reason for the attempted colonoscopy should be reported. Hematochezia is a medical term for blood in stool, which is reported in ICD-10-CM as K92.1, Melena. Hematemesis, melena, and hematochezia are symptoms of acute gastrointestinal bleeding.

CASE STUDY 2

K52.9   Noninfective gastroenteritis and colitis, unspecified

Rationale: The main term in the Alphabetic Index that is referenced is Gastroenteritis—noninfectious and reported as K52.9.

CASE STUDY 3

K85.9   Acute pancreatitis, unspecified

Rationale: Because there is no documentation to indicate the type of acute pancreatitis, which includes billiary, idiopathic, drug induced, or cytomegaloviral, the only code selection possible based on documentation is K85.9, Acute pancreatitis, unspecified. In the clinical setting, it is recommended that the physician is queried for more detail if available to code to the specificity the insurance carriers and contractors desire.

CASE STUDY 4

K21.0   Gastro-esophageal reflux disease with esophagitis

R11.11   Vomiting without nausea

R10.9   Unspecified abdominal pain

Rationale: Because the documentation indicates the patient has gastro-esophageal reflux disease with esophagitis but it cannot be determined if that is the cause of the vomiting and abdominal pain, both are coded. Alphabetic Index, main term: Disease—gastroesophageal reflux (GERD)—with esophagitis (K21.0); Vomiting—without nausea (R11.11); and Pain—abdominal (R10.9). Remember to verify all codes in the Tabular List.

CASE STUDY 5

K59.00   Constipation unspecified

R15.1   Fecal soiling

Rationale: Alphabetic Index, main term: Constipation (K59.00) verified in the Tabular List. Fecal soiling can be a symptom of constipation but because the documentation is unclear, it could be reported. It is recommended that the physician be queried for clarity.

CASE STUDY 6

K92.2   Gastrointestinal hemorrhage, unspecified

E11.9   Type 2 diabetes mellitus without complication

I10   Hypertension

E78.2   Mixed hyperlipidemia

Rationale: The medical term for bleed is hemorrhage. The first-listed diagnosis that describes the reason for the treatment is gastrointestinal hemorrhage. Alphabetic Index: Hemorrhage—gastrointestinal (K92.2). The documentation indicates the patient also has type 2 diabetes (Diabetes—type 2 [E11.9]), hypertension (I10), and hypercholesterolemia with hyperglyceridemia, which is hyperlipidemia mixed.

CASE STUDY 7

R10.13   Epigastric pain

Rationale: Reference the main term in the Alphabetic Index: Pain—epigastric (R10.13).

CASE STUDY 8

K59.00   Constipation unspecified

K62.5   Hemorrhage of anus and rectum

E84.9   Cystic fibrosis unspecified

Rationale: Alphabetic Index, main term: Constipation—unspecified (K59.00);

Hemorrhage—rectum (K62.5); and Fibrosis—cystic (E84.9).

CASE STUDY 9

K80.20   Calculus of gallbladder without cholecystitis without obstruction

Rationale: Alphabetic Index: Calculus—gallbladder—with cholecystitis (K80.20) and verified in the Tabular List.

CASE STUDY 10

K46.9   Unspecified abdominal hernia without obstruction or gangrene

Rationale: Alphabetic Index, main term: Hernia—abdominal (K46.-) and verified in the Tabular List as K46.9, Unspecified abdominal hernia without obstruction or gangrene.

CASE STUDY 11

K80.10   Calculus of gallbladder with chronic cholecystitis without obstruction

Rationale: Alphabetic Index, main term: Cholecystitis—with cholelithiasis, see calculus—gallbladder—cholecystitis (K80.10).

CASE STUDY 12

K40.20   Bilateral inguinal hernia, without obstruction or gangrene, not specified as recurrent

K57.90   Diverticulosis of intestine, part unspecified, without perforation, abscess or bleeding

Rationale: Alphabetic Index, main term: Hernia—inguinal (K40.2-). Verify the code in the Tabular List as K40.20, Bilateral inguinal hernia, without obstruction or gangrene, not specified as recurrent.

CASE STUDY 13

K43.9   Ventral hernia without obstruction or gangrene

K91.62   Intraoperative hemorrhage and hematoma of a digestive system organ or structure complicating other procedure

Rationale: Alphabetic Index, main term: Hernia—ventral (K43.9) and secondary diagnosis; main term

Hemorrhage—intraoperative with cross-reference "*see* Complication, hemorrhage (hematoma), intraoperative (intraprocedural) by site"; Complication—intraoperative (intraprocedural), hemorrhage, digestive system organ, during procedure on other organ (K91.62).

CASE STUDY 14

K43.0   Incisional hernia with obstruction, without gangrene

Rationale: Alphabetic Index, main term: Hernia—incisional—with gangrene (and obstruction) (K43.0).

CASE STUDY 15

B20   Human immunodeficiency virus (HIV) disease

R13.12   Dysphagia, oropharyngeal phase

K92.0   Hematemesis

Rationale: Alphabetic Index: Dysphagia—oropharyngeal phase (R13.12); Hematemesis (K92.0); Human—immunodeficiency virus (B20). Because dysphagia is a symptom/condition related to the HIV virus, code B20 is listed first, followed by the dysphagia and hematemesis.

Chapter 8

CASE STUDY 1

L71.9   Rosacea, unspecified

L21.9   Seborrheic dermatitis, unspecified

L20.9   Atopic dermatitis, unspecified

Rationale: Any of the three diagnoses can be listed as the first-listed diagnosis because there are no guidelines for these conditions that take precedence. Alphabetic Index, main term: Dermatitis—seborrheic (L21.9); Dermatitis—atopic (L20.9); and Rosacea (L71.9). Verify all codes in the Tabular List.

CASE STUDY 2

E10.628   Type 1 diabetes mellitus with other specified skin complications

L03.116   Cellulitis of left lower limb

Rationale: Alphabetic Index, main term: Cellulitis—lower limb (L03.11-). Diabetes mellitus is referenced under the main term: Diabetes.

CASE STUDY 3

L98.9   Other specified disorder of the skin and subcutaneous tissue

Rationale: Alphabetic Index, main term: Dermatosis (L98.9), which is referenced in the Tabular List under other specified disorders of the skin and subcutaneous tissue.

CASE STUDY 4

E10.22   Type 1 diabetes mellitus with diabetic chronic kidney disease

E10.628   Type 1 diabetes mellitus with other skin complications

L03.116   Cellulitis of left lower limb

N18.9   Chronic kidney disease, unspecified

I50.9   Heart failure, unspecified (Congestive Heart Failure)

M19.90   Unspecified osteoarthritis, unspecified site

R41.0   Disorientation unspecified (delirum, NOS)

I10   Hypertension

Rationale: The cellulitis bilateral cannot be reported in category L02.11- with a bilateral code, which is unavailable. Alphabetic Index, main term: Cellulitis—lower extremity (L03.11-). Each side is reported for the cellulitis of the right and left lower extremity. Because there is no documented relationship between the heart and kidney disease, hypertension is reported as I10.

CASE STUDY 5

C44.212   Basal cell carcinoma of skin of right ear and external auricular canal

Rationale: Reference the Neoplasm Table, main term Ear and select the code from the primary malignancy column and verify the code in the Tabular List.

CASE STUDY 6

M06.211   Rheumatoid bursitis right shoulder

Rationale: The reason for the visit is right shoulder pain. However, the physician diagnosed the patient in the assessment with rheumatoid bursitis of the right shoulder. Alphabetic Index, main term: Bursitis—rheumatoid—shoulder—right (M06.21-). The code should be verified in the Tabular List. Laterality is reported with the sixth character "1" for right shoulder.

CASE STUDY 7

S70.911A   Unspecified superficial injury to right hip, initial encounter

W06.xxxA   Fall from bed, initial encounter

Y92.003   Bedroom of unspecified (private residence)

Y99.8   Other external cause status

Rationale: In the Alphabetic Index the main term is referenced as Injury, superficial, hip (S70.9-). However, the fall from the bed must be reported. Review the following excerpt from the ICD-10-CM codebook:

W06.-   Fall from bed

       The appropriate seventh character is to be added to code W06

       A—initial encounter

       D—subsequent encounter

       S—sequela

W06.xxxA   Fall from bed

Y92.003   Bedroom of unspecified (private residence)

Y99.8   Other specified activity status

Note: Placeholders must be added (x) because a seventh character is required.

CASE STUDY 8

M25.511   Pain right shoulder

Rationale: Alphabetic Index: Pain—joint, shoulder—right (M25.511).

CASE STUDY 9

M51.36   Other intervertebral disc degeneration, lumbar region

M48.07   Spinal stenosis, lumbosacral region

M81.0   Osteoporosis age related osteoporosis without current pathological fracture

Z90.710   Acquired absence of both cervix and uterus

Rationale: The documentation indicates the disc degeneration is in the lumbar region, which would be referenced in the Alphabetic Index under main term Degeneration—intervertebral disc NOS—lumbar region, which is coded as M51.36. The spinal stenosis is documented as the lumbosacral region with the L4-5 and L5-Sl region and is coded as M48.07, and the patient has osteoporosis without a pathological fracture and is coded as M81.07. All three diagnosis codes can be supported in the documentation.

CASE STUDY 10

M25.561   Pain in right knee

M25.562   Pain in left knee

I10   Hypertension

Rationale: In ICD-10-CM laterality is crucial in the documentation and coding. Some categories provide one code to identify right/left and bilateral. In this category there is not a code to identify the bilateral condition, so both diagnoses for right knee pain and left knee pain must be reported. In ICD-10-CM the type of hypertension (benign, essential malignant, etc) is not a factor when selecting the diagnosis code. There is one code for hypertension, I10, unless the hypertension is due to another condition, which is coded in another category.

CASE STUDY 11

S72.001A   Fracture of unspecified part of neck of right femur, initial encounter for closed fracture

I10   Hypertension

E03.9   Hypothyroidism, unspecified

R10.13   Epigastric pain, Dyspepsia

M79.7   Fibromyalgia (Note: site not specified in documentation)

F32.9   Major depressive disorder, single episode, unspecified

K59.00   Constipation, unspecified

G47.00   Insomnia, unspecified (NOS)

J30.9   Allergic rhinitis, unspecified

F41.1   Generalized anxiety disorder

E87.1   Hypo-osmolality and hyponatremia

Rationale: Fractures are coded based on type, site, and laterality in most cases. The seventh character "A" is used to report the initial encounter. In ICD-10-CM the type of hypertension (benign, essential malignant, etc) is not a factor when selecting the diagnosis code. There is one code for hypertension, I10, unless the hypertension is due to another condition, which is coded in another category. The documentation supports numerous diagnoses that are either being managed by the provider or contribute to the management of the patient and are reported.

CASE STUDY 12

M19.011   Primary osteoarthritis, right shoulder

Rationale: Alphabetic Index, main term: Osteoarthritis—primary—shoulder—right and verified in the Tabular List as M19.011.

CASE STUDY 13

M25.562   Pain in left knee

Rationale: Osteoarthritis cannot be confirmed based on the stated degenerative changes, so pain is to be reported.

CASE STUDY 14

M17.11   Unilateral primary osteoarthritis, right knee

M21.161   Varus deformity, not elsewhere classified right knee

Rationale: Laterality is important when coding category M21.

CASE STUDY 15

M76.61   Achilles tendinitis, right leg

M76.62   Achilles tendinitis, left leg

Rationale: There is not a bilateral ICD-10-CM code to report Achilles tendinitis bilateral, so the tendinitis for the right and left leg must be reported to support medical necessity for the service provided.

CASE STUDY 16

M17.12   Unilateral primary osteoarthritis, left knee

M25.561   Pain in right knee

Rationale: Because in the provider's impression the left knee is documented as localized osteoarthritis, M17.12 is reported. The pain in the right knee can be reported because it is documented in the history. The knee pain in the left knee should not be reported because osteoarthritis is typically associated with knee pain.

CASE STUDY 17

M23.42   Loose body in knee, left knee

Rationale: Codes in category M23 are selected based on laterality. It is important to identify the right or left knee when reporting this condition.

CASE STUDY 18

M67.431   Ganglion right wrist

Rationale: The Alphabetic Index is referenced as Ganglion—wrist M67.43-. The sixth character identifies the right wrist.

CASE STUDY 19

M84.451A Pathological fracture, right femur

M19.90   Unspecified osteoarthritis, unspecified site

E03.9   Hypothyroidism, unspecified

G90.09   Other idiopathic peripheral autonomic neuropathy

W18.30xA Fall on same level, unspecified, initial encounter

Y92.038   Other place in apartment as the place of occurrence of the external cause

Y99.8   Other external cause status

Rationale: The fall should be reported as well as the place of occurrence, which is referenced in the External Cause of Injuries Index. Because the home is a condominium, it is coded in the category "apartment." The fracture is referenced as Fracture—pathological—femur—right. The seventh character "A" is reported for the initial encounter.

CASE STUDY 20

M72.2   Plantar fascial fibromatosis

M77.32   Calcaneal spur, left foot

Rationale: The Alphabetic Index is referenced under the main term: Fasciitis—plantar (M72.2).

CASE STUDY 21

M65.311 Trigger thumb, right thumb

Rationale: The Alphabetic Index is referenced under the main term Pain—limb, upper, hand (M79.64-). In the Tabular List laterality of right finger is the correct selection (M79.644). For the trigger thumb, the Alphabetic Index reference is Trigger finger (acquired)—thumb (M65.31-). In the Tabular List M65.311 is the correct selection for laterality of the right thumb.

CASE STUDY 22

M62.828   Other muscle spasm

M25.562   Pain in left knee

Rationale: The Alphabetic Index is referenced under the main term spasm, muscle, NEC (M62.838). The Alphabetic Index is referenced under the main term Pain—joint, knee (M25.56-). Laterality is selected in the Tabular List (left knee) M25.562.

Chapter 9

CASE STUDY 1

N83.7   Hematoma of broad ligament

Rationale: Alphabetic Index, main term: Seroma, with a cross-reference to "*see also* Hematoma." Referencing Hematoma; broad ligament (nontraumatic), directs the user to N83.7.

CASE STUDY 2

N10   Acute tubulo-interstitial nephritis

E87.6   Hypokalemia

R11.2   Nausea with vomiting, unspecified

Rationale: The Alphabetic Index is referenced under the main term Pyelonephritis—acute (N10), and main term Hypokalemia (E87.6). All codes should be verified in the Tabular List.

CASE STUDY 3

N92.4   Excessive bleeding in the premenopausal period

D50.0   Iron deficiency anemia secondary to blood loss (chronic)

Rationale: The Alphabetic Index is referenced under the main term Anemia—iron deficiency (D50.0); Menorrhagia—premenopausal (N92.4).

CASE STUDY 4

N76.0   Acute vaginitis

Rationale: Alphabetic Index, main term: Vaginitis—acute (N76.0).

CASE STUDY 5

N81.10   Cystocele, unspecified

N39.3   Stress incontinence (female) (male)

Rationale: Both the cystocele and urethrocele are documented, but based on the Excludes1 instruction under Urethrocele, only N81.10 is reported. Stress incontinence is reported in ICD-10-CM for both male and female.

CASE STUDY 6

N99.3   Prolapse of vaginal vault after hysterectomy

Rationale: In the Alphabetic Index, main term Prolapse, prolapsed—vagina—posthysterectomy (N99.3).

CASE STUDY 7

N20.0   Calculus of kidney

N39.0   Urinary tract infection, site not specified

B95.1   Streptococcus, group B, as the cause of diseases classified elsewhere

F17.210   Nicotine dependence, cigarettes, uncomplicated

R03.0   Elevated blood-pressure reading, without diagnosis of hypertension

Rationale: In the Alphabetic Index, main term: Calculus—kidney (N20.0); Infection—urinary tract (N39.0). An instructional note in N39.0 provides guidance to use an additional code to identify the infectious agent. Documentation does indicate strep is the cause (hemolytic strep is type B, B95.1). Tobacco use is documented and reported in ICD-10-CM as nicotine dependence. The term "uncomplicated" does not indicate control. There is not a code in ICD-10-CM for nicotine dependence uncontrolled, so F17.200 is reported. The elevated blood pressure is not reported as hypertension (I10) but as R03.0 and can be referenced under the main term: Elevated—blood pressure, reading.

CASE STUDY 8

N87.1   Moderate cervical dysplasia

Rationale: The Alphabetic Index can be referenced under the main term Dysplasia—cervix, moderate (N87.1).

CASE STUDY 9

N47.1   Phimosis

Rationale: The Alphabetic Index can be referenced under the main term Phimosis—congenital (N47.1).

CASE STUDY 10

I12.9   Hypertensive chronic kidney disease with stage 1 through 4 chronic kidney disease or unspecified chronic kidney disease

N18.9   Chronic kidney disease, unspecified

N17.0   Acute kidney failure with tubular necrosis

Rationale: For hypertension there is a cause and effect relationship with CKD and hypertension. Alphabetic index is referenced as failure—renal—hypertension—kidney (I12.9). The Alphabetic Index can be referenced under the main term Failure—renal, with tubular necrosis (acute) (N17.0).

CASE STUDY 11

E11.22 Type 2 diabetes mellitus with diabetic chronic kidney disease

N18.3 Chronic kidney disease, stage 3 (moderate)

Z79.4 Long-term (current) use of insulin

Rationale: Several codes are necessary for this encounter. In addition to type 2 diabetes mellitus and chronic kidney disease stage 3, long-term use of insulin should be reported as a tertiary diagnosis because this is a type 2 diabetic patient on insulin.

CASE STUDY 12

O24.012   Pre-existing diabetes mellitus, type 1, in pregnancy, second trimester

E10.69   Type 1 diabetes mellitus with other specified complication

Rationale: The Alphabetic Index can be referenced under the main term Pregnancy—complicated by—diabetes—type 1—second trimester. The sixth character "2" identifies the second trimester in the code description. An instructional note directs the user to report a code from category E10 with O24.012.

CASE STUDY 13

O36.4xx0   Maternal care for intrauterine death (one fetus)

O70.2   Third degree perineal laceration during delivery

Z37.1   Single stillbirth

Z3A.37   37 weeks' gestation of pregnancy

Rationale: The Alphabetic Index can be referenced under the main term pregnancy—complicated (by) fetal death (near term) (O36.4-). The documentation indicates the stillbirth was affected by the compression of the umbilical cord. The outcome of delivery must be reported as a single stillbirth (Z37.1). In addition, the third-degree perineal laceration during delivery is reported as O70.2 and the weeks of gestation should also be reported (Z3A37).

CASE STUDY 14

O69.81x0   Labor and delivery complicated by cord around neck, without compression (one fetus)

Z37.0   Single live birth

Z3A.38   38 weeks' gestation of pregnancy

Rationale: The Alphabetic Index can be referenced under the main term Delivery—complicated by. The seventh character reports fetus 1. The dummy placeholder "x" is built into the code to allow for the seventh character. The single live birth should also be reported on the maternal record to report the outcome of delivery.

CASE STUDY 15

O80   Encounter for full term uncomplicated delivery

O70.1   Second degree perineal laceration during delivery

Z37.0   Single live birth

Z3A.41   41 weeks' gestation of pregnancy

Rationale: The Alphabetic Index can be referenced under the main term Laceration—perineal—second degree (O70.1). The outcome of delivery for the single live birth is also reported as Z37.0. The delivery can be referenced in the Alphabetic Index under main term Delivery—childbirth (labor)—uncomplicated (O80) and should be the first listed diagnosis code.

CASE STUDY 16

Z32.01 Encounter for pregnancy test, results positive

Rationale: The Alphabetic Index can be referenced under the main term Encounter—pregnancy—test—result positive (Z32.01).

CASE STUDY 17

O24.414   Gestational diabetes mellitus in pregnancy, insulin controlled

O09.892   Supervision of other high risk pregnancies, second trimester

Z3A.22   22 weeks' gestation of pregnancy

Z79.4   Long-term (current) use of insulin

Rationale: Four diagnoses should be reported for the gestational diabetes in pregnancy, supervision of the high-risk pregnancy because of the gestational diabetes, the weeks of gestation (22) and the current use of insulin. There is an instructional note under category O24 in the Tabular List, "Use additional code for long-term (current) use of insulin (Z79.4)."

CASE STUDY 18

O80   Encounter for full-term uncomplicated delivery

Z3A.39   Weeks of gestation

Z73.0   Outcome of Delivery, single liveborn

Rationale: In the Alphabetic Index, reference the main term Delivery (childbirth) (labor)—completely normal case (O80). In addition, the weeks of gestation and outcome of delivery should be reported.

Chapter 10

CASE STUDY 1

R06.83   Snoring

Rationale: Signs and symptoms/snoring rule out tonsillitis (R06.83). The Alphabetic Index can be referenced under the main term Snoring (R06.83).

CASE STUDY 2

I10   Hypertension

R51   Headache

Rationale: In ICD-10-CM, the type of hypertension (benign, essential malignant, etc) is not a factor when selecting the diagnosis code. There is one code for hypertension, I10, unless the hypertension is due to another condition, which is coded in another category. For the headache, documentation should indicate whether the headache is vascular or nonvascular and whether the pain is intractable or not intractable to code to the level of specificity the insurance carriers and contractors desire.

CASE STUDY 3

B19.20   Unspecified viral hepatitis C without hepatic coma

M17.0   Bilateral primary osteoarthritis of knee

R65.21   Severe sepsis with septic shock

N39.0   Urinary tract infection, site not specified

R18.8   Other ascites

K83.0   Cholangitis

K70.31   Alcoholic cirrhosis of liver with ascites

F10.21   Alcohol dependence, in remission

F14.21   Cocaine dependence, in remission

D69.6   Thrombocytopenia, unspecified

D89.1   Cryoglobulinemia

Z87.891   Personal history of nicotine dependence

W18.30x1   Fall on same level, unspecified

Rationale: Several codes are necessary to report multiple conditions for this patient. All main terms should be referenced and verified in the Tabular List.

CASE STUDY 4

R10.13   Epigastric pain

Rationale: The Alphabetic Index can be referenced under the main term Pain—epigastric (R10.13).

CASE STUDY 5

R10.30   Lower abdominal pain, unspecified

Rationale: The Alphabetic Index can be referenced under the main term: Pain—abdominal—lower (R10.30).

CASE STUDY 6

R07.9   Chest pain, unspecified

R06.02   Shortness of breath

E11.9   Type 2 diabetes mellitus without complications

E78.5   Hyperlipidemia unspecified

R63.5   Abnormal weight gain

Rationale: The angina may not be coded because it is suspect and not confirmed. Only the signs and symptoms may be reported. The Alphabetic Index can be referenced under the main terms Pain—chest (central) (R07.9) and Breath—shortness (R06.02). The type 2 diabetes is the default when the documentation does not specify which type of diabetes mellitus the patient has. E11.9 is the only choice unless the provider is queried (recommended) to determine actual type and if manifestations are evident; Hyperlipidemia (E78.5) and Weight—gain (abnormal) (excessive) (R63.5) are reported.

CASE STUDY 7

R13.10   Dysphagia, unspecified

M06.9   Rheumatoid arthritis, unspecified

Rationale: The Alphabetic Index can be referenced under the main term Dysphagia—unspecified (R13.10). Even though the dysphagia is the reason for the procedure performed, the rheumatoid arthritis is the cause of the dysphagia and may be reported as the secondary diagnosis.

CASE STUDY 8

R31.2   Other microscopic hematuria

Rationale: The Alphabetic Index can be referenced under the main term Hematuria—microscopic (R31.2).

CASE STUDY 9

R30.0   Dysuria

N91.0   Primary amenorrhea

Z32.02   Encounter for pregnancy test, result negative

Rationale: The Alphabetic Index can be referenced under the main terms Dysuria (R30.0) and Amenorrhea—primary (N91.0). Verify both codes in the Tabular List. The pregnancy test is referenced in the Alphabetic Index under Encounter—pregnancy—test—result negative (Z32.02).

CASE STUDY 10

R19.01   Right upper quadrant abdominal swelling, mass and lump

Rationale: The Alphabetic Index can be referenced under the main term Mass—abdominal—right upper quadrant (R19.01). The flank is located in the upper quadrant of the abdomen.

CASE STUDY 11

R07.9   Chest pain, unspecified

R06.02   Shortness of breath

I73.9   Peripheral vascular disease, unspecified

E78.5   Hyperlipidemia, unspecified

Z86.79   Personal history of other diseases of the circulatory system

Rationale: Only the signs and symptoms may be reported as the reason for the patient encounter since the condition has not yet been confirmed. The Alphabetic Index can be referenced under the main terms Pain—chest (central) (R07.9) and Breath—shortness (R05.03). In addition, the patient has peripheral vascular disease (I73.9) and hyperlipidemia (E78.5), which may also be reported. The personal history of the coronary artery disease may also be reported because it does have relevance to the care of this patient and is referenced under main term History—personal.

CASE STUDY 12

S50.02xA   Contusion of left elbow, initial encounter

S80.02xA   Contusion of left knee, initial encounter

V28.0xxA   Motorcycle driver injured in noncollision transport accident in nontraffic accident

Y99.8   Other external cause status

Rationale: A seventh character is required for the contusion code(s) and the external cause code. The placeholder "x" must be added to meet the seventh character requirement because the specificity for each diagnosis is five characters. In addition, the activity (motorcycle accident) should be reported as an additional diagnosis as well as an external cause status (Y99.8)

CASE STUDY 13

S52.021A   Displaced fracture of olecranon process without intra-articular extension of right ulna

Rationale: A seventh character is required for the fracture code(s). In this scenario, "A" is the correct seventh character because it is the initial encounter. The Alphabetic Index can be referenced under the main term Fracture.

CASE STUDY 14

T22.211A   Burn of second degree of right forearm, initial encounter

Place of Occurrence:

Y92.511   Restaurant or cafe as the place of occurrence of the external cause

X10.2xxA   Contact with fats and cooking oils, initial encounter

Activity Code:

Y93.G3   Activity, cooking and baking (use of stove, oven and microwave oven)

Y99.0   Civilian activity done for income or pay

Rationale: For burns and corrosions the reason for the burn (the contact with cooking oil), the activity taking place (cooking), and the place of occurrence should be reported. Burns are coded based on degree of burn, laterality (site), and the encounter, whether it is initial, subsequent, or sequela. In this encounter the seventh character "A" is reported. An external cause status is also reported (Y99.0) to identify that the injury occurred at work.

CASE STUDY 15

S83.232A   Complex tear of medial meniscus, current injury, left knee, initial encounter

Rationale: The Alphabetic Index can be referenced under the main term Tear; meniscus, medial, complex—left knee (S83.23-) and is reported as the initial encounter with the seventh character "A".

CASE STUDY 16

S42.415A   Nondisplaced simple supracondylar fracture without intercondylar fracture of left humerus, initial encounter for closed fracture

V00.281A   Fall from other gliding-type pedestrian conveyance

Y99.8   Other external cause status

Rationale: The Alphabetic Index can be referenced under the main term Fracture—humerus, supracondylar (displaced) (S42.4-). The seventh character "A" is reported for the initial encounter. In addition to the condition an activity code (V00.281A) to identify the activity that caused the injury as well as the External Cause status should be reported. Since the documentation does not indicate whether the activity was for personal recreation or income, the unspecified external cause status should be reported.

CASE STUDY 17

T81.4xxA   Infection following a procedure, initial encounter

Z98.89   Other specified postprocedural states

Rationale: The Alphabetic Index can be referenced under the main term Infection—due to or resulting from—surgery (T81.4-). The seventh character "A" is reported for the initial encounter. The other postprocedural status is referenced as Status; postoperative (postprocedural).

CASE STUDY 18

G06.0   Intracranial abscess and granuloma

T81.4xxA   Infection following a procedure, initial encounter

G00.9   Other bacterial meningitis (Meningitis due to gram-negative bacteria, unspecified)

G04.90   Ventriculitis (cerebral) NOS

Rationale: The Alphabetic Index can be referenced under the main term Abscess—intracranial (G06.0). The infection is also reported and referenced under the main term Infection—due to or resulting from—surgery (T81.4-). Gram-negative meningitis is an infection of the membranes covering the brain and spinal cord (meninges) from bacteria that turn pink when exposed to a special stain (gram-negative bacteria). G00.9, Other bacterial meningitis (Meningitis due to gram-negative bacteria, unspecified), is also reported.

CASE STUDY 19

First-listed diagnosis:

T23.301A   Burn of third degree of right hand, unspecified site, initial encounter

Second-listed diagnosis:

X04.xxxA   Exposure to ignition of gasoline, initial encounter

Additional diagnosis:

Y92.096   Yard, private residence as the place of occurrence of the external cause

Y99.8   Other external cause status

Rationale: The secondary diagnosis, X04, is a three-character code, but it requires the seventh character. Because a seventh character is required to identify the encounter, the placeholder "x" must be added to the code. The place of the occurrence should also be reported. Burns are reported by site, degree, encounter, and, if third degree, the Total Body Surface Area (TBSA). We don't know the TBSA so it is not reported in this instance. Because this patient encounter is for treatment to re-excise the burns, the seventh character is "A." The seventh character "A" for the initial encounter is reported during the course of treatment for the burn. The ICD-10-CM Official Guidelines for Coding and Reporting indicate that the initial encounter seventh character is used while the patient is receiving active treatment for the condition.

CASE STUDY 20

S52.371A   Galeazzi's fracture of right radius

Rationale: The Alphabetic Index can be referenced under the main term Galeazzi's fracture (S52.37-). The seventh character "A" is reported for the initial encounter.

CASE STUDY 21

S83.231A   Complex tear of medial meniscus, current injury, right knee, initial encounter

S83.281A   Other tear of lateral meniscus, current injury, right knee, initial encounter

M25.461   Effusion, right knee

Rationale: The Alphabetic Index can be referenced under the main term Tear—meniscus, medial, complex—right knee. The seventh character "A" identifies the initial encounter. The tear of the lateral meniscus is also reported with the seventh character "A." The effusion of the joint is referenced as Effusion—joint, knee—right (M25.461).

CASE STUDY 22

S43.421A   Sprain of right rotator cuff capsule, initial encounter

M75.101   Unspecified rotator cuff tear or rupture of right shoulder, not specified as traumatic

Rationale: The Alphabetic Index can be referenced under the main term Sprain—rotator cuff (capsule)—right. The seventh character "A" identifies the initial encounter. In addition, the Alphabetic Index is referenced under the main tear—rotator cuff (nontraumatic) (M75.10-). The code is selected in the Tabular List based on laterality—right versus left shoulder.

Chapter 11

CASE STUDY 1

S83.212A   Bucket-handle tear of medial meniscus, current injury, left knee, initial encounter

Y93.67   Activity, playing basketball

Y92.014   Private driveway of single-family (private) house as the place of occurrence of the external cause

Y99.8   Other external cause status

Rationale: The Alphabetic Index can be referenced under the main term Tear—meniscus—(knee) (current injury), medial, bucket-handle (S83.21-). Remember the (-) indicates additional digits are required and are located in the Tabular List. The sixth character "2" identifies the laterality for the left knee and the seventh character "A" identifies the initial encounter. In additional the activity must be reported and can be referenced in the External Causes of Injuries Index under the main term: Activity—sports played individually (Y93.59). The place of occurrence identifies where the injury occurred and is also referenced in the External Causes of Injuries Index under the main term Place of occurrence—residence—house single family—driveway (Y92.014). Y99.8 is also reported to identify the External Cause status.

CASE STUDY 2

Z21   Asymptomatic human immunodeficiency virus (HIV) infection status

Rationale: The patient is asymptomatic, which is reported with code Z21. Reference the ICD-10-CM Official Guidelines for Coding and Reporting, Chapter 1. The Alphabetic Index can be referenced under the main term Status.

CASE STUDY 3

R10.11   Right upper quadrant pain

Z85.038   Personal history of other malignant neoplasm of large intestine

Z93.3   Colostomy status

Rationale: The Alphabetic Index can be referenced under the main term Pain—abdominal—right upper quadrant (R10.11). The personal history is referenced under main term History—personal.

CASE STUDY 4

Z48.815   Encounter for surgical aftercare following surgery on the digestive system

Rationale: The Alphabetic Index can be referenced under the main term Aftercare—following surgery—digestive system (Z48.815).

CASE STUDY 5

M48.06   Spinal stenosis, lumbar region

M54.89   Other dorsalgia

Z98.1   Arthrodesis status

I25.10   Atherosclerotic heart disease of native coronary artery without angina pectoris

Z95.0   Presence of cardiac pacemaker

Rationale: The Alphabetic Index can be referenced under the main terms Pain—back (M54.9) or Dorsalgia—specified NEC (M54.89); and for the arthrodesis, the main term is referenced in the Alphabetic Index under Arthrodesis—status (Z98.1).

Spinal stenosis is referenced in the Alphabetic Index as Stenosis—spinal—lumbar region.

CASE STUDY 6

Z45.89   Encounter for adjustment and management of other implanted devices

Rationale: The Alphabetic Index can be referenced under the main term Encounter—fitting (of), with a cross-reference to "*see* Fitting (and adjustment) (of)" (Z45.89) for the removal and reinsertion of the pessary.

CASE STUDY 7

Z45.2   Encounter for adjustment and management of vascular access device

Z85.3   Personal history of malignant neoplasm of breast

Rationale: Because the patient has a history of breast cancer, the personal history should also be reported. The encounter for the vascular access device Z45.2 is reported as the first-listed diagnosis followed by Z85.3 for the personal history of the breast cancer.

CASE STUDY 8

N73.9   Female pelvic inflammatory disease, unspecified

Z21   Asymptomatic human immunodeficiency virus (HIV) infection status

Rationale: The Alphabetic Index can be referenced under the main term Disease—pelvic—inflammatory (female)—acute (N73.0). The HIV status must also be reported because the patient is HIV-positive and may be reported as the secondary diagnosis.

CASE STUDY 9

Z45.2   Encounter for adjustment and management of vascular access device

Z47.89   Encounter for other orthopedic aftercare

Rationale: The Alphabetic Index can be referenced under the main terms Removal—vascular access device or catheter (Z45.2) and Aftercare—orthopedic NEC (Z47.89).

CASE STUDY 10

Z23   Encounter for immunization

Rationale: The Alphabetic Index can be referenced under the main term Immunization—encounter (Z23). Because this is the only reason for the visit, this is the first-listed diagnosis and can be reported.

CASE STUDY 11

S79.912A	Unspecified injury of left hip, initial encounter
G89.21	Chronic pain due to trauma
W06.xxxA	Fall from bed, Initial encounter
Y93.84	Activity, sleeping
Y92.122	Bedroom in nursing home as the place of occurrence
Y99.8	Other external cause status

Rationale: When using External Cause codes make sure you identify (if known), what happened (fall from bed), the activity (sleeping), place of occurrence (bedroom in nursing home), and the External Cause status (other external cause status). Make certain the conditions treated are the first-listed diagnosis codes (injury and chronic pain due to trauma). With this encounter because we don't know the specific type of hip injury, unspecified is selected. It is recommended in this type of situation, that the physician is queried for more specificity.

CASE STUDY 12

S00.432A	Contusion of left ear
W50.0xxA	Accidental hit or strike by another person
Y93.71	Activity boxing
Y92.39	Other specified sports and athletic area as the place of occurrence of the external cause
Y99.8	Other external cause status

Rationale: When coding this condition using the External Cause codes, the first-listed diagnosis is referenced in the Alphabetic Index under main term Contusion—ear. Laterality is important as well as the phase of treatment (initial encounter), the external cause (accidental hit or strike), activity (boxing), place of occurrence, and external status code.

CASE STUDY 13

S01.22xA	Laceration with foreign body of nose, initial encounter
S01.03xA	Puncture wound without foreign body of scalp, initial encounter
S01.412A	Laceration without foreign body of left cheek and temporomandibular area, initial encounter
V43.63xA	Car passenger injured in collision with pick-up truck or van in traffic accident
Y92.411	Interstate highway as the place of occurrence of the external cause
Y93.8	Activities, other specified
Y99.8	Other external cause status

Rationale: When coding this condition using the External Cause codes, the first-listed diagnosis is referenced in the Alphabetic Index under main term Laceration—ear—with foreign body (S01.32-). Laterality is important in the code selection. For the puncture wound, the Alphabetic Index is referenced under the main term Puncture—scalp—with foreign body (S01.04-). For coding the laceration of the cheek, the main term is Laceration—cheek (S01.41). For all three conditions, the phase of treatment must be reported as well as laterality. Because this is the initial treatment phase, "A" is the seventh character. The optional External Cause codes are selected based on the external cause activity, place of occurrence, and external status code.

Subject Index

Pneumonia, *continued*
  Methicillin resistant
    Staphylococcus aureus
    infection causing, 9
  ventilator-assisted, 68
Poisonings, adverse effects,
    underdosing, and toxic effects,
    130, 133–134
Postoperative pain, 38
Postpartum period, 114, 117
Pregnancy
  complications of, 114, 115, 116
  first-listed diagnosis for, 115
  high-risk, 115
  incidental, 115
  with pre-existing conditions, 116
  sequelae of complication of, 111
  trimester of, documenting, 115
Pregnancy, Childbirth, and the
    Puerperium (ICD-10-CM
    codebook Chapter 15), 27,
    114–118, 120–122
  case studies for, 120–122
  coding guidelines for, 114–118
  sequencing codes for, 115
Prematurity of newborn, 119
Prenatal visits, 115
Pressure ulcers, 4, 91–92
Psychoactive substance abuse,
    31–32

R

Radiotherapy, adverse effects of, 16
Routine administrative
    examinations, 147

S

Screening, Z codes for, 5, 146
Sepsis and septic shock
    complicating abortion,
    pregnancy, childbirth, and
    puerperium, 116–117

Sepsis, severe sepsis, and septic
    shock
  case studies for, 125–126
  differentiating among, 8–9
  puerperal, 117
Sequelae of cerebrovascular
    disease, 51
Seroma cavity, ablation of, 110
Seventh-character extensions, A,
    D, and S, 4, 28, 95, 130–131,
    132, 133
Sick sinus syndrome, 64
Signs and symptoms, 3
  coding guidelines for, 123–124
  reporting, 118, 123
Skin cancer, 19, 95
Sleep disorders, primary, 68–69
Status codes, 145
ST elevation myocardial infarction
    (STEMI), 51–52
Stillbirth, 119
Stress urinary incontinence, 112
Subsequent encounter for
    condition, D character for,
    95
Surgical procedure, complications
    of, 16, 95
Surgical wounds, healing, 95, 131
Surgery performed in utero, 116
Symptoms, Signs, and Abnormal
    Clinical and Laboratory
    Findings, Not Elsewhere
    Classified (ICD-10-CM
    codebook Chapter 18), 118,
    123–130
  case studies for, 124–130
  coding guidelines for, 123–124
Systemic inflammatory response
    syndrome (SIRS), 124

T

Table of Drugs and Chemicals, 1,
    2, 28, 133

Terrorism, external cause of injury
    from, 144, 145
Therapeutic services, 5
Tobacco use
  during pregnancy, childbirth,
    and puerperium, 117
  history of, 57–58, 82
Total body surface area for burns
    and corrosions, 133
Toxic effects, 133–134
Transfer of newborn, 118
Transplanted organ, neoplasm
    associated with, 17

U

Underdosing, 130, 133–134
  in pregnant patient, 117
"Unspecified" code, 3

V

Vaccinations, 145
Ventilator-associated pneumonia,
    68
Ventricular empyema, 139–140

W

Wounds, 23. *See also* Fractures
  catheter, 150, 151
  infected, 10–11, 13, 125–126
  re-excision of, 140
  superficial, 131
  surgical, 9–11, 38–42, 44–46, 48,
    89–90, 95, 104, 106, 114, 131,
    138–141

Z

Z codes, circumstances for use of,
    145–148
Zika virus infection, 9–10

Index of ICD-10-CM Workbook Codes

6-Character Subclassifications of Anatomic Site, Etiology, or Severity

7-Character Extension Codes